THE

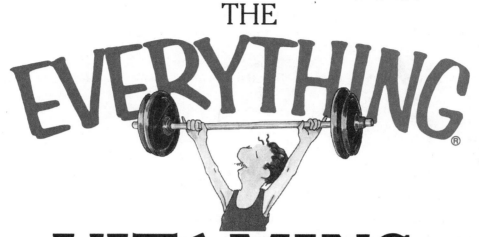

EVERYTHING®

VITAMINS,
MINERALS, AND NUTRITIONAL
SUPPLEMENTS BOOK

All the information you need to make
the right choices for your health

Maureen Ternus, M.S., R.D.,
and Kitty Broihier, M.S., R.D.

A

Adams Media Corporation
Holbrook, Massachusetts

D1412239

An Everything® Series Book.
The Everything® Series is a registered trademark of Adams Media Corporation.

Published by Adams Media Corporation
260 Center Street, Holbrook, MA 02343
www.adamsmedia.com

ISBN: 1-58062-496-0
Printed in the United States of America.

J I H G F E D C B A

Library of Congress Cataloging-in-Publication Data
Ternus, Maureen.
The Everything vitamins, minerals, and nutritional supplements book /
Maureen Ternus and Kitty Broihier.–1st ed.
p.   cm.
ISBN 1-58062-496-0
1. Nutrition. 2. Dietary supplements. I. Broihier, Kitty. II. Title.
RA784 .T465   2001
613.2–dc21   00-065019

Many of the designations used by manufacturers and sellers to distinguish their products are claimed as trademarks. Where those designations appear in this book and Adams Media was aware of a trademark claim, the designations have been printed in initial capital letters.

This publication is designed to provide accurate and authoritative information with regard to the subject matter covered. It is sold with the understanding that the publisher is not engaged in rendering professional medical advice. If assistance is required, the services of a competent professional person should be sought.

Illustrations by Barry Littmann

This book is available at quantity discounts for bulk purchases.
For information, call 1-800-872-5627.

Visit the entire Everything® series at everything.com

Contents

Chapter 4
Amino Acids: The Body's Building Blocks / 157

Chapter 5
Enzymes and Coenzymes / 181

Chapter 6
Essential Fatty Acids / 193

Chapter 7
Fiber / 201

CONTENTS

Introduction

Vitamin and mineral supplements make up the third largest over-the-counter drug category in the United States and are among the most widely used nonprescription products today. According to recent reports, sales of these nutritional supplements increased by about $3.5 billion between 1994 and 1998, to nearly $5 billion.

These supplements—whether vitamins alone, minerals alone, or combinations of the two—are used by many in hopes of preventing the aging process and avoiding chronic diseases including cancer, heart disease, and diabetes. But are these "magic pills" all they're cracked up to be? As public interest in vitamin and mineral supplements has increased, so has research on them. Once recommended solely for the prevention and treatment of particular deficiency diseases, supplements are now being studied for their potential health benefits. A recent example is the recommendation to take folic acid to prevent a certain type of birth defect. The research was so compelling that the U.S. Public Health Service now recommends that all women of childbearing age consume 400 micrograms of folic acid per day via fortified foods and/or supplements.

Still, there are a number of products being sold today that may not be useful to most people, and could, in fact, be dangerous to some. With so many choices, it's sometimes difficult to decide whether or not you need a particular supplement, and if so, which brand to buy. *The Everything® Vitamins, Minerals, and Nutritional Supplements Book* was written to provide you with a better understanding of the research behind some of the more popular vitamin and mineral supplements, and to help you figure out which, if any, supplements are right for you.

There are thousands of different types of supplements available on the market that are not vitamins or minerals. Because readers may also be interested in these, some of the most commonly used supplements—including enzymes, hormones, and probiotics—have been addressed in this book. However, no attempt has been made to be all-inclusive, and no herbal supplements have been included. For a thorough

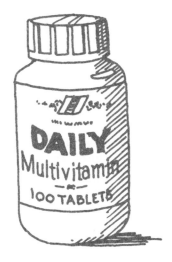

resource on herbal supplements, you might want to check out *The Everything® Herbal Remedies Book.*

When discussing nutrients and the appropriate levels at which to consume them, a number of standards, requirements, and recommendations are invariably mentioned—and with them, an alphabet soup of acronyms. Here is a list of the most common acronyms used in this book:

Food and Drug Administration (FDA). The U.S. Food and Drug Administration is a public health agency in charge of protecting the American consumer. It's FDA's job to see that all food, cosmetics, medicines, and medical devices are safe and effective—and won't hurt us. The FDA also monitors all of these products to ensure that they are labeled truthfully, with useful information that will enable people to use them properly.

Recommended Dietary Allowance (RDA). So how much of each nutrient do you need? We have the Recommended Dietary Allowances, or RDAs, to guide us. The RDAs are the amounts of nutrients that are needed to prevent disease and maintain basic body functions. RDAs are intended to meet the nutrient requirements of nearly all healthy people in certain age and gender groups (as well as during pregnancy and lactation).

The RDAs are set by the Food and Nutrition Board (FNB), a committee of highly regarded nutrition and health professionals who consult to the Institute of Medicine, a section of the National Academy of Sciences (NAS). The NAS is a private, nonprofit group of scholars that was mandated by Congress in 1863 to advise the federal government on scientific and technical matters.

To set the RDAs, the FNB first determines the least amount of the nutrient needed to prevent deficiency, and then determines the "ceiling" amount or the most that can be consumed—above which health problems occur. Then, a number is selected somewhere between the two limits that provides the body with a reserve amount of the nutrient, but not too much.

Many people mistakenly think that they must consume the RDA level of each nutrient each day or risk being deficient. This is *not* true, and that's why the acronym RDA doesn't stand for recommended *daily* allowances. The RDAs allow a cushion, calling for more than the average person really needs to stay healthy. That way, if your intake falls short of the RDA amount—for weeks or even a few months—you won't become deficient. RDAs are supposed to be used as *goals* for dietary intake. People who eat a varied diet generally meet these goals for most nutrients, although there are exceptions, as noted in specific chapters of this book.

Dietary Reference Intake (DRI). The FNB has recently completed a new series of dietary recommendations called Dietary Reference Intakes, or DRIs. The DRIs expand on and replace the RDAs. In developing the DRIs, the FNB carefully reviews each nutrient (and other food components that affect human health) not only to establish how much of a nutrient is needed to prevent classical deficiencies (as is done with RDAs), but to determine the nutrient's role in chronic disease, developmental disorders, and other health problems.

DRIs are groups of values that provide quantitative estimates of nutrient intakes. They're used for planning and assessing diets for healthy people. DRIs are "umbrella" categories, which take into account the RDA values as goals for intake, but also include three new types of reference values: Estimated Average Requirement, Adequate Intake, and Tolerable Upper Intake Level.

Estimated Average Requirement (EAR). The EAR is the amount of a nutrient that is estimated to meet the nutrient needs of *half* (50 percent) of the healthy people in certain age and gender groups. This is done in order to keep the RDA, which meets the needs of nearly all (97 to 98 percent) healthy people, conservatively low. If an EAR cannot be determined, no RDA is proposed.

Adequate Intake (AI). When not enough is known about a nutrient to set an EAR or RDA (as is the case with many trace minerals), an AI is established instead. The AI is based on the observed nutrient intake or experimentally determined estimates of nutrient intake by groups of people. For example, the AI for nutrients for young infants age 4 to 6 months is based on the nutrients supplied in breastmilk. In many ways an AI represents a "judgment call" by experts as to how much of the nutrient is needed. And, like the RDA, the AI is intended to be a goal of intake for healthy people. When an AI is used, it's an indication that further research is needed in order to more accurately determine the human requirements for that nutrient.

Tolerable Upper Intake Levels (UL). The UL is, as one might expect, the highest level of a daily nutrient intake that is likely to pose no risks of adverse health effects to almost all individuals in the general population. The UL is definitely not intended to be a recommended level of intake—there is no established benefit of consuming nutrients at the UL limit. The UL is especially important for people who take supplements or eat fortified foods. *If adverse effects have been observed only from taking supplements or eating fortified foods, this is specified.* For example, the UL for magnesium is from supplement intake only, and for niacin and folate the UL is from fortified food and supplement intake. *In these cases, the amount of each nutrient found naturally in foods is not counted because it would be difficult to reach the UL from food levels only.* In some cases UL values could not be established, such as with infants. Of course, this doesn't mean that the body can tolerate chronic, excessive intakes of these nutrients, only that there is a lack of information. When there is a lack of data, it generally pays to be cautious in terms of consumption of these nutrients.

United States Recommended Daily Allowance (USRDA). These are just simplified versions of the RDAs that were traditionally used for food labeling purposes. These are being phased out and replaced with Recommended Dietary Intake (RDI) values.

Daily Value (DV). The DV recommendations appear on food labels and are a combination of two other standards: the Daily Recommended Values, or DRVs (which cover recommendations for fat, carbohydrate, fiber, protein, cholesterol, sodium, and potassium based on a daily intake of 2,000 calories) and the Recommended Dietary Intakes, or RDIs (which replace the old USRDAs). The DV is not the same as the RDA—it isn't as up-to-date. The government has delayed requiring updated label information on supplements until all scientific reviews on RDAs are completed, which is not expected before the year 2005.

Recommended Dietary Intake (RDI). Considered to be the international version of the RDAs, these standards are set by the World Health Organization.

This book is here to help you understand why certain supplements may or may not be necessary, and to provide guidance on how to purchase and use these products. The book is divided into product categories, and the supplements are then listed alphabetically in each section. Each chapter covers a specific set of nutrients, and within each nutrient description the information is provided in the following format:

- An introduction to the nutrient and its functions.
- *The Benefits of the Nutrient.* Here, the latest research on a particular nutrient and potential health benefits are discussed. Examples include the role of folate in heart disease, or calcium in osteoporosis.
- *The Nutrient in Food.* Because most nutrition experts recommend getting your nutrients through food first, it's important to understand which foods provide particular vitamins and minerals. When

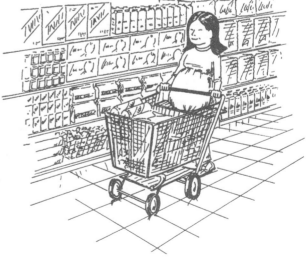

available, we've included charts containing food sources and the amounts of a particular nutrient.

- *When to Supplement with the Nutrient.* Although increasingly popular, supplements are not for everyone. This section discusses the reasons a particular nutrient may or may not be needed above and beyond what is provided in a balanced diet. Where appropriate, symptoms of deficiency and toxicity are also discussed, and a "bottom line" recommendation is provided in each chapter.

- *What to Know about Taking the Nutritional Supplement.* The various forms and dosages of a particular supplement are listed here, as well as the recommended upper limits for each nutrient, when available.

- *Caution!* Lists health alerts to be aware of when taking the nutrients.

- *Adequate Intakes (AIs)* or *Recommended Dietary Allowances (RDAs).* When available, the AIs and RDAs are listed in chart form for each nutrient.

At the end of the book you will find a list of additional resources and a glossary of terms to help you make informed choices regarding vitamin and mineral supplementation.

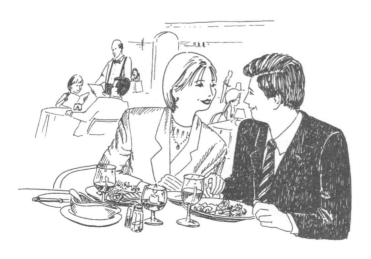

CHAPTER 1

Supplements: An Overview

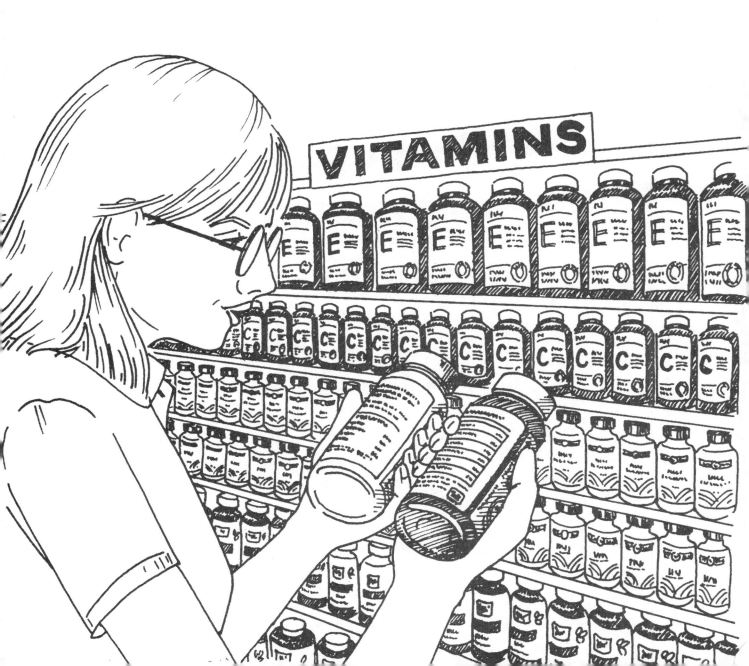

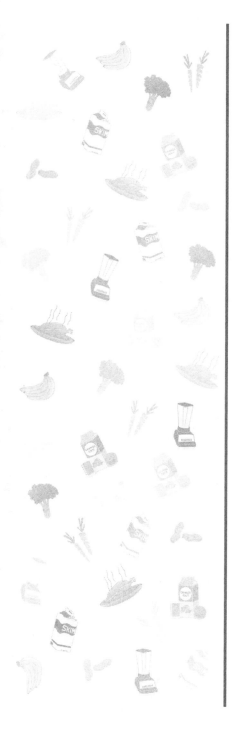

With so many different **vitamin** and **mineral** supplements on the market, and so many advertisements for these products in newspapers and magazines, and on television and radio, you might think supplements were essential for good health. The fact of the matter is, although vitamins and minerals are necessary for good health, the majority can be obtained from a well balanced diet.

The key is deciding whether or not you do, in fact, eat a well balanced diet, and if not, which **nutrients** you may be short on. First, take a look at your diet. For several days, jot down on a piece of paper everything you eat. Next, compare your intake with the Food Guide Pyramid recommendations outlined here:

Food Guide Pyramid

- 2–3 servings from the *Milk, Yogurt, and Cheese Group* (1 serving = 1 cup (8 ounces) milk or yogurt; 1½–2 ounces cheese)
- 2–3 servings from the *Meat, Poultry, Fish, Dry Beans, Eggs, and Nuts Group* (1 serving = 2½–3 ounces cooked lean meat, poultry, or fish; ½ cup cooked beans; 1 egg; ⅓ cup nuts; 2 tablespoons peanut butter count as 1 ounce lean meat)
- 3–5 servings from the *Vegetable Group* (1 serving = ½ cup chopped, raw, or cooked; 1 cup of leafy raw vegetables)
- 2–4 servings from the *Fruit Group* (1 serving = 1 piece of fruit or melon wedge; ¾ cup (6 ounces) juice; ½ cup canned fruit; ¼ cup dried fruit)
- 6–11 servings from the *Bread, Cereal, Rice, and Pasta Group* (1 serving = 1 slice bread; ½ cup cooked rice, cereal, or pasta; 1 ounce of ready-to-eat cereal)

Are you getting the minimum number of servings a day from each food group? If not, you're not alone. Although most nutrition experts recommend getting all of your **essential nutrients** through a healthy diet, few people actually *eat* a healthy diet! According to the 1994–96 Continuing Survey of Food Intakes by Individuals (CSFII), the average number of servings from the fruit, dairy, and meat groups were below the minimums recommended in the Pyramid. The average intakes were 1½ fruit servings; 1½ servings of dairy foods; and 4¾ servings from the meat group. Servings from the grain and vegetable groups were near the bottom of recommended ranges: 6⅔ servings of grains and 3½ servings of vegetables. In addition, the average dietary fiber intake was 15 grams—well below the recommended 25 to 30 grams per day.

And what about specific nutrients? Adult females failed to meet the RDA for five nutrients: calcium, vitamin E, vitamin B_6, magnesium, and zinc. Adult males fell short of the RDA for vitamin E, magnesium, and zinc. Other studies have shown that the average American diet is low in iron and vitamins B_{12} and D.

So, can a supplement or two make up for missed nutrients in the diet? Not according to the experts, many of whom believe that supplements won't fix a bad diet. Unfortunately, many consumers disagree. A number of surveys indicate that roughly 72 percent of those who take vitamin and mineral supplements do so as a type of "insurance." In the American Dietetic Association's national public opinion survey, *Nutrition and You: Trends 2000*, 38 percent of Americans agreed with the statement, "Taking vitamin supplements is necessary to ensure good health." This is up 11 percent from 1993.

In another survey, more than 11,000 people interviewed (the statistical equivalent of about 40 percent of the U.S. population) reported taking at least one vitamin or mineral supplement any time in the previous month.

The most popular groups of supplements were vitamin–mineral combinations and single vitamins. Only 29 percent of those surveyed, and 33 percent of women of childbearing age, reported taking at least one supplement containing folic acid any time in the previous month. This despite the fact that the U.S. Public Health Service recommends that all women in their reproductive years get 400 **micrograms** of folic acid per day (via **fortified** foods and/or supplements) to reduce the risk of **neural tube defects**.

Reasonably Safe?

Under DSHEA, new dietary ingredients in supplements are exempted from the safety requirements that apply to food additives. Instead, companies must have a reason for concluding that a supplement containing a new dietary ingredient is *reasonably* expected to be safe under normal use (use recommended by the product's label). In addition, DSHEA requires that companies notify FDA of their evidence for determining the safety of a new dietary ingredient in a supplement 75 days before marketing the supplement. However, the companies do not have to obtain FDA's approval of their supplements before marketing them. In other words, if FDA decides there is a problem with the new ingredient, it might be after the company has already marketed the supplement!

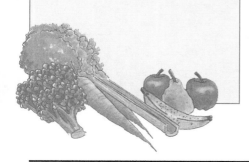

On the flip side, some people take supplements, or quantities of supplements, that they don't need—the old "more is better" way of thinking. For instance, many people consume megadoses of vitamin C in hope of warding off colds. Unfortunately, there have been no studies to date that show vitamin C prevents colds. Furthermore, since vitamin C is a **water-soluble vitamin**, any excess in the body is merely excreted in the urine . . . literally, money down the drain. Moreover, taking large doses of supplements can be dangerous, since many nutrients can be toxic in large amounts.

So what's a person to do? Are supplements really necessary? Yes and no—it depends on the situation. A couple of nutrients, for instance, are better absorbed in the synthetic, or man-made, forms than from foods. Folic acid is one example. Folate, the version of the B vitamin found in food, is 50 percent less absorbed by the body than folic acid, which is the form found in fortified foods and supplements. In the case of vitamin B12, up to one-third of people over the age of 50 have trouble absorbing this vitamin from food. Therefore, the National Academy of Sciences recommends that both of these nutrients come from fortified foods and/or supplements (for people in these age groups).

Given the current information on food intakes in this country, it's safe to say that most people could stand some improvements to their diets—especially in the fruit and vegetable area. And while it's best to get nutrients from food first, you might want to consider the following:

- A *multivitamin* providing no more than 100 to 200 percent of the RDA for most nutrients is probably not a bad idea. In fact, some research shows that a basic multi can help strengthen the immune system and reduce infections in older people.
- Many people, especially women, should consider taking a *calcium* supplement (most multivitamins do not contain enough—if any—calcium because it would make the pill too large) if they're not consuming the equivalent of four cups of milk per day. And, since vitamin D is necessary for calcium absorption, be sure to take a multivitamin with D.

- *Folic acid* is a must for women of childbearing age. Get it either through fortified foods or a supplement—most multivitamins contain the recommended 400 micrograms.
- Everyone over the age of 50 should consider supplementing with *vitamin B$_{12}$*. Some experts recommend 25 micrograms per day; however, most multivitamins only provide 6 micrograms. Be sure to look for one that meets the higher B$_{12}$ level, or think about taking a separate B$_{12}$ supplement.
- An estimated 30 to 40 percent of adults over the age of 50 have borderline *vitamin D* **deficiency**. Look for a multivitamin that provides 400 **International Units (IU)**. If you're over 70 and get little or no sun, make sure you're getting 600 IU a day of vitamin D.
- Some experts suggest taking 200 to 400 IU a day of *vitamin E*.

Supplement Label Claims: Buyer Beware

Once you've decided you need to take a supplement, the next step is buying it. Of course, these days we're all bombarded with a variety of claims for hundreds of different supplement products, both at home (on the television and radio) and at the local market. Have you ever wondered if these supplement label claims are true, or if anyone in the government is regulating these claims? If so, you're not alone. Health professionals and many supplement manufacturers have asked the same questions. In fact, many in the industry want to see stricter regulation of dietary supplements.

Under the Federal Food, Drug and Cosmetic Act (FFDCA), the U.S. Food and Drug Administration (FDA) was named the federal agency responsible for regulating the safety and claims made in the labeling of dietary supplements (including vitamins, minerals, herbs, amino acids, and other dietary substances). FDA regulates dietary supplements under the guidelines set in the Dietary Supplement Health and Education Act (DSHEA) of 1994. The DSHEA was an amendment to the FFDCA that created a new regulatory category, safety standards, and other rules for supplements.

Who's Taking Vitamins?

In general, white adult females take the most vitamin and mineral supplements. The average supplement-taker in the United States is 37 years old with more than 12 years of education, lives in the West, and has a middle to upper income.

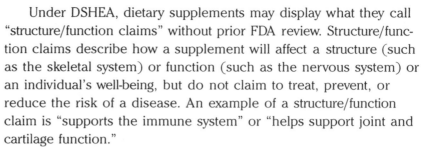

Supplements—More Popular Than Ever

According to industry sources, the market for dietary supplements is growing dramatically. Sales of supplements (including vitamins, minerals, herbs, and others) increased from $9.8 billion in 1995, to an estimated $14.7 billion in 1999. And, the market is expected to continue to grow for several reasons:

1. The aging baby boomers are looking for ways to stay healthy and feel younger longer.
2. Consumers are taking their health into their own hands and are looking for ways to prevent chronic diseases.
3. The science of nutrition has been making great strides in identifying new relationships between diet and disease.

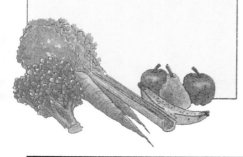

Under DSHEA, dietary supplements may display what they call "structure/function claims" without prior FDA review. Structure/function claims describe how a supplement will affect a structure (such as the skeletal system) or function (such as the nervous system) or an individual's well-being, but do not claim to treat, prevent, or reduce the risk of a disease. An example of a structure/function claim is "supports the immune system" or "helps support joint and cartilage function."

Under FFDCA, structure/function claims cannot be misleading or false. However, the law does not define the source or quantity of evidence needed to support these claims. Moreover, FDA has not instructed the industry on what constitutes appropriate documentation—one study or dozens of studies? Add to this the fact that some ingredients or nutrients have been thoroughly studied and others have not. Take, for instance, the numerous studies showing the positive role of calcium in preventing **osteoporosis**, compared to the limited research available on pine bark extract and its supposed role in reducing arthritis pain. And, some structure/function claims, such as "cleanses the blood," are so vague that they have little or no scientific meaning and would be very difficult to prove.

Unlike "structure/function" claims, labels cannot, however, bear a "health claim" without FDA review. What's the difference? Health claims state that a supplement may reduce the risk of a specific disease such as cancer or heart disease. For example, after FDA review, a folic acid supplement label can have a health claim stating that a certain amount of folic acid may reduce the risk of brain and spinal cord defects.

Before a health claim can be made for a supplement, it must go through a rigorous FDA review of the scientific evidence supporting the claim. To date, only four health claims—for soy, calcium, folic acid, and psyllium husk—have been approved for use on dietary supplements (see "FDA Authorized Health Claims" on page 8).

Although FDA is required to review health claims before authorizing their use on product labels, the same is not true for structure/function claims. Companies must notify FDA of their supplement's structure/function claim within 30 days *after* marketing the product. FDA then reviews these notifications to determine whether the claim is a true structure/function claim as opposed to a claim to prevent, treat, or reduce the risk of a disease.

If the FDA decides the claim is actually a health claim, a letter is sent to the company objecting to the claim. FDA does not review the claim to see if there is scientific evidence for that claim in the first place. In other words, if a company made a claim that product X "reduced the risk of **diabetes**," they would get a letter from FDA saying they had made a health claim rather than a structure/function claim. FDA would not, however, go a step further and ask them if they had the scientific evidence to show that product X reduced the risk for diabetes. This has raised concerns that because of the limited amount of research and FDA review, many claims on supplements may not be supported by scientific data. This has led many in the supplement industry to push FDA to take enforcement actions against unsupported claims. FDA has stated that one of its priorities for 2000 is to develop enforcement procedures to respond to some of these labeling issues.

While FDA regulates supplement labels, the Federal Trade Commission (FTC) regulates advertising on television, radio, the Internet, and print media such as newspapers and magazines. Unfortunately, these two agencies operate under different rules for regulating claims on product labels and advertising. This has enabled some claims that were denied by FDA for supplement labels (the body of data may not be large enough to meet FDA requirements) to be permitted by FTC for use in advertising—provided the claim is truthful and not misleading, and supported by scientific data.

So what's the consumer to do? *Research.* Consumers have to educate themselves when it comes to dietary supplements. Read up on the supplements you're interested in. Talk to your doctor, pharmacist, or registered dietitian, and check out some of the additional resources listed in the back of this book.

Health Claim vs. Structure/Function Claim: What's the Difference?

There are a few basic differences between health claims and structure/function claims. While a health claim requires a rigorous FDA review of the scientific evidence *prior* to approval, a structure/function claim does not. In fact, manufacturers can use a structure/function claim without prior FDA approval as long as it's not misleading or false—they don't have to "prove" the supplement's efficacy with a certain amount and type of research. Additionally, health claims can claim to reduce, prevent, or treat a specific disease. Structure/function claims, on the other hand, may only describe how the supplements may affect a structure (the skeleton) or function ("supports the immune system").

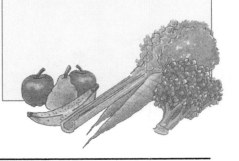

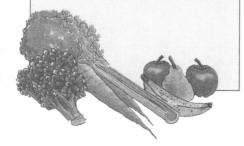
FDA Authorized Health Claims*

Supplement Ingredients	Health Claims
Calcium	Helps maintain healthy bones and may reduce risk of osteoporosis
Folic acid	May reduce the risk of brain and spinal cord birth defects
Soluble fiber from psyllium husks	May reduce the risk of heart disease
Soy protein	May reduce the risk of heart disease

*These are simplified claims. The actual claims used on the supplement labels may differ slightly.

Buying a Supplement

This book provides the reader with general reference information regarding the use and benefits of many different supplements. Once you've become familiar with which supplements might be appropriate for you, you might be tempted to run right out and purchase them. However, it pays to do a little preparation first, so that you'll be sure the supplements you select will be the right ones for you.

> **NOTE:** The first step to take before actually purchasing supplements is to see your doctor. See "Discuss It with Your Doctor" on page 14 for specific questions to ask your doctor about your health and the supplements you're interested in taking.

Where to Buy Supplements

Supermarkets, drug stores, health food stores, mail-order catalogs, and online outlets are all good sources of dietary supplements, though the selection may be better online or through mail-order. Comparison shopping for the most inexpensive supplement (all other things being equal) is wise, as prices can vary widely, and the most expensive supplement isn't necessarily the best. In fact, most manufacturers obtain their vitamins and minerals from the same few sources, so they're all comparable. What may differ is the quality of manufacture, the form, and the extras included in the supplement, such as herbs, **enzymes**, and **phytochemicals**—which may or may not be effective or desirable (see "A Word about Combination Multivitamin/Botanical Supplements" on page 18).

In general, store-brand supplements—especially those from larger chains—are often the best bargain and are equal in quality to the higher-priced supplements advertised on television or available from specialty outlets. The least you can expect to pay for a multivitamin and mineral supplement is $1 to $5 for a one-month supply (one tablet per day). When comparing prices online, be sure to factor in shipping and handling charges.

Check that the supplement manufacturer uses Good Manufacturing Practices (GMPs) before purchasing their products. GMPs ensure that the product and the potency level match what's indicated on the label. If the label has the seal of the National Nutritional Foods Association, it means that the manufacturer meets the association's standards for quality.

ConsumerLab.com, an independent testing lab, tests products for the presence and the levels of compounds that have been proven effective in clinical research. Those that pass the test are published on their Web site. Also, manufacturers of passing product brands can print the ConsumerLab quality seal on their labels and accompanying product literature.

Choosing a Supplement Form

This book lists the most common forms available for each supplement. Capsules and tablets are the preferred form for most people since they're easily stored and easily consumed. They're also the most widely available, but there are a variety of other supplement forms that you may want to investigate.

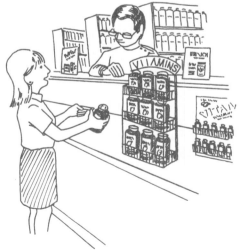

- *Tablets.* Tablets, or their capsule-shaped cousins called "caplets," contain the nutrient itself plus some additives that provide color, help the tablet keep its shape, and break down easily in the body. Talc is a

A Word about Placebos

A placebo is a "fake" treatment designed to look, smell, and taste like the real treatment. In a double-blind placebo-controlled study, neither the study participant nor the researcher knows whether the test substance or a placebo has been given. This ensures that the results won't be affected by the personal beliefs of the participant or the researcher. The researcher in a non-placebo-controlled study would be influenced—he or she will be looking harder at those who received the test supplement, expecting to find some effect. Observed results from a placebo-controlled study are much more meaningful, or valid, than those obtained from a study where no placebo was used.

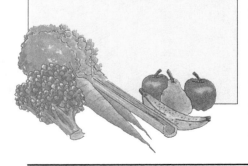

common additive that keeps the ingredients flowing easily during the tableting (or encapsulation) stage of production. In the tiny amounts added to the supplement, talc should not pose any health threat. Tablets are sometimes available in chewable form—for children or those who can't swallow easily. **Sublingual** tablets are made to be held in the mouth under the tongue until dissolved. Tablets can be stored for long periods of time in a cool, dry location.

- *Capsules.* Capsules tend to have fewer additives because the ingredients don't have to hold their shape as tablets and caplets do. The **fat-soluble vitamins** A, D, and E are frequently available in "softgel" capsules, which are essentially liquid-containing capsules. Capsules are easily stored for long periods of time in a cool, dry location.

- *Powders.* Powdered supplements are ideal for those who have a hard time swallowing pills, as they can be mixed with beverages or food. However, not many supplements are available in this form. Powders have fewer additives than tablets and capsules. For this reason, people who are allergic to some additives find powdered supplements more agreeable. Powders are frequently less expensive than tablets or capsules. Storage time varies on powder, but be sure to keep all powders covered tightly so they're not affected by humidity in the air.

- *Liquids.* Liquid vitamins can be swallowed as is, or mixed with beverages or food. Liquids are common for infants' and young children's supplements. Liquid supplements may be more quickly absorbed by the body, but that doesn't mean the nutrients they contain are better absorbed or more available to the body. Isotonic liquid products supposedly provide the nutrients in a similar concentration to that found in the body's cells, which makes them better absorbed. However, there is no scientific evidence that isotonic liquids are absorbed any better than regular liquids, tablets, or capsules.

- *Lozenges.* Although not a very popular form, lozenges are available for some supplements, such as zinc. Lozenges are supposed to be held in the mouth to dissolve slowly.

About the National
Nutritional Foods Association

Founded in 1936, the National Nutritional Foods Association (NNFA) represents the interests of approximately 4,000 member companies including manufacturers, suppliers, retailers, and distributors of health foods, dietary supplements, natural ingredient cosmetics, and other natural products. Headquartered in Newport Beach, California, the NNFA has a strong lobbying presence in Washington, D.C., and is very involved in helping to shape legislation that affects their members.

In 1994, the passing of the Dietary Supplement Health and Education Act gave the Food and Drug Administration (FDA) the authority to issue good manufacturing practice regulations for the dietary supplements industry. FDA has yet to issue these regulations, so the NNFA went ahead and initiated its own GMP standards, which are modeled after guidelines proposed by FDA. Launched in July 1999, the Good Manufacturing Practices (GMP) Certification Program is designed to review standards for all elements of manufacturing in order to provide reasonable assurance that quality control measures are in place and being followed. These standards include specifications for staff training, cleanliness, equipment maintenance, record keeping, and the receiving of raw materials. Earning an "A" compliance rating on a GMP audit entitles the company to be certified and use the NNFA's GMP seal on their products.

Since the launch of the program, products with the GMP seal have begun to appear on the shelves of health food stores around the country. To locate an NNFA health food retailer, visit the NNFA Web site (*www.nnfa.org*) and use the "Find-A-Store" feature by entering your zip code.

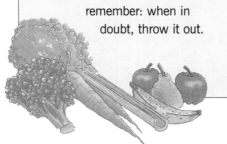

How to Read a Supplement Label

Until recently, reading supplement labels was often an exercise in frustration. Some labels gave lots of information and others gave little or no information, which made evaluating and comparing products next to impossible. In March 1999, a new supplement label ruling by the Food and Drug Administration went into effect. All dietary supplements, including vitamins, minerals, and herbs, must have a "Supplement Facts" panel on the label. This panel lists ingredients by weight and gives the percent Daily Value (DV) for those nutrients with an established Dietary Reference Intake (DRI). (For information about DV and DRI, see the Introduction to this book.)

The "Supplement Facts" panel must also contain serving size/dosage information, the common or usual name for the supplement, and the name and place of business for the manufacturer, packer, or distributor. The ruling also defined the terms "high potency" and specified when the term **antioxidant** can be used. Although complete information such as that on the "Supplement Facts" panel doesn't guarantee that the supplement is high quality, it does help consumers make informed supplement choices.

Following are some terms you'll need to be familiar with in order to understand supplement labels and compare products:

- *Disease claim.* A statement that links the supplement to a disease or health condition, such as calcium and osteoporosis. These are rarely found on labels, since FDA only allows a few supplements to carry these claims.
- *Directions.* Guidelines for when and how to take the supplement, and how much to take.
- *Expiration date.* The date when the supplement may start to lose its potency. Though not required by law, it's common practice to list an expiration date so consumers have an idea of how "fresh" the supplement is and how long it will last. It's a good idea to finish the product before the expiration date, although it isn't dangerous to take a product that's passed its expiration date (unless the manufacturer indicates otherwise on the label).

- *High potency.* This term may be used to describe a single nutrient when it is present at 100 percent or more of the Daily Value. For multi-ingredient or combination products, two-thirds of the nutrients for which the DV is known must be present at 100 percent or more of the DV, and these nutrients must be specifically named on the label.

- *Ingredients.* Everything that's contained in the supplement will be listed in order of decreasing weight. However, if an ingredient is cited in the "Supplement Facts" panel, it does not have to be included in the ingredients list.

- *Lot number.* A number or combination of letters and numbers that appears on the label or is stamped into the container of some supplements. Reputable manufacturers always include a lot number on their products because it allows the manufacturer to trace the product on its journey through production to sale. It's useful for checking product quality or for product recalls. Lot numbers are usually coded and indicate when the product was made and at which production facility.

- *Miscellaneous certification insignia.* There are a few patented certification insignia owned by specific manufacturers that may appear on labels. These insignia generally indicate that the products have passed tests for consistency between batches and pills.

- *Serving size.* The manufacturer's suggested serving expressed in terms of the supplement's form, such as "1 tablet." All numerical values listed on the "Supplement Facts" panel are for that specified serving size.

- *Statement of identity.* A description of the type of supplement; it must include the words "dietary supplement" or "supplement," such as "iron supplement."

- *Storage advice.* A proper storage place for most supplements is a cool, dry location—not in the bathroom (too hot and damp) or the refrigerator (too cold and damp). Any unusual directions for storage will be stated on the label.

- *Structure/function claim.* This statement indicates the benefit of taking the product and relates it to the body or general health status, such as "aids digestion" or "helps maintain

What Is "Chelated"?

The term "chelated" applies to minerals and refers to the chemical structure of the nutrient. The **chelation** process, in which a mineral is bonded to another substance (usually an **amino acid**), protects the mineral from things in food that may inhibit absorption, such as phytates (or **phytic acid**) or even other nutrients. This is supposed to increase the body's absorption of the mineral, but there's little or no evidence that chelated minerals are absorbed any better or quicker than nonchelated minerals. Even if chelated minerals are better absorbed, the increase is minimal and not worth the higher cost of these products.

Natural vs. Synthetic Vitamins

In general, natural and synthetic nutrients are equally absorbed and equally effective in the body, so there's no reason to pay more for **"natural" vitamins**. Nearly every supplement, whether it's from a natural or synthetic source, is processed and refined in a laboratory anyway—and some "natural" vitamins even contain additives. There is some evidence that natural vitamin E (called d-alpha tocopherol) may be better retained and used by the body than synthetic E (called dl-alpha tocopherol); however, the differences are minimal. What's more, the unit of measurement for vitamin E (the International Unit, or IU) takes this into account, so a capsule that provides 400 IU will have that potency whether it's natural or not.

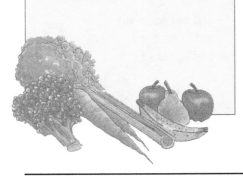

flexible joints." Such claims must also be accompanied on the label by a disclaimer that says that FDA has not evaluated the claim and that the product is not intended to diagnose, treat, cure, or prevent any disease.

- *USP.* The acronym for the United States Pharmacopeia, an independent body of experts that sets the standards for purity and potency for drugs, supplements, and some herbs. A product that says "USP" on the label indicates that the manufacturer has voluntarily tested the product and found it to comply with USP standards for purity, strength, disintegration, and dissolution. (Dissolution is the portion of an ingredient, usually expressed as a percentage, that dissolves in the digestive tract.) The product will also have an expiration date. Products without the "USP" designation are not necessarily inferior—there may be no standards for that supplement, or the manufacturer may choose not to do the required testing for the designation. Keep in mind that no one checks to make sure that manufacturers who do use the "USP" designation actually meet the standards. However, the chance that the standards have been met are greater if a well known brand carries the "USP" designation.

Discuss It with Your Doctor

When it comes to dietary supplements, it pays to be cautious. Supplements provide the body with extra nutrients that for some people are beneficial, but for others may be harmful—even deadly. Schedule a physical and use the appointment time to ask your doctor's advice about supplements. Come prepared—make a list of your questions. Don't be embarrassed to bring a written list or take notes during your discussion. It shows you are serious about getting the information you need to make an informed decision.

In particular, be sure to discuss:

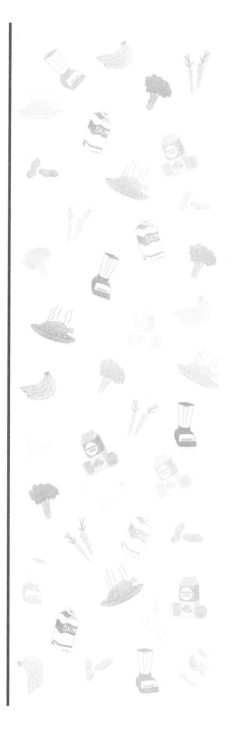

- *Any symptoms you may have that suggest a health problem or illness.* Getting a professional diagnosis of your problem is of utmost importance. **Never self-diagnose.**
- *Any specific health problems or conditions you have that may cause certain supplements to be dangerous to you.* Although this book gives caution statements and warnings regarding certain health conditions and supplement use, it's wise to clarify these issues with your personal physician. Be as specific as possible about which supplements you are interested in taking.
- *Medications.* Both prescribed and over-the-counter medications may interact with supplements in ways that can be dangerous. Be sure your doctor knows about all of the medications you are taking—no matter how trivial they seem to you or how infrequently you take them. In addition, tell your doctor if you're taking any herbal products or supplements, if you regularly drink herbal tea, or if you take any other dietary supplements. Your doctor needs to have a complete picture of your situation in order to give you good advice about supplements.
- *Continuation of current medications or treatments.* In some instances supplements will allow you to decrease dosages of medications, or even stop taking them. However, this isn't always the case, and serious problems could occur if you alter or discontinue medications or treatments. **Never stop taking a prescribed medication or treatment, or alter medication dosage, without discussing it with your doctor first.**
- *Timing of supplements.* Are there certain times when it isn't advisable to take the supplements you're interested in, because of a medical treatment or health condition? Are there specific times of day when you should take supplements because of potential interactions with medications or other supplements?
- *Dosage.* You'll notice that in many cases this book gives general dosage recommendations, and in others it's suggested that you ask your doctor. In either case, it's wise to ask your doctor's advice about dosage. Dosages can vary

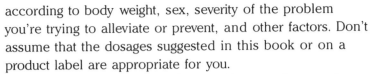

When to Take Your Supplements

Experts generally recommend taking vitamin and mineral supplements with meals because some vitamins are better absorbed with food (such as fat-soluble vitamins) and the digestive system is already primed to receive nutrients. However, some nutrients interfere with the absorption of others. With a multivitamin and mineral supplement there's not much you can do about this, but single nutrient supplements can be taken separately so interactions are avoided. Also, to prevent or discourage any adverse interactions, avoid taking supplements at the same time as medications— leave a couple of hours between them if possible.

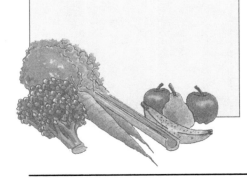

according to body weight, sex, severity of the problem you're trying to alleviate or prevent, and other factors. Don't assume that the dosages suggested in this book or on a product label are appropriate for you.

- *Duration of supplement use.* Depending on what supplements you're interested in taking and why, you may be advised to limit the length of time that you take a supplement or combination of supplements.

Although the number of doctors who believe that dietary supplements are "useless and a complete waste of money" seems to be slowly dwindling, there are still many who take this view and advise their patients to avoid supplements completely. Most medical schools teach students very little about nutritional therapy, so your doctor may just be uninformed about supplements and their uses. In either case, don't go it alone. Seek out a doctor who is more receptive or informed about supplements.

Naturopathic doctors (they use the initials "N.D." after their names) are not licensed in most states but do undergo extensive graduate-level training in nutrition, supplements, and herbal medicine. If you want to consult with an N.D., it's best to choose one who has graduated from an accredited school. (Check with the American Association of Naturopathic Physicians.)

Registered Dietitians (they use the initials "R.D." after their names) are another good source of information and guidance regarding dietary supplements. Although nutritionists do not undergo the same level of training that R.D.s do, and there are no licensing requirements for them, some are still good sources of information. You may want to look for those with doctorate degrees; these use the initials "Ph.D." after their names. A pharmacist with a doctorate degree ("Pharm.D.") can also provide information about side effects and interactions, but may not be well versed in the benefits and uses of dietary supplements.

Checking Up
on Your Supplement

Confused by the growing number of supplements on the market? Not sure which brand to buy? Check out the Web site *www.consumerlab.com*. Founded by a physician, ConsumerLab provides independent reviews and consumer information about health, wellness, and nutrition products, and conducts the largest independent testing of dietary supplements sold in the United States. Privately held and headquartered in New York, the company has developed preset criteria that supplements must pass in order to carry the CL certification seal for a fee. Specific testing criteria vary by product and are selected on the basis of importance to consumers and whether or not the information is already available elsewhere. Products are tested on the following criteria:

- *Identity and potency.* Does the product meet recognized standards of quality, and does the label accurately reflect what's in the product?
- *Purity.* Is the product free of contaminants?
- *Bioavailability.* Can the product be used properly by the body?
- *Consistency.* Does each dose have the same identity, potency, and purity?

How does the process work? ConsumerLab selects a product to test, and then randomly chooses various brands to send to one of 12 different labs for testing. Companies that submit their products for testing can either pay a fee to carry the CL label on their product and/or simply have their product(s) listed on the ConsumerLab Web site. To date, the supplements that have fared the best are glucosamine—10 out of 10 products passed the test—and vitamin C supplements—85 percent of which passed the test. SAMe and chondroitin have fared the worst to date—40 percent of the brands failed to pass. ConsumerLab continually tests and updates its analysis of categories of dietary supplements.

Guidelines for Using Supplements

You've consulted with your doctor and purchased your supplements; now you need a few pointers about using supplements safely and effectively.

Don't exceed the recommended dosage

This book gives recommended dosages for some supplements and suggests that you consult your doctor about the appropriate dosages for others. Erring on the side of caution and taking less of a supplement is always wiser than taking more in hopes that it will work better. In general, start with the lowest effective dosage and work up from there if necessary. Megadoses, or extremely high dosages of supplements, should not be taken unless advised and supervised by a physician.

Check your reaction to the supplement

Some supplements (or ingredients contained in them) may disagree with you or cause an adverse or allergic reaction. Be aware of how you feel, taking note of any symptoms that might be related to the supplement you're taking. If an adverse reaction occurs, stop taking the supplement immediately and contact your doctor. Remember to inform your doctor of all supplements, medications, and herbal products that you are taking—interactions between them could be the source of your problem.

Evaluate your progress

Not all supplements work for everyone. If you've taken the supplement for the recommended amount of time and you still haven't noticed improvement of your symptoms or health problem, stop taking it and consult your doctor. Perhaps a different dosage, a combination of supplements, or a completely different treatment is needed. It's also a good idea to temporarily stop taking a supplement even if you think it's working—the break gives you a chance to see if your symptoms or condition worsens when you're not on the supplement. That way you can confirm whether the supplement does indeed help you.

A Word about Combination Multivitamin/Botanical Supplements

Some new products on the supplement scene combine various vitamins and minerals with herbs or botanical ingredients that may or may not be needed. The amounts of the botanical ingredients added are often insignificant, rendering their presence more of a marketing gimmick than a real benefit. What's more, some of these ingredients have the potential to harm. Before spending money on these combination products, check all the ingredients—do they all provide a benefit without risk? If not, find another multivitamin and mineral supplement.

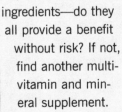

Children and Vitamins

Like adults, children need a wide variety of vitamins, minerals, and other nutrients in order to be healthy. And, as with adults, food is the primary source of these nutrients. According to the American Academy of Pediatrics, a healthy child who eats a balanced diet based on the Food Guide Pyramid should meet all requirements for essential vitamins and minerals. Periods of rapid growth, such as infancy and adolescence, usually require a little more food but don't necessitate supplements.

Pediatricians may prescribe supplements for children who have medical conditions that decrease nutrient absorption, or for children who follow strict vegetarian diets. Occasionally a liquid iron supplement will be prescribed for children who are iron-deficient. *But for most kids—even those who seem to eat unbalanced meals or little food at all—vitamin and mineral supplements are seldom necessary.* Over time, children manage to get the nutrients they need, provided that they're given a variety of foods from which to choose.

Sometimes parents give children a daily multivitamin as a form of nutritional "insurance." Generally, a multivitamin supplement that provides no more than 100 percent of the RDA for nutrients for the child's age is considered safe. It's important to realize, however, that if a child's diet isn't healthy to begin with, supplements won't make it right—they can't make up for too much sugar, too little fiber, or too much fat.

Never give a child any supplement (even a regular multivitamin) designed for adults—they contain too much of certain nutrients that can be dangerous for children. Children's vitamin formulas contain the appropriate amounts of nutrients for them, but to be safe, check with the child's pediatrician before giving a child any type of vitamin or mineral supplement. If your child can't chew the vitamin, crush it into smaller pieces to avoid choking. Finally, keep *all* supplements out of reach of children—preferably in a locked cabinet. Young children can mistake them for candy, or may like the taste so much that they overdose on it. If you suspect your child has overdosed on any supplement, call for medical assistance immediately.

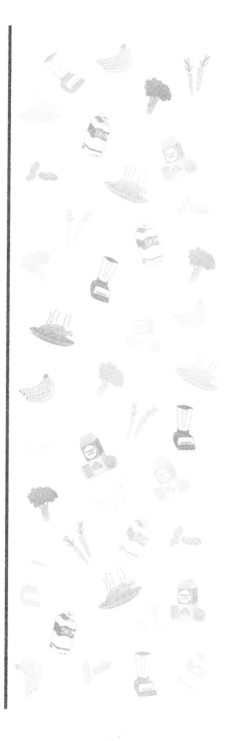

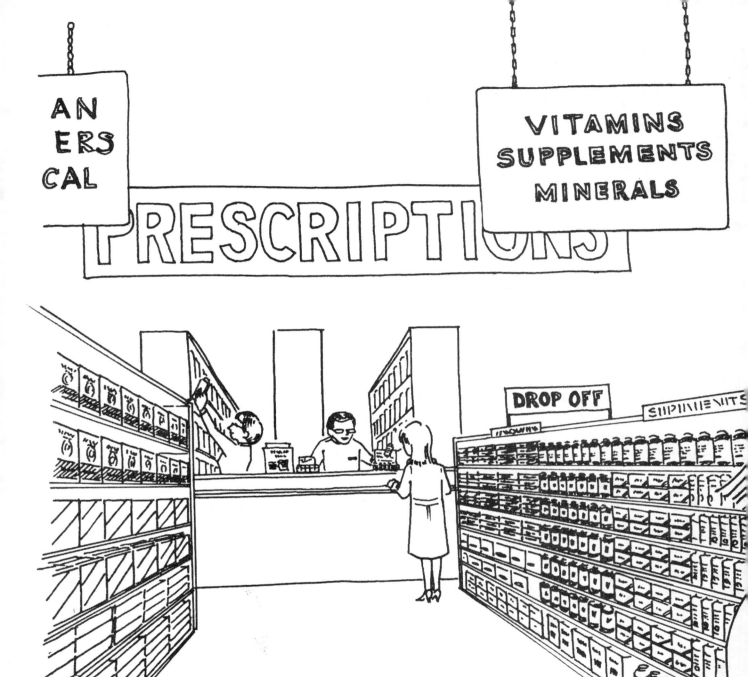

CHAPTER 2

Vitamins: Essential Nutrients for Life

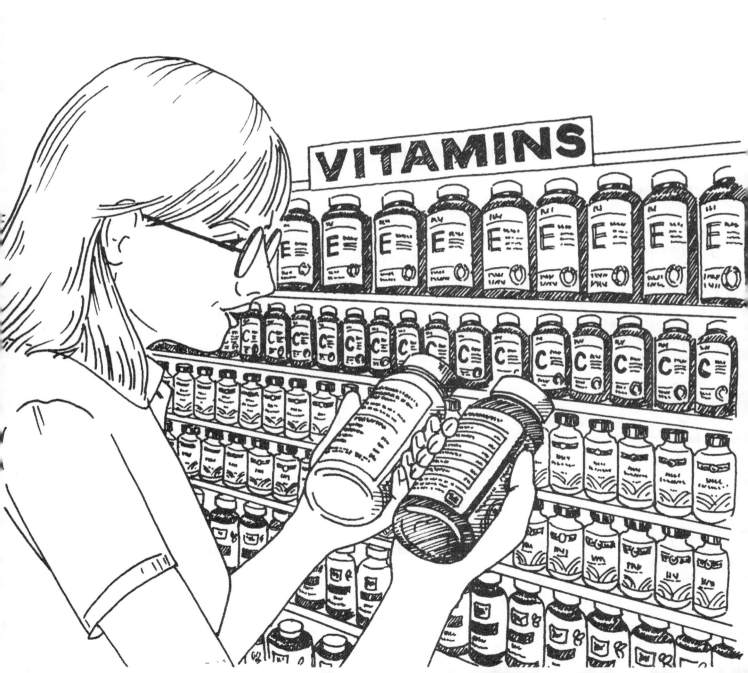

Vitamins at a Glance

Fat-Soluble Vitamins
  Vitamin A
  Vitamin D
  Vitamin E
  Vitamin K

Water-Soluble Vitamins
  Vitamin B₆, or pyridoxine
  Vitamin B₁₂, or cobalamin
  Biotin
  Vitamin C
  Choline*
  Folic acid
  Inositol**
  Niacin
  Pantothenic acid
  Riboflavin
  Thiamin

*Although these nutrients are not true B vitamins, they are often referred to as such.

**Because there is no Recommended Dietary Allowance or Adequate Intake for inositol, we have not covered it in this book.

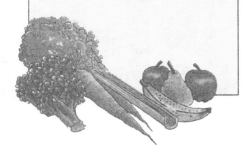

itamins and minerals—we've heard about them since we were kids. In fact, they are an important part of how we choose our milk, breakfast cereals, and almost everything we eat that we consider "healthful" or "good for us." In recent years there have been many different studies and news reports on the health benefits of vitamins C, E, etc. Many of these reports suggest megadoses of certain vitamins. But how much do we really need, and what are the best sources of these important nutrients?

First, vitamins are compounds that are generally much smaller in size than carbohydrates, proteins, or fats. Vitamins do not provide any energy but are necessary for a number of bodily processes. Many act as **coenzymes** or as parts of enzymes responsible for promoting essential chemical reactions. Unlike amino acids (the building blocks of proteins—see the introduction to Chapter 4 for more information), vitamins are never strung together to make other compounds in the body (although they are sometimes attached to proteins). And, although they are needed and consumed in very minute amounts (micrograms—millionths of a gram, and **milligrams**—thousandths of a gram), they are essential for life.

Vitamins are vulnerable both in and out of the body. For instance, certain vitamins are easily destroyed by sunlight and heat. Therefore, manufacturers must take care during production and processing of foods and supplements. In many cases, food manufacturers have to put back into foods some of the vitamins that are lost during the production process. An example is the enrichment of bread with the B vitamin thiamin.

Water-Soluble vs. Fat-Soluble

Vitamins can be water-soluble (water-loving) or fat-soluble (water-avoiding). The B vitamins and vitamin C are water-soluble, while vitamins A, D, E, and K are fat-soluble. The differences between the two groups can affect vitamin absorption, transport, storage, and excretion.

- *Absorption.* Water-soluble vitamins cross the intestinal and vascular (blood vessel) walls directly into the bloodstream.

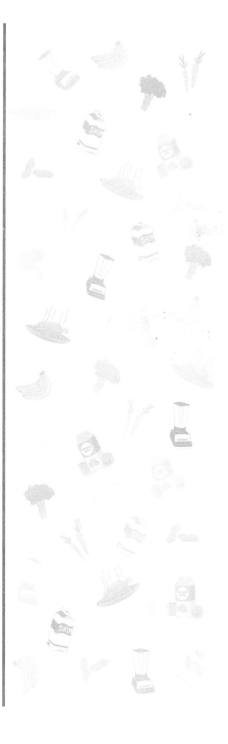

If you're taking them as a multivitamin, take the supplement with or following a meal. Fat-soluble vitamins, on the other hand, must be carried with fat by way of lymph (the bodily fluid found between cells and outside of the bloodstream), before reaching the bloodstream. They must be taken with a food source that contains fat or oil.

- *Transport.* Water-soluble vitamins travel freely throughout the bloodstream, while fat-soluble vitamins must be made water-soluble by being attached to protein carriers.

- *Storage.* Fat-soluble vitamins have a tendency to stay put once reaching the various cells of the body. Water-soluble vitamins have more freedom. When not in use, they circulate among all the organs in the body, including the kidneys.

- *Excretion.* The kidneys are the main excretion tools for the body. They are sensitive to high concentrations of substances in the blood. When particular substances are in excess in the blood, the kidneys remove them and pass them into the urine. This goes for the water-soluble vitamins as well. High doses of most of these vitamins are simply passed into the urine. Fat-soluble vitamins, however, don't accumulate in the blood since they're stored in various places throughout the body. Therefore, high levels of these vitamins are not as easily excreted from the body.

- This can be good and bad. The body does not store extra water-soluble vitamins since they are so readily excreted in the urine. Therefore, you need to make sure you're getting these vitamins on a regular basis through your diet or via supplements. Fat-soluble vitamins, on the other hand, are stored for much longer periods of time. For instance, consuming relatively large amounts of vitamin A once in a while can "hold you over" for quite some time. Although in general this is beneficial, it also increases the likelihood that toxic accumulations of these vitamins may occur. Water-soluble vitamins are less risky, except for vitamin B_6. The National Academy of Sciences recently set a tolerable upper limit for this B vitamin because higher daily doses can cause nerve toxicity.

Vitamin A

Vitamin A, the first fat-soluble vitamin to be discovered (in 1913), is the general name given to a family of compounds called retinoids (i.e., retinol, retinal, and retinoic acid). We obtain the vitamin A we need primarily through the diet. However, the body can also convert some **carotenoids**—yellow, orange, and red pigments in foods—into vitamin A. There are more than 600 different carotenoids in nature, but not all are **provitamins**—carotenoids that turn into vitamin A in the body (see the section on beta-carotene in Chapter 9). Approximately 90 percent of the vitamin A in the body is stored in the liver.

Vitamin A is believed to be one of the most versatile fat-soluble vitamins because of its role in a number of important body processes. It is important for growth, reproduction, proper bone development, healthy skin, and the immune system. It's also necessary for healthy mucous membranes (the smooth linings of the mouth, stomach, intestines, lungs, etc.). Too little vitamin A, for instance, can lead to a lack of mucus in the eye, causing drying and hardening of the cornea, which can result in blindness.

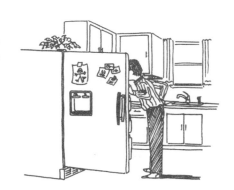

The Benefits of Vitamin A

Vitamin A and Vision

Although many of us know that vitamin A is important for vision, most people don't know why. Vitamin A makes up the visual pigments in the eye. One of the earliest signs of vitamin A deficiency is night blindness—or the slow recovery of vision after flashes of bright lights at night. This occurs because there is an insufficient amount of retinal (vitamin A) available to regenerate the pigments bleached by the light.

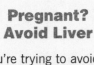

**Pregnant?
Avoid Liver**

If you're trying to avoid too much vitamin A, especially if you're pregnant, you might want to steer clear of liver. Three ounces contain more than 9,000 IU of vitamin A.

Vitamin A and Skin

Vitamin A also plays a role in healthy skin. Both natural and synthetic forms of the vitamin, such as isotretinoin (trade name Accutane), are regularly used in the treatment of skin disorders including acne and **psoriasis**. Individuals undergoing retinoid, or vitamin A, therapy are monitored closely to avoid side effects of vitamin A toxicity such as abnormal blood **lipid** levels, liver toxicity, and birth defects.

Vitamin A and Other Potential Benefits

There are a number of alleged benefits of vitamin A supplements, but the scientific research to support such claims is preliminary, contradictory, or significantly lacking at this time. Examples of such uses include the treatment of breast cancer with a retinoid derivative called 4-hydroxyphenylretinamide (4-HPR, Fenretinide) and the use of vitamin A in skin creams to reduce or prevent wrinkling.

When to Supplement with Vitamin A

Most Americans get enough vitamin A from the diet. The USDA Continuing Survey of Food Intakes by Individuals in 1994–96 showed an average intake of 1,133 micrograms RE (**Retinol Equivalent**) of vitamin A for males aged 20 and older, and 982 micrograms RE for females aged 20 and older. The recommended intake for vitamin A for adult males is 900 micrograms per day, and 700 micrograms for adult females (see "Recommended Dietary Allowances for Vitamin A").

Vitamin A deficiency is not a common problem in the United States. For that reason, vitamin A is not recommended for children in the U.S. However, children, especially those in undeveloped countries, are at an increased risk because they have not yet built up their stores of vitamin A in the liver.

One of the earliest signs of too little vitamin A is night blindness—because of its role in vision. It is estimated that of the 500,000 children worldwide who become blind each year, as many as 70 percent do so because of a vitamin A deficiency. Symptoms

The Many Measurements of Vitamin A

Vitamin A is often discussed in terms of retinol equivalents, milligrams, and International Units. Are they all the same? No. The following list will help you compare the numbers you see on different food and supplement labels:

1 Retinol Equivalent (RE)
= 1 microgram retinol (vitamin A)
= 6 micrograms beta-carotene
= 3 1/3 International Units (IU) vitamin A activity from retinol

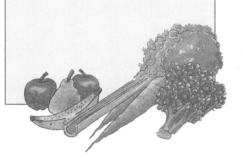

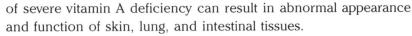

What to Know about Taking Vitamin A Supplements

- Vitamin A is sold in tablet, capsule, softgel, and liquid forms. Multivitamins contain about 5,000 IU (or 1,500 RE) of vitamin A, and a single vitamin A supplement may provide 10,000 IU or 3,000 RE.
- Vitamin A toxicity can occur with sustained intakes (from both food and supplements) of more than 50,000 IU per day for adults and 20,000 IU for infants and young children.
- Since dietary supplements (or claims for them) are not reviewed by the Food and Drug Administration, quality control and potency problems may exist with vitamin A supplements.

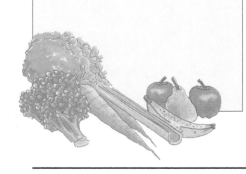

of severe vitamin A deficiency can result in abnormal appearance and function of skin, lung, and intestinal tissues.

Although too little vitamin A can pose a problem, too much can be just as devastating. Symptoms of extremely high doses of vitamin A (greater than 200,000 micrograms RE in adults) can include nausea, vomiting, dizziness, blurred vision, muscular uncoordination, and increased cerebrospinal pressure. Chronic high intakes (as much as 10 times the RDA), on the other hand, can result in hair loss, liver damage, bone and muscle pain, headache, and increased blood lipid (fat) levels.

Vitamin A Toxicity and Osteoporosis

The highest incidence of osteoporotic fractures (fractures due to bones that are brittle and porous) in humans is in Northern Europe, where dietary intake of vitamin A is unusually high. The average dietary intake of vitamin A in the Swedish adult population is 1.3 to 1.6 milligrams per day. And in Norway, intakes can average 1.5 to 2.0 milligrams per day. As a result, researchers studied a group of 422 women in Sweden, between the ages of 28 and 74 years. Interestingly, they found that vitamin A intake was negatively associated with bone mineral density. In other words, for every 1-milligram increase in daily intake of dietary retinol, the risk of hip fractures increased by 68 percent. When comparing intakes greater than 1.5 milligrams per day to intakes less than 0.5 milligrams per day, those with higher intakes had 10 percent less bone mineral density in the neck, 14 percent less at the lumbar spine, and 6 percent less for the whole body. Additionally, the risk of hip fractures was doubled in the higher intake group. The researchers concluded that consuming double the recommended daily amount of vitamin A may dramatically increase the risk of osteoporosis.

Vitamin A Toxicity and Birth Defects

Women who are pregnant and take supplements containing more than two and a half times the RDA for vitamin A (more than 10,000 IU a day) have two and a half times the risk of having a baby with defects, compared to women who don't overdose.

Moreover, the women who take large amounts of vitamin A are five times more likely to have a baby with a cranial neural crest defect— or a defect resulting in a cleft palate, heart abnormalities, and brain damage. Because vitamin A is involved in the growth and development of a healthy fetus, too much A, even stored in the mother's body just before she becomes pregnant, can wreak havoc. In fact, excess vitamin A poses the most danger two weeks *before* conception and during the first two months of pregnancy. The RDA for pregnant women is 750–770 RE or approximately 2,500 IU. A single vitamin A supplement, and some multivitamins, can easily contain more than 10,000 IU. Prenatal vitamins contain as much as 5,000 IU per dose.

FOOD SOURCES OF VITAMIN A

FOOD SOURCES	SERVING SIZE	VITAMIN A (RE)*
Liver, beef	3 ounces	9,011
Sweet potato, baked	1 small	2,488
Carrots, raw	1 large	2,025
Spinach, cooked	½ cup	737
Squash, butternut	½ cup	717
Cantaloupe	¼ melon	444
Apricots, dried	8 large halves	203
Milk, 2% fat	1 cup	139
Broccoli, cooked	½ cup	108
Egg yolk	1	97
Cheese, cheddar	1 ounce	79
Peach	1 medium	53
Halibut, baked	3 ounces	46
Butter	1 teaspoon	38
Margarine, fortified	1 teaspoon	37

Source: USDA Nutrient Database for Standard Reference, Release 13, 1999.
*RE = Retinol Equivalents.

Caution!

- Because of the risk of toxicity, fractures, and birth defects, do *not* exceed recommended levels of vitamin A unless under a doctor's supervision.
- If you have a medical condition or are pregnant or lactating, talk to your doctor before taking any supplement.

RECOMMENDED DIETARY ALLOWANCES (RDA) IN MCG* FOR VITAMIN A

AGE	VITAMIN A (MCG)
Males	
9–13 years	600
14+ years	900
Females	
9–13 years	600
14+ years	700
Pregnancy	
14–18 years	750
19+ years	770
Lactation	
14–18 years	1,200
19+ years	1,300

Source: The National Academy of Sciences, 2000.
*mcg = micrograms.

Vitamin A in Food

Preformed vitamin A (or the active form) can be obtained by consuming foods such as liver, eggs, and fortified foods. Provitamin A carotenoids, such as beta-carotene, are found in dark, leafy greens and in orange and yellow fruits and vegetables (see "Food Sources of Vitamin A" on page 27).

TOLERABLE UPPER INTAKE LEVEL (UL)[a] FOR VITAMIN A

AGE	VITAMIN A (MCG)*
Males	
9–13 years	1,700
14–18 years	2,800
19+ years	3,000
Females	
9–13 years	1,700
14–18 years	2,800
19+ years	3,000
Pregnancy	
14–18 years	2,800
19–50 years	3,000
Lactation	
14–18 years	2,800
19–50 years	3,000

Source: The National Academy of Sciences, 2000.
[a] = The maximum level of daily nutrient intake that is likely to pose no risk of adverse effects. Unless otherwise specified, the UL represents total intake from food, water, and supplements.
*mcg = micrograms.

Vitamin B₆ (Pyridoxine)

Vitamin B₆, or pyridoxine (peer-i-DOX-een), was first discovered in 1938. A water-soluble vitamin, B₆ is found primarily in muscle and exists in three interchangeable forms—pyridoxine, pyridoxal, and pyridoxamine. It is one of the most versatile enzyme **cofactors**, or components, of about 120 enzymes. Vitamin B₆ is essential for glucose (blood sugar) production, fat and protein metabolism, and the production of both niacin (another B vitamin) and hemoglobin.

The Benefits of Vitamin B₆

Vitamin B₆ and Heart Disease

Vitamin B₆, in conjunction with folate (another B vitamin) and vitamin B₁₂, helps to lower blood levels of **homocysteine**, a risk factor for heart disease. In the Framingham Heart Study, individuals with the lowest vitamin B₆ intakes had higher levels of blood homocysteine.

Also, findings from the Nurses' Health Study showed that women with the highest intakes of vitamin B₆ and folate had a lower risk of coronary heart disease than women with lower intakes of these vitamins.

Vitamin B₆ and Carpal Tunnel Syndrome

Over the past twenty years or so, a number of case reports and small studies have suggested that vitamin B₆ deficiency might lead to carpal tunnel syndrome (CTS), a painful wrist condition usually linked to repetitive motion injuries. Some researchers believe vitamin B₆ may be involved in CTS because of its important role in nerve function.

Although many doctors and CTS sufferers became B₆ advocates, no controlled studies have tested the B₆ theory. The first study to do so, involving 125 factory workers, found no connection between blood levels of the vitamin and wrist symptoms. Moreover, deficiency of vitamin B₆ is rare, and too much of the vitamin can cause severe nerve damage. People with CTS who take the recommended megadoses of B₆ (as much as 1,000 milligrams per day)

Caution!

- Because of the risk of toxicity, large doses of vitamin B₆ are *not* recommended. A varied diet and a multivitamin or B-complex supplement should provide most people with the levels they need.
- If you have a medical condition or are pregnant or lactating, talk to your doctor before taking any supplement.

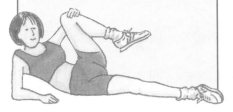

may be putting themselves at risk, since studies have shown that nerve damage can occur with doses as low as 200 milligrams per day.

Vitamin B₆ and Premenstrual Syndrome

For years many women have taken vitamin B₆ supplements to relieve **premenstrual syndrome (PMS)**. However, in a recent review of 25 published studies, although B₆ fared better than a **placebo**, researchers found that there was not enough evidence to warrant a recommendation for using megadoses of B₆ in the treatment of PMS. Furthermore, because of the potential for toxicity, the researchers concluded that at the moment, there is no rationale for giving vitamin B₆ in doses greater than 100 milligrams per day. It may turn out that doses as low as 50 milligrams per day can relieve premenstrual symptoms.

Vitamin B₆ and Other Potential Benefits

In a study of 70 healthy middle-to-older-age men, those with the highest blood levels of vitamin B₆ (similar to that seen with a healthy diet) performed the best on memory tests. Although the results are promising, more research is needed. A number of studies have also looked at the effects of exercise on vitamin B₆ status, **metabolism**, and physical performance, but effects, if any, have been small.

Finally, researchers are also looking at a potential role for vitamin B₆ in the treatment of autism. Many children with the disease have been given large doses of vitamin B₆ and magnesium. In one study researchers observed positive responses in children receiving as much as 3,000 milligrams of B₆ per day. Unfortunately, no other studies have shown similar results. Children being treated with large levels of B₆ should be closely monitored by a physician, because toxicity is a concern.

Vitamin B₆ in Food

Data from the USDA Continuing Survey of Food Intakes by Individuals 1994–96 shows that the greatest contribution of vitamin B₆ to the American diet comes from fortified, ready-to-eat cereals; mixed foods whose main ingredient is fish, meat, or poultry; white potatoes and other starchy vegetables; and noncitrus fruits. Foods especially rich in B₆ include highly fortified cereals and soy-based meat substitutes, beef liver, and other organ meats (see "Food Sources of Vitamin B₆").

When to Supplement with Vitamin B$_6$

National food surveys show that the median daily intake of vitamin B$_6$ in the United States by men is nearly 2 milligrams, and for women it's about 1.5 milligrams—well within the recommended levels (see "Recommended Dietary Allowances for Vitamin B$_6$" on page 33). B$_6$ is not recommended for children.

While extreme B$_6$ deficiency is rare (it's never been seen with intakes of 0.5 milligrams or more per day), marginal deficiencies are more likely. Certain groups are at a greater risk of deficiency, including the elderly, alcoholics, and women on high-dose oral contraceptives—although the studies done with contraceptives were conducted when the level of estrogen in the pill was three to five times higher than the oral agents used today.

When deficiencies occur, they are usually associated with other nutrient deficiencies. For example, since riboflavin is needed for the production of B$_6$, a deficiency in riboflavin could lead to low levels of B$_6$. The earliest symptoms of vitamin B$_6$ deficiency are changes in the nervous system, which can be seen on an EEG (electroencephalogram). Severe deficiency may result in seizures, dermatitis, glossitis (smooth tongue), cheilosis (cracking of corners of the mouth), stomatitis (inflammation of the mouth), irritability, and **anemia**.

Vitamin B$_6$ supplementation has been used in the treatment of, or in an attempt to prevent, a number of diseases, including **Down's syndrome**, autism, gestational diabetes (diabetes during pregnancy), premenstrual syndrome, CTS, and **diabetic neuropathy**. However, B$_6$ supplementation has been of limited benefit in these circumstances. And in some cases, such as the treatment of premenstrual syndrome, supplementing with B$_6$ has resulted in a small number of cases of neurotoxicity (which can cause a loss of sensation in hands and feet and an inability to walk) and photosensitivity. These symptoms are usually seen when doses above 500 milligrams per day are used on a chronic basis.

"B-complex" Vitamins

The B vitamins (folic acid, biotin, niacin, pantothenic acid, riboflavin, thiamin, vitamin B$_6$, and vitamin B$_{12}$) work together as a team, so it makes sense to take them together. Most multivitamins contain varying amounts of most or all of the B vitamins. "B-complex" supplements contain only B vitamins.

What to Know about Taking Vitamin B₆ Supplements

- Vitamin B₆ is sold in tablet, capsule, and liquid forms. Multivitamins contain about 2 milligrams of B₆; B-complex supplements contain about 25 to 50 milligrams; and a single B₆ supplement may provide as much as 100 milligrams.
- The National Academy of Sciences recommends no more than 100 milligrams of supplemental B₆ per day (unless under a doctor's supervision). No cases of B₆ toxicity have been reported from food sources.
- Since dietary supplements (or claims for them) are not reviewed by the Food and Drug Administration, quality control and potency problems may exist with vitamin B₆ supplements

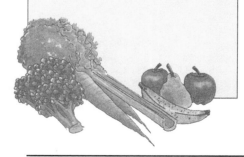

FOOD SOURCES OF VITAMIN B₆

FOOD SOURCES	SERVING SIZE	VITAMIN B₆ (MG)*
Liver, beef	3 ounces	0.77
Banana	1 medium	0.68
Chicken, white meat	3 ounces	0.51
Pistachios	1 ounce	0.48
Avocado, California	1	0.48
Potatoes, mashed	1 cup	0.47
Halibut, baked	3½ ounces	0.39
Chicken, dark meat	3 ounces	0.30
Pork chop, baked	3 ounces	0.30
Sunflower seeds, kernels	¼ cup	0.28
Rice, brown, cooked	1 cup	0.28
Prunes, dried	10	0.22
Milk, 2% fat	1 cup	0.11
Orange juice	1 cup	0.10
Oatmeal	¾ cup	0.03
Bread, white	1 slice	0.01

Source: USDA Nutrient Database for Standard Reference, Release 13, 1999.
*mg = milligrams.

TOLERABLE UPPER INTAKE LEVEL (UL)[a] FOR VITAMIN B₆

AGE	VITAMIN B₆ (MG)*
0–½ year	ND[b]
½–1 year	ND
1–3 years	30
4–8 years	40
9–13 years	60
14–18 years	80
19+ years	100
Pregnant women	
≤18 years	80
19–50 years	100
Lactating women	
≤18 years	80
19-50 years	100

Source: The National Academy of Sciences, 1998.
[a] = The maximum level of daily nutrient intake that is likely to pose no risk of adverse effects. Unless otherwise specified, the UL represents total intake from food, water, and supplements.
*mg = milligrams.
[b] = Not determinable due to lack of data or adverse effects in this age group and concern with regard to lack of ability to handle excess amounts. Source of intake should be from food only to prevent high levels of intake.

RECOMMENDED DIETARY ALLOWANCES (RDA)
FOR VITAMIN B6

AGE/SEX	VITAMIN B6 (MG)*
Males	
9–13 years	1.0
14–50 years	1.3
51+ years	1.7
Females	
9–13 years	1.0
14–18 years	1.2
19–50 years	1.3
51+ years	1.5
Pregnant women	1.9
Lactating women	2.0

Source: The National Academy of Sciences, 1998.
*mg = milligrams.

Vitamin B12 (Cobalamin)

Vitamin B_{12}, or cobalamin (pronounced co-BALL-uh-min), was first discovered in 1948. Roughly 50 percent of this water-soluble vitamin is stored in the liver and the other half is transported to other tissues. Vitamin B_{12} serves as a cofactor (an essential component of enzymes) for two different enzymes. It is necessary for normal blood formation and neurological function. Vitamin B_{12} also maintains the sheath, or covering, that surrounds and protects nerve fibers and promotes their normal growth.

The Benefits of Vitamin B12

Vitamin B12 and Heart Disease

Vitamin B_{12}, in conjunction with folate (another B vitamin) and vitamin B_6, helps to lower blood levels of the amino acid homocysteine, a risk factor for heart disease.

Vitamin B12 and HIV/AIDS

There is a high prevalence of low vitamin B_{12} levels in people with HIV. In one study, researchers found that individuals with low B_{12}

Vitamin B12 Cooking Tip

Few studies have reported cooking losses of B_{12}. However, one study found that boiling milk for just 10 minutes reduced its B_{12} content by 50 percent. Such cooking losses may pose a problem for vegetarians, who don't consume the best sources of B_{12}—animal products—or for those who regularly boil milk in their cooking. Fresh pasteurized fluid milk, which contains about 0.9 micrograms of vitamin B_{12} per cup, may be an important source of this nutrient for vegetarians. Interestingly, reconstituted evaporated milk contains 75 percent less B_{12} than fluid whole milk.

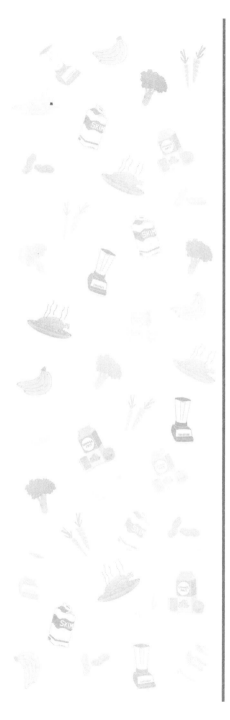

blood levels had a faster progression from HIV to AIDS, compared to those with adequate B_{12} blood levels. In fact, low blood levels of vitamin B_{12} were associated with a nearly twofold increase in risk of progression to AIDS. However, whether or not B_{12} supplementation would slow the progression of the disease is not yet known.

Vitamin B_{12} and Depression

In new research from the Women's Health and Aging Study, older women with vitamin B_{12} deficiency appear to be more prone to depression. Experts studied 700 women aged 65 and older, and those with a B_{12} deficiency were more than twice as likely to suffer from severe depression than women without a deficiency. Evidently, a lack of B_{12} may cause a buildup, or alter chemicals in the brain involved with mood.

Vitamin B_{12} and Other Potential Benefits

There are a number of other potential benefits of B_{12} supplements, including the treatment of Alzheimer's disease and dementia, sleep disorders, and diabetic neuropathy. However, further research is needed in these areas.

When to Supplement with Vitamin B_{12}

National food surveys indicate that the median daily intake of vitamin B_{12} in the United States by men is approximately 5 micrograms and the median intake of women is about 3.5 micrograms—well within the recommended levels (see "Recommended Dietary Allowances for Vitamin B_{12}"). B_{12} is not recommended for children.

There are, however, a number of conditions that may cause deficiencies of vitamin B_{12}. Individuals who suffer from malabsorption syndrome of any cause will most likely need extra vitamin B_{12}. Diseases/conditions requiring supplementation under a doctor's care include post stomach surgery, pernicious anemia, post gastric bypass surgery, **Crohn's disease**, and HIV patients with chronic **diarrhea**. Treatment usually involves monthly intramuscular injections of 100 micrograms of vitamin B_{12}. In addition, the National Academy of Sciences has recommended that individuals over the age of 50 meet their RDA mainly by consuming foods fortified with the synthetic form of B_{12} or a supplement containing vitamin B_{12}.

Vitamin B_{12} and Pernicious Anemia

Vitamin B_{12} requires an "intrinsic factor"—a compound made inside the body—for absorption from the intestinal tract into the bloodstream. This intrinsic factor is made in the stomach, where it attaches itself to the vitamin and carries it to the small intestine to be absorbed.

Certain people have a defective gene for intrinsic factor in their genetic makeup, so they can't make it in their bodies. This defect usually becomes evident in midlife. If the intrinsic factor is missing, vitamin B_{12} cannot be absorbed from the diet and deficiency occurs. When this happens, or when the stomach has been injured and cannot produce enough intrinsic factor, B_{12} must be provided via injections in order to bypass the stomach.

Vitamin B_{12} deficiency, or pernicious anemia, is a type of anemia characterized by large, immature red blood cells identical to those seen in folate deficiency. Symptoms include decreased energy and exercise tolerance, shortness of breath, fatigue, and palpitations. Left untreated, pernicious anemia can lead to a creeping paralysis of the nerves and muscles that begins at the extremities and works up the spine.

Although the symptoms—including the paralysis—can be reversed with vitamin B_{12} treatment, the anemia can be misdiagnosed as a folate deficiency. Folic acid supplements will correct the anemia, but not the damage to the nervous system. For this reason, people over the age of 50 who take folic acid supplements should also take at least 25 micrograms of B_{12} per day, since excess folic acid could mask a potential B_{12} problem.

It is estimated that 10 to 30 percent of people over the age of 50 may develop vitamin B_{12} deficiency due to an inability to absorb the naturally occurring form of B_{12} found in food. Why? Many older people have inadequate gastric (stomach) acid production, which can limit the amount of vitamin B_{12} absorbed. They can, however, absorb synthetic forms of the vitamin, which are found in fortified foods and supplements.

What to Know about Taking Vitamin B_{12} Supplements

- Vitamin B_{12} is sold in tablet and capsule forms. Multivitamins contain about 6 micrograms of B_{12}; B-complex supplements contain about 50 to 100 micrograms, and a single B_{12} supplement may provide as much as 2,500 micrograms.

- No cases of vitamin B_{12} toxicity have ever been reported from food and supplement sources in healthy individuals.

- Since dietary supplements (or claims for them) are not reviewed by the FDA, quality control and potency problems may exist with vitamin B_{12} supplements.

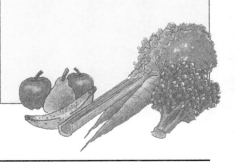

Vitamin B$_{12}$ in Food

Unlike most other nutrients, vitamin B$_{12}$ is only found in animal products. Excellent sources include organ meats, clams, and oysters. Moderate sources include egg yolks, muscle meats and poultry, fish, fermented cheeses, and dry milk (see "Food Sources of Vitamin B$_{12}$").

Data from the USDA Continuing Survey of Food Intakes by Individuals 1994–96 shows that the greatest contributors of B$_{12}$ in the American diet are mixed foods whose main ingredients are meat, fish, or poultry. Milk and milk drinks are the second most important source for women, while beef ranks number two for men. Fortified ready-to-eat cereals are also an important source of vitamin B$_{12}$ for women—more so than for men.

Vitamin B$_{12}$ and Smoking

Cigarettes have a high cyanide content that can interfere with B$_{12}$ metabolism. In one study, vitamin B$_{12}$ loss in urine was significantly higher among smokers than nonsmokers. However, in other studies the difference has been negligible.

Vitamin B$_{12}$ and Vegetarians

Because B$_{12}$ comes from animal products, people who follow a strict vegetarian, or **vegan**, diet are at risk for vitamin B$_{12}$ deficiency. This also holds true for babies who are breastfed by vegan mothers. These infants begin to show signs of deficiency at about four months of age. Therefore, infants at risk of B$_{12}$ deficiency should be supplemented with the Adequate Intake (AI) for vitamin B$_{12}$ from birth.

FOOD SOURCES OF VITAMIN B$_{12}$

FOOD SOURCES	SERVING SIZE	VITAMIN B$_{12}$ (MCG)*
Clams, canned	½ cup	80
Liver, beef	3 ounces	60
Oysters, raw, Pacific	½ cup	20
Crab, Dungeness	3 ounces	9
Tuna, canned	3 ounces	2.5
Beef, hamburger	3 ounces	1.5
Halibut, baked	3½ ounces	1.35
Milk, 2% fat	1 cup	0.89
Yogurt, low fat, plain	½ cup	0.69
Pork chop, baked	3 ounces	0.60
Frankfurters	1	0.59
Egg	1	0.50
Chicken, white meat	3 ounces	0.27
Ice cream	½ cup	0.26

Source: USDA Nutrient Database for Standard Reference, Release 13, 1999.
*mcg = micrograms.

RECOMMENDED DIETARY ALLOWANCES (RDA) FOR VITAMIN B12

AGE/SEX	VITAMIN B12 (MCG)*
Males	
9–13 years	1.8
14+ years	2.4[a]
Females	
9–13 years	1.8
14+ years	2.4[a]
Pregnant women	2.6
Lactating women	2.8

Reprinted by permission of The National Academy of Sciences, 1998. Courtesy of the National Academy Press, Washington, D.C.

[a] = Because 10–30 percent of older people may have trouble absorbing the form of vitamin B12 found in food, it is advisable for those over 50 years to meet their RDA mainly by consuming foods fortified with the synthetic form of B12 or a supplement containing vitamin B12.

*mcg = micrograms.

Biotin

Biotin (pronounced BY-o-tin), also known as vitamin H and coenzyme R, is found largely in the liver, kidney, and muscle. Biotin works together with the B vitamins and is a coenzyme (a small molecule that works with an enzyme to promote the enzyme's activity) involved in carbohydrate, protein, and fat metabolism. Biotin is also important for cellular function and growth, and is essential for fetal development.

The Benefits of Biotin

Research has shown that biotin may play a positive role in treating skin disorders such as dermatitis. It may also be effective in the treatment of brittle nails. Veterinary medicine has long shown that biotin can improve hoofs on horses and pigs by making them stronger, so researchers decided to see if a similar effect could be achieved on human nails. After supplementing with 2.5 milligrams of biotin per day for six months, two-thirds of the study participants saw an improvement in their brittle nails. However, since the study was small, more research is needed.

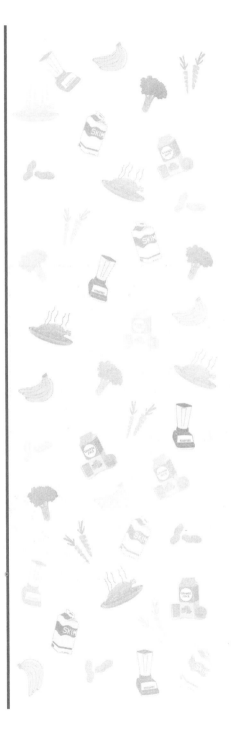

Biotin in Food

Biotin is found in a variety of foods and a large amount is made in the intestine, by bacteria, then absorbed by the body.

FOOD SOURCES OF BIOTIN	
FOOD SOURCES	BIOTIN (MCG/100G OF FOOD)*
Yeast, brewer's	200
Liver, chicken	170–210
Liver, beef	96
Egg yolk, raw	60
Walnuts	37–39
Bran, wheat	22–33
Oatmeal	22–31
Fish and shellfish	3–24
Vegetables	0.2–4

Source: *Krause's Food, Nutrition, and Diet Therapy,* Revised by L.K. Mahan, R.D., C.D., M.S., and M.T. Arlin, R.D., M.S., 8th ed., 1992.
*mcg = micrograms.

When to Supplement with Biotin

Severe biotin deficiency causes thinning and eventual loss of hair; a scaly red rash around the eyes, nose, and mouth; and nervous system problems such as lethargy, depression, and hallucinations. Although biotin deficiency is rare, there are certain groups who are at greater risk.

Individuals who are on total intravenous (by the veins) feedings without added biotin may develop *biotin deficiency facies,* characterized by an unusual distribution of facial fat along with a rash and hair loss. Chronic consumption of raw egg whites can also cause biotin deficiency.

Low biotin levels have been seen in people on long-term antibiotic therapy, or who take anticonvulsants, which may increase the rate of biotin breakdown in the body and interfere with biotin absorption.

Finally, pregnancy may also increase biotin breakdown, so adequate intakes for pregnant women may need to be increased in the future. However, to date there have been no proven problems from marginal biotin status in pregnancy.

Caution!

- Since biotin deficiency is rare, most people do not need to supplement beyond a multivitamin or B-complex.
- If you have a medical condition or are pregnant or lactating, talk to your doctor before taking any supplement.

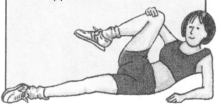

What to Know about Taking Biotin Supplements

- Biotin is often sold in 300- to 1,000-microgram tablets, capsules, softgels, and liquid forms. Special "hair and nail" formulas can contain as much as 2,500 micrograms per supplement.
- A multivitamin or B-complex supplement should provide most people with the extra biotin they need.
- Though toxicity levels from supplemented biotin are unknown, if you are considering taking an individual biotin supplement it's probably wise to stay under 50 milligrams (50,000 micrograms) per day.
- Since dietary supplements (or claims for them) are not reviewed by the Food and Drug Administration, quality control and potency problems may exist with biotin supplements.

ADEQUATE INTAKES (AI) FOR BIOTIN

AGE/SEX	BIOTIN (MCG)*
Males	
9–13 years	20
14–18 years	25
19+ years	30
Females	
9–13 years	20
14–18 years	25
19+ years	30
Pregnant women	30
Lactating women	35

Reprinted by permission of The National Academy of Sciences, 1998. Courtesy of the National Academy Press, Washington, D.C.

*mcg = micrograms.

Biotin Cooking Tips

- If you, or someone you know, likes to start the day consuming a lot of raw egg whites (15 or more per day), you're not only putting yourself at risk for food poisoning, but you may be cheating your body of biotin. Egg whites contain a substance called avidin. In large amounts, avidin combines with biotin in the intestine and prevents its absorption. Cooking egg whites alleviates this problem—and is better from a food safety standpoint as well.
- Biotin is a water-soluble vitamin, so when you boil a food containing this nutrient, much will be lost into the water. Try to steam vegetables in as little water as possible and avoid overcooking foods.

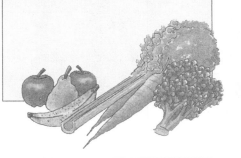

Vitamin C

Vitamin C, also known as ascorbic acid, is a water-soluble vitamin that aids in wound healing and iron absorption and helps maintain bones, blood vessels, and teeth. Vitamin C helps form **collagen**, a protein that gives structure to bones and other connective tissues such as gums and blood vessel walls. It also plays an important role in the production of hormones and the amino acid carnitine.

Vitamin C has long been heralded for its antioxidant properties. Antioxidants are special compounds that protect against **oxidation**, or cellular damage caused by **free radicals**. Common examples of oxidation in everyday life include the rusting of metal and the browning of fruit. In the human body, oxygen-derived free radicals are highly reactive molecules that are normally produced as a byproduct of metabolism in cells. However, free radicals can also be generated in the body as a result of exposure to sunlight, x-rays, tobacco smoke, car exhaust, and other environmental pollutants. Excessive free-radical formation can overwhelm the body's antioxidant defense mechanisms and may lead to a number of chronic diseases such as cancer, stroke, diabetes, heart and lung disease, and **cataracts**.

The Benefits of Vitamin C

Vitamin C and Heart Disease

As an antioxidant, vitamin C may improve immune function and reduce the risk of heart disease by preventing the oxidation of LDL (**low-density lipoprotein** or "bad" **cholesterol**). A lipoprotein is a molecule that carries fat through the blood. Research indicates that LDL oxidation increases the risk for plaque formation, which can clog **arteries** and lead to a heart attack or stroke. Vitamin C also protects vitamin E from oxidation. Research has shown that vitamin E protects against heart disease, too.

Vitamin C may also affect heart health by preventing blood vessels from constricting and thus cutting off blood supply to the heart. This benefit may even be seen in people who already have cardiovascular disease. In one study of individuals with diseased arteries, taking 500 milligrams of supplemental vitamin C per day for

Vitamin C in Food

Roughly 90 percent of the vitamin C in the United States diet comes from fruits and vegetables, especially citrus fruits, tomatoes and tomato juice, and potatoes (see "Food Sources of Vitamin C"). Five servings of most fruits and vegetables per day will provide more than 200 milligrams of vitamin C.

Ascorbic acid is very sensitive to water, heat, and air, so it can be easily destroyed by boiling or prolonged storage, cooking, and processing of foods. Vitamin C is often added to processed foods as an antioxidant.

a month completely normalized the blood flow in their arteries. A number of studies have also shown that supplementing with 1,000 to 2,000 milligrams of vitamin C per day can help block the dangerous artery-destroying effects of the amino acid homocysteine.

Vitamin C and Blood Pressure

Supplementing with 500 milligrams of vitamin C per day may lower blood pressure according to a recent study. Evidently, vitamin C increases the activity and levels of nitric oxide, which relaxes arteries and lowers blood pressure. Nitric oxide also helps prevent clot formation and plaque buildup on artery walls.

Vitamin C and Cancer

There is growing evidence that vitamin C may have a protective effect in cancers of the esophagus, mouth, pharynx, stomach, pancreas, cervix, rectum, breast, and lung. The most promising evidence, however, is with stomach cancer. High doses of vitamin C in animals inhibit *H. pylori*, the bacterium that is responsible for most ulcers and possibly an increased risk of stomach cancer. Vitamin C may also protect against cancer by neutralizing free radicals or blocking the formation of nitrosamines. These carcinogenic compounds form when nitrates (found naturally in foods and as food additives) or nitrites (found naturally in saliva) combine with substances called amines in the digestive juices of the stomach.

Interestingly, a recent study suggested that individuals with cancer who take megadoses of vitamin C may actually be hurting themselves rather than helping. It seems that cancer cells contain vitamin C, which may protect them from oxidation. Many cancer treatments, especially radiation, work by causing oxygen damage to cancer cells. Thus, vitamin C may be working against some forms of cancer treatment. Although these findings are preliminary, the researchers advise that cancer patients avoid supplementing with more than the RDA for vitamin C.

Vitamin C and Cataracts

In its role as an antioxidant, vitamin C is believed to help protect against cataracts. Researchers at Tufts and Harvard Universities

Caution!

- Those with a history of renal stones or diseases related to excess iron accumulation may want to avoid vitamin C supplementation above the RDA.
- If you have a medical condition or are pregnant or lactating, talk to your doctor before taking any supplement.
- Research has shown beneficial effects from vitamin C supplementation up to 1,000 milligrams per day. Supplementing above this level may not be worth the extra money, since excess vitamin C is lost in the urine.

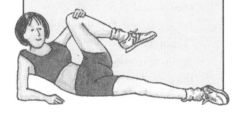

What to Know about Taking Vitamin C Supplements

- Vitamin C is sold as ascorbic acid, calcium ascorbate, sodium ascorbate, or a combination of these forms in tablet, capsule, powder, and liquid forms. Multivitamins contain about 400 milligrams, and a single supplement provides as much as 800 milligrams.
- The National Academy of Sciences recommends no more than 2,000 milligrams of vitamin C per day (from supplements). Megadoses can cause diarrhea, nausea, and abdominal cramps.
- Since dietary supplements (or claims for them) are not reviewed by the FDA, quality control and potency problems may exist with vitamin C supplements.
- Vitamin C chewable tablets may destroy the tooth's protective enamel coating.

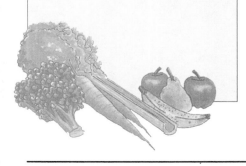

studied nearly 250 women with no history of cataracts. Those who had been supplementing with vitamin C for at least 10 years had 77 percent fewer early-stage opacities (the first sign of cataracts) and 83 percent fewer moderate opacities than women who did not supplement. Although there is much debate among the experts regarding how much vitamin C is necessary for this protective effect, 150 to 200 milligrams is the amount needed to saturate eye tissues.

Vitamin C and Iron Deficiency

Vitamin C can increase iron absorption, which can be helpful for those with an iron deficiency, or for women, who generally have higher iron needs and low intakes. However, it can be a problem for men, who tend to take in too much iron. In fact, some researchers suspect that iron overload among men may contribute to heart disease and several types of cancer. Too much iron in the body may lead to oxidative reactions that can damage tissues and DNA. More research is needed in this area.

Vitamin C and Gallbladder Disease

A recent study indicates that women who don't get enough vitamin C may be at a greater risk for gallbladder disease. **Gallstones** are often formed when **bile**, a liquid formed by the liver to help break down fats during digestion, becomes saturated with cholesterol. Vitamin C helps break down cholesterol, preventing it from hardening into gallstones. These stones can grow as large as one inch across and cause severe abdominal pain. In some cases treatment involves removing the gallbladder altogether.

Gallstones affect many more women than men. This may be due, in part, to the fact that estrogen increases the concentration of cholesterol in bile—and most gallstones are made up of cholesterol. The findings from this latest study indicate that women who have higher blood levels of vitamin C and those who take vitamin C supplements have a lower risk of gallstones and gallbladder disease.

Vitamin C and Asthma

Vitamin C may help people with exercise-induced asthma (EIA) breathe more easily. In a well controlled study from Israel, individuals with EIA were given a single dose of 2,000 milligrams of vitamin C one hour before exercising on a treadmill. The researchers found that ascorbic acid prevented or decreased the severity of wheezing attacks and lung discomfort in over half of the study participants. It appears that vitamin C may protect against damaging oxidants in the lungs.

Vitamin C and Other Potential Benefits

There are a number of alleged benefits of vitamin C supplements that have not been proven by scientific research or are still under investigation. One of the more infamous claims for vitamin C is that it prevents colds. Unfortunately, there has not been a study to date that has shown that supplementing with vitamin C can reduce the risk of catching a cold, although it may shorten the duration and/or severity of the cold.

Lead poisoning is a major public health problem in this country. In a recent study, researchers found that high blood levels of ascorbic acid were associated with a decreased prevalence of elevated blood lead levels in adults. If vitamin C does truly affect blood lead levels, vitamin C intake could have public health implications for control of lead toxicity.

Preliminary research has also suggested that supplementing with vitamin C may protect against mental declines following a stroke or other circulatory problems, although much more research is needed. Finally, researchers are also looking at a potential role for vitamin C in the prevention of osteoporosis and periodontal disease.

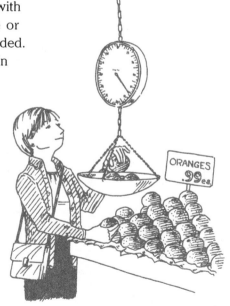

When to Supplement with Vitamin C

As long ago as the 1700s, sailors realized that consuming foods with vitamin C could prevent **scurvy**, or vitamin C deficiency. Although scurvy is rarely seen in developed countries, certain people are at greater risk, including those who consume few fruits and vegetables or abuse alcohol or drugs. In the United States, low vitamin C levels in the blood are more common in men—especially the elderly—than in women and are more prevalent in lower socioeconomic groups.

Symptoms of scurvy include swollen, bleeding gums; loosening of the teeth; hemorrhaging, including bleeding into the

joints; tender and painful extremities; poor wound healing; weakness and fatigue; and psychological disturbances.

For many years experts thought the only use for vitamin C was to prevent scurvy. However, although as little as 10 milligrams of vitamin C per day will prevent deficiency, much higher levels are needed for stress situations such as trauma, wound healing, and infection. Over the years more and more research has shown that vitamin C may be necessary for the prevention of *disease*—not just deficiency.

As a result, the RDA for vitamin C was recently increased (see "Recommended Dietary Allowance for Vitamin C"). The higher levels were set to achieve maximum saturation of vitamin C in the body without excess loss in the urine. It was also recommended that smokers take in an additional 35 milligrams per day to offset some of the oxidative damage from cigarettes. However, some experts argue that these new levels are not high enough. In a report published in 1999, researchers at the National Institutes of Health suggested raising the recommended intake of vitamin C to 100 to 200 milligrams per day.

The USDA Continuing Survey of Food Intakes by Individuals in 1994–96 showed an average daily intake of 109 milligrams of vitamin C for males aged 20 and older, and 91 milligrams for females aged 20 and older.

Although vitamin C toxicity is not a problem for most people, there are certain groups that are at risk of getting too much of this nutrient. Individuals with kidney disease, for instance, should avoid getting more than the RDA. Additionally, intakes above 250 milligrams per day can cause false-negative results in tests for stool and gastric blood. Therefore, high-dose supplementation with vitamin C should be stopped at least two weeks before physical exams because they may interfere with blood and urine tests.

FOOD SOURCES OF VITAMIN C

FOOD SOURCES	SERVING SIZE	VITAMIN C (MG)*
Peppers, hot chili, raw	½ cup	182
Cantaloupe	½ melon	116
Peppers, sweet	1 medium	106
Kiwi	1 medium	74
Orange	1 medium	70
Orange juice, fresh	½ cup	62
Mango	1 medium	57
Cranberry juice cocktail (vitamin C added)	½ cup	45
Grapefruit	½	44
Papaya	½ cup	43
Strawberries	½ cup	41
Tomatoes, raw	1 (3" diameter)	35
Lemon	1	31
Broccoli, raw	1 spear	29
Watermelon	1 wedge (¹/₁₆ of a melon)	27
Cauliflower, cooked	½ cup	27
Collards, cooked	½ cup	22
Potato, baked, peeled	1 medium	20
Spinach, raw	½ cup	8

Source: USDA Nutrient Database for Standard Reference, Release 13, 1999.
*mg = milligrams.

ADEQUATE INTAKES (AI) FOR VITAMIN C*

AGE/SEX	VITAMIN C (MG)**
Infants	
0–½ year	40
½–1 year	50

*There is no RDA for infants due to insufficient information.
**mg = milligrams.

Rating the Supplements

In a May 2000 testing of 26 brands of vitamin C supplements by ConsumerLab.com, 15 percent either did not contain all of the claimed ingredient, or failed to break down as needed for absorption in the body. Check the ConsumerLab Web site (*www.consumerlab.com*) to see how specific brands fared in tests before purchasing a vitamin C supplement. For more information on ConsumerLab.com see the "Buying a Supplement" section of Chapter 1.

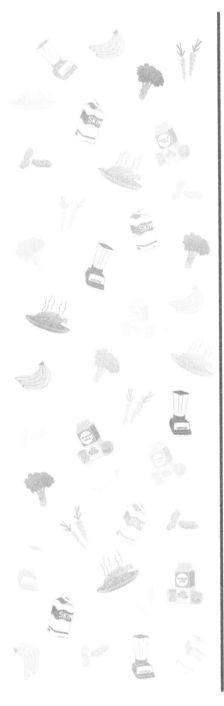

RECOMMENDED DIETARY ALLOWANCES (RDA)* FOR VITAMIN C

AGE/SEX	VITAMIN C (MG)**
Children	
1–3 years	15
4–8 years	25
Males	
9–13 years	45
14–18 years	75
19+ years	90
Females	
9–13 years	45
14–18 years	65
19+ years	75
Pregnant Women	
≤18 years	80
19–50 years	85
Lactating Women	
≤18 years	115
19–50 years	120

Reprinted with permission of The National Academy of Sciences, 2000. Courtesy of the National Academy Press, Washington, D.C.

*There is no RDA for infants due to insufficient information.

**mg = milligrams.

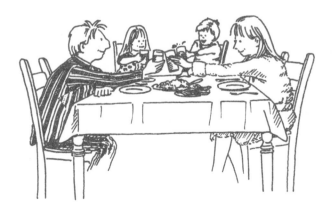

TOLERABLE UPPER INTAKE LEVEL (UL)[a] FOR VITAMIN C

AGE	VITAMIN C (MG)*
0–½ year	ND[b]
½–1 year	ND
1–3 years	400
4–8 years	650
9–13 years	1,200
14–18 years	1,800
19+ years	2,000
Pregnant women	
≤18 years	1,800
19–50 years	2,000
Lactating women	
≤18 years	1,800
19–50 years	2,000

Reprinted with permission of The National Academy of Sciences, 2000. Courtesy of the National Academy Press, Washington D.C.

[a] = The maximum level of daily nutrient intake that is likely to pose no risk of adverse effects. Unless otherwise specified, the UL represents total intake from food, water, and supplements.

*mg = milligrams.

[b] = Not determinable due to lack of data or adverse effects in this age group and concern with regard to lack of ability to handle excess amounts. Source of intake should be from food only to prevent high levels of intake.

Vitamin D

Vitamin D has long been known as "the sunshine vitamin" because the body can make it when the skin is exposed to sunlight. Actually, what we know as vitamin D really isn't a vitamin at all—it's a steroid **hormone**. Long ago it was misclassified as a fat-soluble vitamin and the name just stuck. It does have some of the same characteristics of a vitamin; namely, that people who are not exposed to sunlight need to get vitamin D from food or supplements just as they do for other vitamins. To make matters even more confusing, vitamin D is actually a general term for the many forms of the vitamin. The two major forms are vitamin D_2 and vitamin D_3, which were discovered in the 1930s.

Don't Rely on Milk Alone

Although fortified milk is considered to be the major food source of vitamin D, three studies have shown that less than 20 percent of the milk samples from all sections of the United States and western Canada contained the amount of vitamin D indicated on the label (usually 400 IU). One study even showed that 14 percent of samples had no measurable vitamin D at all! To be sure you're getting enough, take a multivitamin that contains vitamin D, or get some sun.

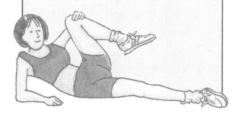

What to Know about Taking Vitamin D Supplements

- Vitamin D is available in tablet, capsule, liquid, and softgel forms. Multivitamins generally contain about 200 IU of vitamin D. Combination products, such as vitamin A and D supplements, also contain 200 IU of vitamin D. A single vitamin D supplement contains about 400 IU, as do some high-potency multivitamins.
- Vitamin D supplements can be taken with or without food.
- People who take glucocorticoids (an anti-inflammatory medication) may require vitamin D supplements. Check with your doctor.
- Seizure medications can decrease the amount of vitamin D in the body. People who take these medications should check with their doctors about taking vitamin D.
- Strict vegetarians are known to have low vitamin D intakes, so a supplement is warranted.
- Since dietary supplements (or claims for them) are not reviewed by the FDA, quality control and potency problems may exist with vitamin D supplements.

Vitamin D_2 (also called ergocalciferol) is the plant form of the vitamin—the form found in some foods and used most often in supplements. Vitamin D_3 (also called cholecalciferol) is the form that's produced when the skin is exposed to sunshine. Some vitamin D_3 is stored in the liver and kidneys, some goes to the bones, and the rest goes to the intestines to aid in calcium absorption from food.

The Benefits of Vitamin D

Vitamin D's most important function is to regulate the body's absorption and use of calcium and phosphorus, thereby making this vitamin essential for bone and tooth formation and strength. Since calcium is also necessary for muscle contraction (including the heart muscle) and sending messages along the nerves, vitamin D is important in these areas, too.

Vitamin D and Osteoporosis

Osteoporosis is a progressive condition characterized by decreased bone density. That is, the mineral content of the bones is diminished, making them brittle, weak, and more likely to break. The condition is most common in women who have gone through menopause, but older men get osteoporosis, too, though it's generally less severe. Although most people think of calcium as being the anti-osteoporosis nutrient, vitamin D's role is also essential.

Bone fractures (often of the hip or spine) in older people are increasingly recognized to be a result of osteoporosis. And for more than twenty years, experts have known that vitamin D deficiency is associated with an increased risk of hip fracture. A recent study conducted at Brigham and Women's Hospital in Boston found that half of the women with hip fractures were deficient in vitamin D.

In some regions of the United States, where sunshine is less abundant and weaker during the winter, researchers have documented measurable loss of bone mineral density in the hips and spines of older people. This is especially troublesome for those who may not be getting adequate amounts of vitamin D from milk products. Researchers from Tufts University found that daily supplements of 500 milligrams of calcium plus 700 IU of vitamin D, taken for three years, decreased the risk of bone fractures in older men and women by 50 percent. A previous study with the same supplements taken over a two-year period resulted in a 43 percent reduction of hip fractures in older women. Experts believe that the main way vitamin D contributes to bone density is by increasing calcium absorption in the small intestine. This ensures an adequate level of calcium in the blood, which can then be deposited in the bone.

Vitamin D and Other Potential Benefits

There is some preliminary evidence that vitamin D supplements may slow the progression of **osteoarthritis** in the knees. A study of 556 participants showed that, among those people who already had arthritic knees, those who also had low blood levels of vitamin D were three times more likely to experience a worsening of their arthritis than those with higher levels of the vitamin.

There are some reports that link vitamin D deficiency to colon and breast cancers. These two types of cancers are more common among people who live in northern climates, where there's less opportunity to get the vitamin from sunshine. Although these studies are still speculative, what is known is that vitamin D inhibits the growth of cancer cells in test tubes. Currently, a government funded study called the Women's Health Initiative is looking into the potential role of vitamin D in cancer.

Psoriasis, a chronic disease that results in itchy, red, flaky patches on the skin, can be treated with sunshine and a prescription cream called Dovonex, which contains a form of vitamin D. However, taking vitamin D supplements alone, or using nonprescription creams with vitamin D, won't work.

When to Supplement with Vitamin D

Surveys indicate that the usual dietary intake of vitamin D in the United States is low—50 to 70 IU per day. Presumably, vitamin D stores are enriched in most people by regular exposure to sunlight, at least during certain times of the year. Recommended intake for vitamin D for males and females aged 51 to 70 is 400 IU, or 600

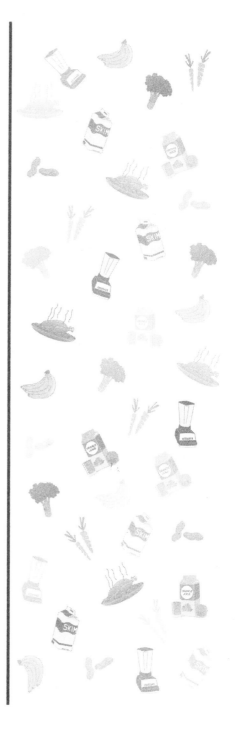

IU per day if over age 70. Vitamin D is not recommended for infants and children unless supervised by a doctor.

Vitamin D Deficiency

The symptoms of vitamin D deficiency include muscle twitching, cramps, and convulsions, as well as aching bones. Conditions that would cause a vitamin D deficiency include severe liver failure, Crohn's disease, and **celiac sprue** (a malabsorption disorder caused by an intolerance to a protein found in wheat, rye, oats, and barley).

Children who are vitamin D deficient get **rickets**, which is characterized by short stature, bowlegs or "knock-knees," and deformities of the skull. In the United States, rickets was virtually eliminated by the 1930s because of the fortification of milk with vitamin D. In Europe, however, foods are not fortified with vitamin D, which is why rickets continues to be a health problem in some European countries. Adults who are vitamin D deficient develop **osteomalacia**, sometimes called "adult rickets." Osteomalacia doesn't cause bone deformities, but it does result in a decrease of the mineral content of the bones, leaving them more prone to fractures. Some people with osteomalacia complain of deep bone pain. Adults over age 50 should consider getting a blood test for vitamin D levels (the form called 25-hydroxyvitamin D) because until a deficiency is quite severe, it's hard to detect. Women should also consider getting a bone mineral density test.

Older People Need More Vitamin D

The recommended amounts of vitamin D are difficult to get if one doesn't drink milk or get regular exposure to the sun. Older people who are housebound or living in nursing homes and rarely spend any time outside in the sun are particularly at risk for vitamin D deficiency. In fact, experts estimate that up to 40 percent of Americans over the age of 50 are vitamin D deficient. Compared to adults aged 20 to 30, those over age 65 produce four times less vitamin D in their skin. It's recommended that people over age 50 take a multivitamin that contains 400 IU of vitamin D per day, as well as a calcium supplement with added vitamin D (200 IU).

Caution!

- People with high intakes of fatty fish or fortified milk may be at risk for vitamin D toxicity.
- Too much vitamin D can be extremely dangerous; taking more than the recommended levels is not advised.
- If you have a medical condition or are pregnant or lactating, talk to your doctor before taking any supplement.
- Because of the extreme importance of adequate vitamin D in developing and maintaining bone, and considering the fact that most diets are generally low in vitamin D, a multivitamin containing 400 IU is recommended for most people.

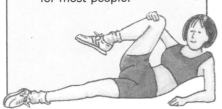

People in Northern Climates Need More Vitamin D

The body can store vitamin D (in the fatty tissues and liver) for a long time, so for most people who are outside a lot during sunny months, body stores of the vitamin are probably sufficient to last the winter. However, people who live in the northern United States or other northern regions and consume little vitamin D may be at increased risk for developing vitamin D deficiency. In northern climates, a multivitamin containing 200 IU of vitamin D is recommended to supplement dietary intake in the winter months. Those who reside year-round in cloudy climates such as Seattle or London may also be deficient and should take the same supplement all year long. And, if the diet contains no fortified milk, a higher-dose vitamin D supplement may be necessary to bring intake up to the recommended levels (see "Adequate Intakes (AI) for Vitamin D").

Vitamin D Toxicity

Reports of vitamin D toxicity from food sources are extremely rare since very few foods contain much of the vitamin. However, high intakes of fatty fish or milk may put one at risk for vitamin D toxicity. With supplements, the chance of getting too much vitamin D is much greater, especially in people who take more than one vitamin D–containing supplement per day (such as a multivitamin and a calcium-plus-vitamin-D supplement).

The upper limit for vitamin D is 1,000 IU per day for infants and 2,000 IU per day for everyone else, including pregnant or lactating women. At an intake of 3,800 IU per day, hypercalcemia (too much calcium) can occur, since vitamin D facilitates calcium absorption. This condition can cause calcification of the soft tissues including the kidneys, blood vessels, heart, and lungs. In infants, intakes greater than 45 micrograms per day may reduce growth.

Other symptoms of vitamin D toxicity include loss of appetite, nausea, vomiting, thirst, joint pains, muscular weakness, and disorientation. Ironically, getting too much vitamin D can cause bone demineralization and bone loss. Severe vitamin D toxicity can be fatal.

Vitamin D in Food

Only fatty fish, fish liver oils (such as cod liver oil), and eggs from hens fed vitamin D supplements are good sources. Fish can contain anywhere from 200 to 1,600 IU of vitamin D per 100 grams. Most of us get our vitamin D from fortified milk.

The body can also make vitamin D, given adequate exposure to the sun. Experts say you only need to expose your face and hands to the sun for 5 to 15 minutes, two or three times a week. It's estimated that this exposure is about equal to consuming 200 IU of vitamin D. You're better off getting exposure during early morning or late afternoon hours to avoid a sunburn. Also, the pigment in the skin is a factor (darker-skinned people may not make as much vitamin D), as well as the time of year and location.

Unlike water-soluble vitamins, fat-soluble vitamins such as vitamin D are not as easily destroyed during cooking. Research has shown that less than 10 percent of the vitamin D in food is lost during cooking.

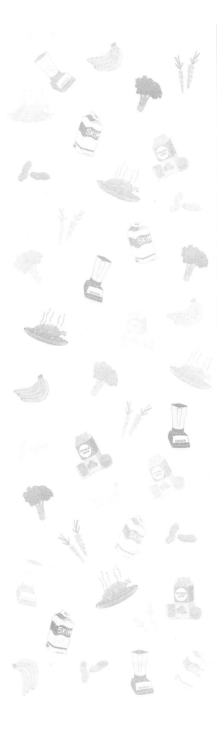

FOOD SOURCES OF VITAMIN D

FOOD SOURCES	SERVING SIZE	VITAMIN D (IU)*
Salmon, canned with bones	1 ounce	177
Milk, 2% fat	1 cup	98
Sardines, canned with bones	1 ounce	77
Egg yolk	1	25
Cheese, cheddar	1 ounce	3
Butter	1 teaspoon	1.4

Source: USDA Nutrient Database for Standard Reference, Release 13, 1999.
*IU = International Units.

ADEQUATE INTAKES (AI)* FOR VITAMIN D

AGE/SEX	VITAMIN D (MCG AND IU)[a,b],**
Males	
19–50	5 (200 IU)
51–70	10 (400 IU)
71+	15 (600 IU)
Females	
19–50	5 (200 IU)
51–70	10 (400 IU)
71+	15 (600 IU)
Pregnant women	5 (200 IU)
Lactating women	5 (200 IU)

Reprinted with permission of The National Academy of Sciences, 1997. Courtesy of the National Academy Press, Washington, D.C.
*There is no RDA due to insufficient information.
**mcg = micrograms; IU= International Units.
[a] = Microgram amounts are for the cholecalciferol form. 1 microgram cholecalciferol = 40 IU vitamin D.
[b] = In the absence of adequate exposure to sunlight.

TOLERABLE UPPER INTAKE LEVELS (UL)[a] OF VITAMIN D

AGE/SEX	VITAMIN D (MCG)*
0–1 year	25
1+ years	50
Pregnancy	50
Lactation	50

Reprinted with permission of The National Academy of Sciences, 1997. Courtesy of the National Academy Press, Washington, D.C.
*mcg = micrograms.
[a] = The maximum level of daily nutrient intake that is likely to pose no risk of adverse effects. Unless otherwise specified, the UL represents total intake from food, water, and supplements.

Vitamin E

Vitamin E, discovered in 1922, is the general name for eight different forms of the vitamin: four tocopherols and four tocotrienols. The tocopherols are the most important, and these are designated alpha, beta, delta, and gamma (i.e., beta-tocopherol). Alpha-tocopherol has the highest biological activity. The tocotrienols are active in the body, but are usually considered less nutritionally important. Tocopherols and tocotrienols are the general names for the two primary chemical structures of vitamin E. Within each group are four forms of the vitamin that differ from each other slightly in chemical structure.

Vitamin E is generally considered the major fat-soluble antioxidant in the blood and body tissues. As such, it is the first line of defense against free radicals—unstable oxygen molecules that can damage body cells and may lead to heart disease, cancer, stroke, and other health problems. (For more information about free radicals, see the vitamin C section.) Vitamin E, which is stored mainly in fat tissue and the liver, is particularly important in the brain and nervous system.

The Benefits of Vitamin E

Vitamin E and Heart Disease

Vitamin E could well be considered the nutrient of the 1990s. That was the decade when the popularity of the vitamin soared as a result of evidence from almost 20 population studies that suggested that people who had a high intake of vitamin E had a reduced risk of heart disease. But, population studies can only draw associations—they don't prove true cause and effect. Intervention trials (also called clinical trials, where particular treatments are specifically investigated with carefully selected participants in a controlled setting) are needed for that—and there haven't been many.

A study in China showed heart benefits from vitamin E supplementation, but the supplements contained more than just vitamin E, so it's unclear which of the ingredients was the most helpful. The Cambridge Heart Antioxidant Study, an intervention trial with 2,002 people, demonstrated that supplementing with vitamin E reduced nonfatal heart attack risk by 77 percent compared to a placebo.

Caution!

- Because of its blood-thinning effect, stop taking vitamin E several days before and for two weeks after surgery.
- People taking anticoagulant medications (i.e., heparin, warfarin) should not take vitamin E supplements.
- The National Academy of Sciences has set intake limits for vitamin E (see "Tolerable Upper Intake Levels of Vitamin E"). Do not routinely exceed the UL. Vitamin E supplement use is high in the United States, and as long as consumption stays below the 1,000 milligram level, it's safe.
- If you have a medical condition or are pregnant or lactating, talk to your doctor before taking any supplement.

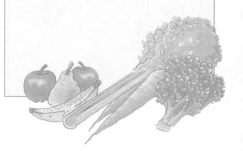

Recently, however, the Heart Outcomes Prevention Evaluation in Canada failed to show that vitamin E supplements decrease the risk of heart disease or stroke. In this study, 9,500 people aged 55 and up who were diagnosed with cardiovascular disease or diabetes (a major risk factor for cardiovascular disease) received either a placebo or a 400 IU supplement of vitamin E daily. After four and a half years, those who took vitamin E were no less likely than the placebo-takers to have had a heart attack or stroke, or to have died from cardiovascular disease. There was also no difference between the groups in frequency of other heart problems such as **angina**. Another study in Italy concluded that 300 IU of supplemental synthetic (man-made) vitamin E, taken daily for three and a half years, did not significantly reduce risk of heart attack or stroke in more than 11,000 men and women.

Why the discrepancy? It may be that vitamin E only offers *protection* from cardiovascular disease in otherwise healthy people—not a reversal of the condition or cure. Perhaps, as the researchers acknowledge, vitamin E may work best when taken in conjunction with other antioxidants. Also, the form of vitamin E may be causing the conflicting results. Some animal studies have shown that gamma-tocopherol (the type found primarily in foods) may be more effective in preventing free radical damage than alpha-tocopherol, the form used most frequently in supplements. In any case, a number of other trials with vitamin E are currently underway, and the overall body of research does indicate some probable benefit from vitamin E supplements.

Vitamin E and Alzheimer's Disease

There is a good amount of evidence to suggest that free radical damage to the **neurons** (nerve cells) is at least partially responsible for the development of Alzheimer's disease. Studies have also shown an association between vitamin E and the risk of, or progression of, Alzheimer's disease.

Vitamin E has been shown to prevent free radical damage and delay memory deficits in animal studies. And, a recent human study in which participants took 2,000 IU of vitamin E per day showed that the supplement may slow the functional deterioration that frequently leads to placement in a health-care or long-term care facility. In a two-year study of people with Alzheimer's disease, progression of the disease was slowed when either 2,000 IU of vitamin E (alpha-tocopherol), a drug (10 milligrams Selegiline), or a combination of the two was taken daily. The researchers noted that, compared to those taking a placebo, those in the treatment groups took seven months longer to reach severe dementia, institutionalization, loss of the ability to perform basic activities of living, and death. The combined treatment (drug plus vitamin E) appeared to be just as effective as either component alone.

Although the evidence for vitamin E is promising, it's important to note that such large doses of vitamin E, when taken by healthy people, have not been shown to *prevent* Alzheimer's disease. What's more, the safety and efficacy of supplemental vitamin E taken over many years has not been adequately studied. Whether the risks associated with large doses of vitamin E are worth any possible benefit is a decision that should be made with the help of a personal physician.

Vitamin E and Cancer

A number of epidemiological studies suggest that low blood levels or intakes of vitamin E are associated with increased risk of certain types of cancer. Occurrence of cancer of the stomach, esophagus, and cervix seems to be reduced when antioxidant supplements (including vitamin E) are taken for a period of years. Vitamin E supplements have also been associated with lower risk of oral, colon, breast, thyroid, prostate, gastrointestinal tract, lung, and bladder cancers. In many cases, at least 100 IU of vitamin E per day is needed. And, studies seem to indicate that vitamin E is not effective if a person already has cancer. In other words, it doesn't cure or reverse cancer progression, but it may delay or prevent it. However, since most results only show associations between vitamin E and cancer outcomes—not true cause-and-effect relationships—some researchers think it's premature to recommend supplements for the prevention of cancer. What's more, many of these studies used supplements containing a mixture of antioxidants, so it's impossible to say that vitamin E supplements alone will produce similar effects.

Natural vs. Synthetic Vitamin E

A number of animal studies have shown that supplements containing natural vitamin E are absorbed and retained in the body longer than synthetic vitamin E. This has led to considerable debate about whether this is true for people as well. Some human studies confirm the animal study results, indicating that when natural vitamin E is taken only half as much is needed. However, a recent study done at the Center for Human Nutrition at the University of Texas Southwestern Medical Center indicates that, when given equivalent amounts, humans appear to absorb both forms of alpha-tocopherol equally well. Natural vitamin E supplements cost more than synthetic ones, so if cost is an issue, look for labels that specify "dl-alpha-tocopherol" (the synthetic version) instead of "d-alpha" (the natural version).

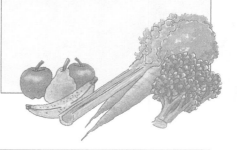

Vitamin E and Cataracts

A cataract starts off as a cloudy spot on the lens of the eye, which may or may not interfere with vision. As it gets worse, or as more of them develop on the lens, blurred vision, sensitivity to light, and changes in color perception may occur. Although cataract surgery is performed on an outpatient basis and is very successful, preventing cataracts in the first place is even better. Age is still considered the major risk factor in cataract development, which is caused by exposure to ultraviolet radiation (sunlight) that causes oxidation, or free radical damage.

A number of epidemiological studies have suggested an association between cataract development and low blood levels of vitamin E and other antioxidants. For example, in a U.S. study of 112 people, high blood levels of at least two of the three antioxidant nutrients (vitamins E, C, and carotenoids) were associated with a significantly reduced risk of cataract development compared to people with low levels of at least one of the nutrients. Two studies conducted in Finland have shown an association between low vitamin E levels and cataract risk, or the development of cortical lens opacities (cloudy spots on the lens that lead to cataract formation).

Experts suggest that vitamin E will not prevent cataracts, but supplements may delay the onset and slow the progression of cataract development. A few animal studies have shown this to be true, but clinical trials with humans are necessary in order to firmly establish vitamin E's efficacy in cataract prevention.

Vitamin E and Immunity

Aging is associated with a decline in immune status, which leads to more infections, cancers, and other chronic diseases. A study conducted at the Human Nutrition Research Center on Aging at Tufts University examined the effects of various vitamin E supplements on 78 healthy people aged 65 and older. After four months, those who took 200 milligrams of vitamin E per day had stronger responses to vaccines for hepatitis B and tetanus than those who took the placebo. That is, they created more antibodies to fight off future attacks of the illnesses. Responses for other doses (60 or 800 milligrams) were not as good. The vitamin E takers also experienced

30 percent fewer infections, and other indicators of immunity were also improved by the supplements. Finally, immune effects were confirmed in people under age 30 as well, with six months of supplementation with 400 IU of vitamin E.

Vitamin E and Other Potential Benefits

There are many additional areas of vitamin E research, including male infertility, diabetes, skin disorders, circulatory problems, and physical performance (both in athletes and in people who live at high altitudes). Vitamin E supplementation appears somewhat promising for each of these areas, but at the current time the research is preliminary. The use of topical (applied to the skin) vitamin E in treating skin wounds has been investigated for years, with conflicting results. A recent study of 15 people who had skin cancers removed and were treated with either topical vitamin E or a placebo showed that there was no benefit to using the vitamin (the wounds didn't heal faster or scar less). What's more, a third of the participants developed inflamed skin from the vitamin E treatment.

When to Supplement Vitamin E

For adults, the recommended amount of daily vitamin E intake is 15 milligrams (22 IU of natural-source vitamin E or 33 IU of the synthetic form) of alpha-tocopherol. (For more information about natural and synthetic vitamin E sources, see "Natural vs. Synthetic Vitamin E.") According to the USDA Continuing Survey of Food Intakes by Individuals 1994–96, the average reported dietary intake of vitamin E for people aged 31 to 50 years is 7.5 milligrams alpha-tocopherol per day for men and 5.4 milligrams for women—significantly below the recommended amounts (see "Recommended Dietary Allowances for Vitamin E"). However, this survey probably underestimated actual vitamin E intake because of measurement errors that are common with vitamin E. According to the National Academy of Sciences, real vitamin E intake in the United States and Canada is likely to meet or even exceed the RDA level.

Vitamin E supplements are not recommended for children.

Vitamin E in Food

By far, the richest sources of vitamin E in the U.S. diet are vegetable oils (including soybean, corn, cottonseed, and safflower) and products made from these oils, such as shortening and margarine. Wheat germ, nuts, and grains also provide some vitamin E, but meats, fish, and most fruits and vegetables (except leafy greens) contain little (see "Food Sources of Vitamin E").

Alpha-tocopherol is the only form of vitamin E that's counted toward the recommended daily intake amounts (such as the RDA). It's the only form that human blood can maintain and transfer to cells. The other forms of the vitamin, however, may provide health benefits.

At least half of the tocopherol content of wheat germ, sunflower, cottonseed, safflower, canola, and olive oils is in the form of alpha-tocopherol. Palm and rice bran oils also contain appreciable amounts of alpha-tocopherol. Soybean and corn oils contain about 10 times as much delta-tocopherol as alpha-tocopherol.

Vitamin E Deficiency

A deficiency of vitamin E causes reproductive problems; neurological abnormalities, including diminished reflexes, limb weakness, sensory loss in the arms and legs, and difficulty walking; immunological abnormalities; and hemolytic anemia (breakdown of red blood cells).

Deficiency is not common, but is known to occur in premature infants with very low birth weights and in people suffering from malnutrition. The most common cause of vitamin E deficiency is fat malabsorption. People who can't absorb fat properly cannot absorb vitamin E well either, since it's a fat-soluble vitamin. Therefore, **cystic fibrosis**, chronic liver disease, chronic diarrhea, celiac sprue (a condition where food absorption is impaired due to an intolerance to gluten, a protein found in certain grains), short bowel syndrome, and Crohn's disease hamper vitamin E absorption. For people with these conditions, a water-soluble vitamin E supplement is suggested. People who follow a very low-fat, low-calorie diet and those who take cholesterol-lowering drugs may also be at risk for deficiency.

Because vitamin E is stored in the body for long periods of time, it takes several years in adults before blood levels of the vitamin decrease to a deficient range. Neurologic abnormalities may take five to 10 years to appear. However, in children with vitamin E malabsorption from infancy (such as those born with liver diseases), vitamin E deficiency can develop rather early in life, rapidly producing neurologic symptoms if the deficiency is untreated. If corrected in the first few years of life, all symptoms can be reversed or prevented. Once neurologic damage has occurred, vitamin E can produce only limited improvement.

Vitamin E Toxicity

Compared with the other fat-soluble vitamins, oral vitamin E supplements produce few side effects and are relatively nontoxic. In adults, large doses may interfere with the absorption of vitamins A and K and cause fatigue, gastrointestinal upset, breast soreness, and thyroid problems. The biggest concern with large amounts of vitamin E relates to the vitamin's blood-thinning effect. Intakes of more than 1,200 milligrams per day, combined with anticoagulant medications, can cause dangerous bleeding. Even on its own, vitamin E can lead to postsurgery bleeding when taken in doses greater than 800 to 1,200 milligrams per day. In premature infants, large doses of vitamin E have caused a number of problems, including an increased risk of infection and gastrointestinal problems.

FOOD SOURCES OF VITAMIN E

FOOD SOURCES	SERVING SIZE	VITAMIN E (MG ALPHA-TOCOPHEROL)*
Wheat germ oil	1 tablespoon	26.94
Sunflower oil	1 tablespoon	7.08
Almonds	1 ounce	7.28
Hazelnuts	1 ounce	6.78
Safflower oil	1 tablespoon	6.03
Cottonseed oil	1 tablespoon	5.36
Wheat germ, toasted	1/4 cup	5.26
Corn oil	1 tablespoon	2.96
Canola oil	1 tablespoon	2.93
Turnip greens, boiled	1/2 cup	2.39
Salad dressing, Italian	1 tablespoon	1.55
Spinach, canned	1/2 cup	1.39
Anchovy, in oil	5 anchovies	1.00
Beans, navy	1 cup	1.00
Egg, fried	1	.75

Source: *Pennington, Bowes & Church's Food Values of Portions Commonly Used*, 17th Ed., Revised by Jean Pennington, Ph.D., R.D., 1998.
*mg = milligrams.

RECOMMENDED DIETARY ALLOWANCES (RDA)* FOR VITAMIN E IN MG**

Males
9–13 years	11
14+ years	15

Females
9–13 years	11
14+ years	15
Pregnant women	19
Lactating women	19

Reprinted with permission of The National Academy of Sciences, 2000. Courtesy of the National Academy Press, Washington D.C.
*There is no RDA for infants due to insufficient information.
**mg = milligrams.

The Many Measurements of Vitamin E

Vitamin E is often discussed in terms of International Units (IU) and milligrams (mg). An IU is a standardized unit of measurement for vitamin potency, whereas a milligram is a unit of measurement for weight. Before 1980, the conversion equation for vitamin E was:

1 milligram alpha-tocopherol = 1.49 IU vitamin E

Since then, more specific conversions are used to differentiate between natural and synthetic (man-made) vitamin E. To convert the IU measurements found on supplement labels into milligrams of alpha-tocopherol, use the following equations.

- For vitamin E labeled as "natural" or "d-alpha-tocopherol":

IU × 0.67 = 1 milligram alpha-tocopherol

- For vitamin E labeled as "dl-alpha-tocopherol" (synthetic):

IU × 0.45 = 1 milligram alpha-tocopherol

Tolerable Upper Intake Levels (UL)[a] of Vitamin E[b]

Age	Vitamin E (mg supplementary alpha-tocopherol)*
0–1 year	Not possible to establish; intake should be from food and formula only
1–3 years	200
4–8 years	300
9–13 years	600
14–18 years	800
19+ years	1,000
Pregnancy	
14–18 years	800
19+ years	1,000
Lactation	
14–18 years	800
19+ years	1,000

Reprinted with permission of The National Academy of Sciences, 2000. Courtesy of the National Academy Press, Washington D.C.

[a] = The maximum level of daily nutrient intake that is likely to pose no risk of adverse effects.

[b] = The UL for vitamin E pertains to supplementary alpha-tocopherol only—not that consumed in food.

*mg = milligrams.

Folic Acid

Folic acid, or folate, is a B vitamin that appears to be protective against certain birth defects, cancer, and heart disease. Folate is the form found naturally in foods, and folic acid is the synthetic form found in fortified foods and supplements. Folate is needed to make DNA, the carrier of genetic information in all cells. Rapidly dividing cells, especially in the blood, the developing fetus, and the lining of the colon, need folic acid the most. Folate is also necessary for the production of red blood cells and protein metabolism, and to convert the amino acid homocysteine into another amino acid, methionine.

The Benefits of Folic Acid

Folic Acid and Birth Defects

In recent years researchers have discovered that folic acid reduces the risk of neural tube defects (NTDs), one of the most serious and common birth defects in the United States. These defects occur in the neural tube, which develops into the spinal cord. If the defect occurs at the top of the tube, the result is fatal, since the baby is born with anencephaly (no brain). If the defect occurs farther down on the tube, the baby is born with spina bifida (an open spine). Damage to the exposed spinal cord usually results in a child who is either wheelchair bound or on crutches.

Each year, an estimated 2,500 babies are born with these defects, and many additional affected pregnancies result in miscarriage or stillbirth. Since these birth defects occur within the first month of pregnancy—before many women even know they're pregnant—it is important for a woman to have enough folic acid in her system prior to conception. Folic acid, when consumed in adequate amounts by women at least one month prior to and for 6 weeks after conception, can prevent up to 70 percent of these birth defects. The benefits are so great that in 1992 the U.S. Public Health Service recommended that all women of childbearing age consume 400 micrograms of folic acid every day.

Folic Acid and Down's Syndrome

In a recent study, researchers found that supplementing with folic acid may also help prevent Down's syndrome, one of the most common developmental disorders in the United States. This syndrome affects nearly 1 in 150 conceptions every year. Although the age of the mother has long been recognized as a risk factor for Down's syndrome, most children with the disorder are born to women under the age of 30.

Down's syndrome is caused by a genetic mutation resulting in an extra chromosome. Previous research suggests that insufficient folate leads to some genetic mutations. The theory is that low folate levels may increase the risk of a genetic mutation leading to Down's syndrome. Although more research is needed, consuming

Caution!

- Talk to your physician before supplementing with folate if you are taking any kind of anticonvulsant drugs.
- If you have a medical condition, talk to your doctor before taking any supplement.
- Intakes higher than the RDA may be needed by women pregnant with more than one fetus, mothers nursing more than one infant, alcoholics, and individuals on chronic anticonvulsant or methotrexate therapy.
- Synthetic folic acid, in addition to a folate-rich diet, is recommended for all women of childbearing age.

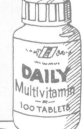

enough folic acid to meet the RDA is the prudent thing to do for all women of childbearing age.

Folic Acid and Heart Disease

Folate may also play an important role in reducing the risk for cardiovascular disease. It is involved in controlling blood levels of homocysteine by converting this amino acid into methionine. High levels of homocysteine may increase the risk of heart disease and stroke. In the Physicians' Health Study, men who started out with elevated homocysteine levels were three times as likely to have a heart attack over the next five years.

Previous research indicates that folic acid intakes of 400 micrograms (the current RDA) or more per day may keep homocysteine at stable low levels. The same research suggests that possibly 88 to 90 percent of the population is not consuming enough folate to keep homocysteine levels low. Findings from the Nurses' Health Study showed that women with the highest intakes of folate and vitamin B6 had a lower risk of coronary heart disease than women with lower intakes of these vitamins.

Folic Acid and Colon Cancer

A growing body of clinical studies suggests a possible association between low folate status and an increased risk for cancer, with the strongest evidence for colorectal cancer—one of the leading causes of death by cancer in the United States. In findings from the U.S. Nurses' Health Study, women who had been taking a multivitamin with folic acid for at least 15 years had 75 percent less risk of developing colon cancer than those who didn't take multivitamins. Folate from foods also appeared to be protective, but not significantly. Similar findings were also seen in men in the U.S. Health Professionals Follow-up Study. Men who reported eating the most folate-rich foods were less likely to develop colon cancer over the next few years. Researchers suspect that folate protects against DNA damage—which can cause cancer.

Researchers are also investigating the protective effects of folate against lung, esophagus, uterine, cervix, and liver cancers. Here, however, more research is needed.

Folic Acid and Alcohol

In a recent study of 90,000 women, those who consumed less than 300 micrograms of folate per day and regularly drank alcohol (at least one drink per day) increased their risk of breast cancer by 30 percent, compared to those who drank less than one drink per day. However, breast cancer risk increased by only 5 percent in those who regularly drank alcohol while consuming more than 300 micrograms of folate per day. Apparently, alcohol interferes with folate metabolism, preventing the vitamin from reaching tissue cells, thereby leaving them vulnerable to cancerous changes. Consuming adequate folate helps counteract this effect.

Folic Acid and Other Potential Benefits

There are a number of alleged benefits of folic acid supplements, but the evidence to support such claims is very preliminary. One example is the possible use of folic acid to treat depression. Several studies have shown individuals suffering from depression may have low folate levels.

When to Supplement with Folic Acid

Folate in food is nearly 50 percent less bioavailable than folic acid in fortified foods and supplements. In fact, folate is one of the few nutrients that is more beneficial in the man-made form than the natural form.

Folate deficiency is one of the most common nutrient deficiencies in the United States and can result in megaloblastic anemia, which is characterized by a reduced number of red blood cells. Side effects of the anemia include weakness, fatigue, headache, irritability, difficulty concentrating, and shortness of breath.

It is not recommended that children take folic acid supplements.

Folate and Vitamin B_{12} Deficiency

Folate and vitamin B_{12} work closely together, and a deficiency of either nutrient leads to anemia. However, in the case of vitamin B_{12}, deficiency can bring about not only anemia, but nerve damage as well. If a B_{12} deficiency is misdiagnosed as a folate deficiency,

---

What to Know about Taking Folic Acid Supplements

- Folic acid is sold in tablet, capsule, powder, and liquid forms. Multivitamins and B-complex supplements contain about 400 micrograms, and a single folic acid supplement may provide as much as 800 micrograms.

- The National Academy of Sciences recommends no more than 1,000 micrograms of folic acid per day (unless under a doctor's supervision) to avoid masking a vitamin B_{12} deficiency.

- Since dietary supplements are not reviewed by the FDA, quality control and potency problems may exist.

- The synthetic form of folate (folic acid) is better absorbed than the folate found naturally in foods. When synthetic folate is consumed in a supplement without food, nearly 100 percent is absorbed. Folic acid in fortified foods had an absorption rate of about 85 percent. Only half of the folate found naturally in foods is absorbed.

Folic Acid in Food

Although folate is found naturally in a variety of foods, it is difficult to meet the RDA through diet alone (see "Food Sources of Folate"). Therefore, the Department of Health and Human Services (DHHS) and the FDA announced in 1997 that U.S. food manufacturers would be required, as of January 1998, to add folic acid to most **enriched** breads, rolls, buns, flours, cornmeals, pastas, rice, and other grain products. Prior to mandatory fortification, U.S. adults consumed an average of 250 micrograms of folate per day. However, after 1998, the average intake was expected to increase by about 100 micrograms of folate per day for women and by more for men.

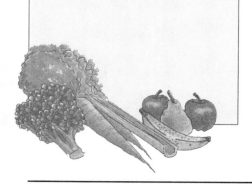

folic acid supplements will correct the anemia but not the damage to the nervous system. For this reason, people over the age of 50 who take folic acid supplements should also take at least 25 micrograms of B_{12} per day, since excess folic acid could mask a potential B_{12} deficiency.

Folate and Alcohol

Surveys of chronic alcoholics suggest that inadequate intake is a major cause of folate deficiency in this group. Additionally, ethanol intake may impair folate absorption and increase folate loss in the urine.

Folate–Drug Medications

Methotrexate is an "anti-folate" medication that has been used successfully with people suffering from rheumatoid arthritis, inflammatory bowel disease, asthma, psoriasis, and certain liver diseases. Patients with rheumatoid arthritis are often deficient in folate, and folate stores are decreased in rheumatoid arthritis patients who take methotrexate. Moreover, some of the side effects of the drug, including gastrointestinal distress, mimic folate deficiency. Therefore, patients are often put on high-folate diets or given supplemental folic acid to reduce the side effects with no reduction in the drug's effectiveness. It is recommended that patients with rheumatoid arthritis who are undergoing methotrexate therapy increase folate consumption or supplement with 1,000 micrograms of folic acid per day.

High doses of folate may also interfere with certain anticonvulsant medications used to treat epilepsy, by competing with them for absorption in the intestine. This in turn could interfere with the drugs crossing the barrier to the brain and could lead to seizures.

FOOD SOURCES OF FOLATE

FOOD SOURCES	SERVING SIZE	FOLATE (MCG)*
Beef liver	1 slice	185
Lentils, cooked	½ cup	180
Cereal, ready-to-eat, fortified	½–1 cup	170
Rice, white enriched, processed, cooked	1 cup	170
Macaroni, enriched, cooked	1 cup	140–160
Noodles, enriched, cooked	1 cup	160
Beans, black, cooked	½ cup	130
Spinach, raw	1 cup	110
Asparagus, cooked	5 spears	100
Spinach, cooked	½ cup	100
Mustard greens, cooked	½ cup	90
Orange juice, ready-to-drink	1 cup	80
Bagel, enriched	1, 3" diameter	70
Avocado	½ medium	55
Broccoli, raw	½ cup	30
Potato, baked, with skin	1 medium	25
Egg	1 large	25

Copyright ©The American Dietetic Association. Reprinted by permision from the *Journal of the American Dietetic Association*, 2000, Vol. 100, pp. 88–94.
*mcg = micrograms.

RECOMMENDED DIETARY ALLOWANCES (RDA) FOR FOLATE (MCG)[a],*

SEX/AGE	FOLATE (MCG)
Males	
9–13 years	300
14+ years	400
Females	
9–13 years	300
14+ years	400[b]
Pregnant women	600[c]
Lactating women	500

Reprinted with permission of The National Academy of Sciences, 1998. Courtesy of the National Academy Press, Washington D.C.

[a] = As dietary folate equivalents (DFE). 1 DFE = 1 microgram food folate = 0.6 microgram of folic acid from fortified food or as a supplement consumed with food = 0.5 microgram of a supplement taken on an empty stomach.
*mcg = micrograms.

[b] = In view of evidence linking folate intake with neural-tube defects in the fetus, it is recommended that all women capable of becoming pregnant consume 400 micrograms from supplements or fortified foods in addition to intake of folate from a varied diet.

[c] = It is assumed that women will continue consuming 400 micrograms from supplements or fortified food until their pregnancy is confirmed and they enter prenatal care, which ordinarily occurs after the end of the periconceptional period—the critical time for formation of the neural tube.

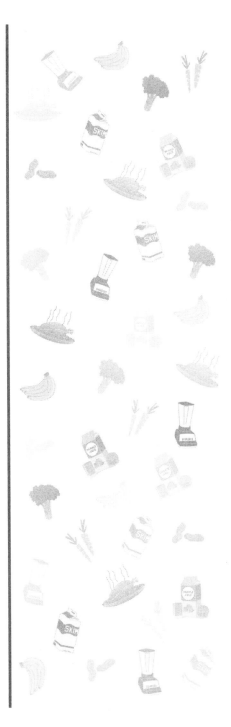

Vitamin K

Vitamin K was only discovered about 50 years ago, and like vitamin D, it is made within the human body. Vitamin K is stored in the liver and then distributed throughout the body. It's necessary for the production of proteins found in blood, bones, and kidneys.

There are at least three different forms of vitamin K, all belonging to a group of chemical compounds called quinones. The naturally occurring, fat-soluble forms are K_1 (*phylloquinone*), which occurs in green plants, and K_2 (*menaquinone*), which is formed in the intestinal tract in the body as a result of the action of intestinal bacteria. The fat-soluble synthetic vitamin K_3 (*menadione*) is nearly twice as potent in the body as the naturally occurring K_1 and K_2.

The Benefits of Vitamin K

Vitamin K and Blood Clotting

Vitamin K is best known for its important role in blood clotting. At least 13 different proteins are involved in making a blood clot, and vitamin K is essential for the production of at least six of them—especially the protein thrombin. If any of these important proteins are missing, blood cannot clot, which results in hemorrhagic disease. In other words, if an artery or vein is cut the bleeding will not stop.

Hemorrhagic disease is caused by a vitamin K deficiency, which can occur as a result of fat malabsorption (from liver disease, Crohn's disease, or ulcerative **colitis**) or *destruction of the intestinal bacteria by prolonged use of antibiotics*. Prior to surgery, patients are sometimes given vitamin K to prevent excess bleeding during an operation, but only if a known vitamin K deficiency exists.

Vitamin K and Bone Health

Until recently, researchers believed that the body made all of the vitamin K it needed. But new studies indicate that even

---

Caution!

- Most people do not need to supplement with vitamin K.
- Individuals who take aspirin regularly as a blood thinner should consult their physician before supplementing with vitamin K.
- People who take anticoagulant medications such as Coumadin need to monitor their vitamin K intake. The purpose of these drugs is to prevent blood clotting (too much clotting can lead to a heart attack or stroke), so if you have too much vitamin K, you defeat the purpose of the medication.
- If you have a medical condition or are pregnant or lactating, talk to your doctor before taking any supplement.

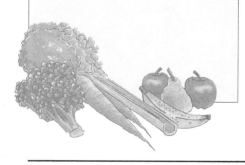

though the body may make enough vitamin K for blood clotting, it's not necessarily enough for good bone health. In fact, the current RDAs for vitamin K may be too low.

In a 10-year study, part of the Nurses' Health Study at Harvard, researchers looked at the diets of women aged 38 to 63. They found women whose diets contained the most vitamin K (at least 109 micrograms per day) had a 30 percent decreased risk of hip fracture than those who consumed less. This finding supports other data correlating low concentrations of vitamin K in the body with low bone mineral density and bone fractures. This may, in part, be due to the fact that vitamin K is needed to make osteocalcin, the active form of bone protein necessary for bone strength.

When to Supplement with Vitamin K

Vitamin K deficiency is rare in humans, since we get it through diet and our bodies can make it. However, newborn babies are often susceptible to vitamin K deficiency. Why? First, they're born with a sterile intestinal tract. As they pass through the birth canal they come in contact with the mother's intestinal bacteria, but it often takes the bacteria a day or so to become established in the baby's intestines. Second, babies who are breastfed may not get enough vitamin K, since human milk is a poorer source of the vitamin than infant formula or cow's milk. Infants are at risk of severe cerebral hemorrhage (bleeding in the brain) the first three to four months of life if they do not get enough vitamin K. Therefore, in the United States and in many other countries, newborn babies routinely receive a vitamin K injection at the hospital. People taking sulfa drugs such as the antibiotic Septra may also need extra vitamin K, since these medications can destroy the intestinal bacteria that produce the vitamin. Children, however, do not need vitamin K supplements.

What to Know about Taking Vitamin K Supplements

- Vitamin K supplements are usually available in 100-microgram capsules and tablets.
- Vitamin K should be taken with a meal containing some fat in order to enhance absorption.
- Since dietary supplements (or claims for them) are not reviewed by the FDA, quality control and potency problems may exist with vitamin K supplements.

FOOD SOURCES OF VITAMIN K

FOOD SOURCES	SERVING SIZE	VITAMIN K (MCG*)
Seaweed, dulse or rockweed, dried	3½ ounces	1,700
Tea, green, dried	1 ounce	199
Turnip greens, raw	½ cup, chopped	182
Spinach, frozen	½ cup	131
Liver, beef, cooked	3½ ounces	104
Cauliflower, raw	½ cup pieces	96
Soybean oil	1 tablespoon	76
Chickpeas (garbanzo beans), dried	1 ounce	74
Lentils, dried	1 ounce	62
Broccoli, raw	½ cup chopped	58
Tomato, green, raw	1 medium	58
Lettuce, iceberg, raw	1 leaf	22
Strawberries, raw	1 cup	21

Source: *Pennington, Bowes & Church's Food Values of Portions Commonly Used,* 17th Ed., Revised by Jean Pennington, Ph.D., R.D., 1998.
*mcg = micrograms.

ADEQUATE INTAKES (AI) FOR VITAMIN K

AGE/SEX	VITAMIN K (MCG)*
Males	
9–13 years	60
14–18 years	75
19+ years	120
Females	
9–13 years	60
14–18 years	75
19+ years	90
Pregnancy	
14–18 years	75
19+ years	90
Lactation	
14–18 years	75
19+ years	90

Source: The National Academy of Sciences, 2000.
*mcg = micrograms.

Vitamin K in Food

Vitamin K is found in large amounts in green leafy vegetables. Other vegetables, fruits, cereals, eggs, dairy products, and meat contain smaller amounts (see "Food Sources of Vitamin K"). It's believed that the average American diet provides about 300 to 500 micrograms of vitamin K per day. This estimate may be high since much of the population does not eat leafy greens every day.

Vitamin K is fairly heat-resistant and is not destroyed by ordinary cooking methods. Because vitamin K is fat-soluble, it is not leached into the cooking water. It is, however, unstable in light.

Niacin

Niacin (pronounced NIGH-uh-sin), or Vitamin B$_3$, was discovered in 1867, but it wasn't until 1937 that scientists realized it was necessary to prevent the disease known as **pellagra**. Pellagra is characterized by diarrhea, dry/scaly skin, anemia, and eventually, disorientation, memory loss, and confusion. Pellagra is caused by niacin deficiency.

Actually, niacin could be considered the "generic" name for two similar substances: nicotinic acid and niacinamide (or nicotinamide—not related to nicotine found in tobacco). Both nicotinic acid and niacinamide can prevent niacin deficiency. Interestingly, the amino acid tryptophan can also prevent niacin deficiency because the body can convert tryptophan to niacin.

The main function of niacin is as a cofactor (an essential component of an enzyme) for two enzymes (substances that speed up chemical reactions in the body) that are necessary for the body to convert carbohydrates, proteins, and fats in food into energy. It also helps mobilize calcium from cells and maintains the body's energy supply by controlling how much glucose (blood sugar) is circulating. Other roles for niacin include keeping skin healthy and helping the digestive and nervous systems function properly.

The Benefits of Niacin

Niacin and Heart Disease

The heart-healthy aspect of niacin stems from its ability to significantly lower blood cholesterol levels, an effect that was first reported in 1955. Nicotinic acid taken in extremely large doses of 1.5 to 3 grams per day has been shown to decrease total cholesterol, LDL ("bad" cholesterol), and **triglyceride** levels, and increase **high-density lipoprotein**, or HDL ("good" cholesterol). Some studies show that this ability to simultaneously affect both HDL and LDL cholesterol in beneficial ways makes nicotinic acid more effective than prescription cholesterol-lowering drugs that just lower LDL cholesterol. In fact, the National Cholesterol Education Program recommends niacin as one of the primary treatments for high cholesterol. Under a doctor's supervision, niacin therapy can also be

combined with some prescription cholesterol-lowering drugs for added effectiveness.

Niacin and Circulatory Disorders

Niacin is known to relax and loosen blood vessels, and therefore may be useful in treating some circulatory disorders such as **intermittent claudication**, or a limp in one's walk. This disorder is the result of poor circulation and is characterized by painful cramping in the calf that frequently occurs after walking. Raynaud's disease, a disorder in which numbness or pain is experienced in the hands or feet when they're exposed to cold, is another circulatory problem that may be helped by niacin.

Niacin and Other Potential Benefits

Although research into additional uses for niacin therapy is preliminary, supplementing with the vitamin may one day prove beneficial for other health problems. For example, people suffering from either **rheumatoid arthritis** or osteoarthritis may benefit from niacinamide's anti-inflammatory effect. One research study in New Zealand suggests that large doses of niacinamide given to children who are at risk for developing Type 1 diabetes (the insulin-dependent type) may reverse the progression of the disease. And finally, there is limited evidence that niacinamide can ease premenstrual headaches, depression, anxiety, and insomnia. Much more research needs to be completed before niacin is recommended for any of these problems.

When to Supplement with Niacin

Most of us get all the niacin we need from the food we eat. Data from the USDA Continuing Survey of Food Intakes by Individuals 1994–96 reveals that the average intake of niacin for Americans is 21.7 milligrams per day—slightly above the current recommended amounts (see "Recommended Dietary Allowances for Niacin"). Children do not need niacin supplements. Additional survey data indicate that most of our niacin is coming from poultry; mixed dishes that contain a lot of meat, fish, or poultry;

enriched and whole-grain breads and bread products; and fortified breakfast cereals.

Niacin is a unique vitamin because, theoretically, it's possible to maintain an adequate amount of it in our bodies without eating niacin-containing foods. Why? Because about half of the tryptophan (an amino acid) we eat is converted to niacin. Since tryptophan is found in many common foods, including milk and turkey, a diet containing at least 100 grams of protein could supply us with enough niacin. In fact, when estimating and calculating the required amounts of niacin, the experts took the tryptophan conversion factor into account, which is why the requirements are nearly always expressed in niacin equivalents (NE). A niacin equivalent is equal to 1 milligram of preformed niacin or 60 milligrams of tryptophan. Milk and other dairy foods are good sources of niacin because they're high in tryptophan.

Niacin and Pellagra

Pellagra (Italian for "raw skin") is a niacin deficiency disease that was first observed in the mid-18th century in Spain, although at the time the cause wasn't known. In 1920, experts realized that some dietary component lacking in corn was causing pellagra in populations that largely subsisted on corn. It wasn't until 1937 that nicotinic acid was found to be the lacking nutrient.

In scientific experiments with humans, signs of pellagra develop within 50 to 60 days after beginning a niacin-deficient diet. The most common and recognizable signs of a niacin deficiency are changes in the skin. A red rash that looks similar to a sunburn develops in areas exposed to sunlight. Vomiting, constipation, or diarrhea are the classic digestive symptoms of a deficiency, and the tongue becomes bright red. Depression, headache, fatigue, and neurological problems, including loss of memory, also occur.

In the early 1900s, when highly refined cornbread was the main food of poor Americans in the South, asylums were full of patients whose neurological problems were traced to pellagra. Niacin supplements were the cure, and ultimately cornmeal was required to be enriched with niacin (much as the Enrichment Act of 1942 required food processors to restore the iron, thiamin, riboflavin, and niacin

Caution!

- If you have diabetes, low blood pressure, bleeding problems, glaucoma, gout, liver disease, or ulcers, see your doctor before taking niacin supplements. All of these conditions can be made worse by niacin supplementation.
- People taking medication for high blood pressure should not take niacin supplements.
- Healthy people don't need niacin supplements, although the amount contained in a multivitamin is safe. If you want to take niacin for cholesterol-lowering purposes, be sure to talk to your doctor about the possible risks.
- If you have a medical condition or are pregnant or lactating, talk to your doctor before taking any supplement.

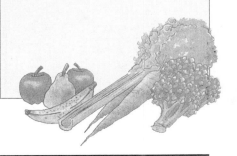

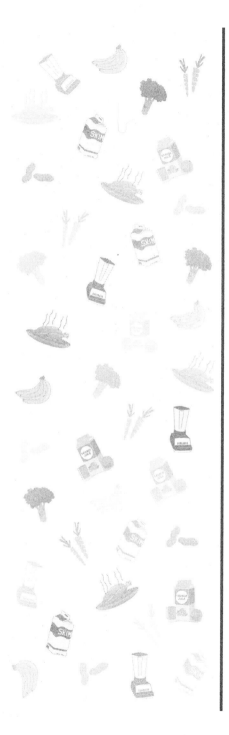

lost in the milling of wheat). Although pellagra has now virtually disappeared from the United States and Europe, it still appears in India and parts of China and Africa.

There is evidence that niacin deficiency isn't the only thing that can cause pellagra or pellagra-like symptoms. Deficiencies of other nutrients required in the tryptophan-to-niacin conversion (such as riboflavin, pyridoxine, and iron) may also be involved in the development of pellagra. Other conditions, such as the reduction in the conversion of tryptophan to niacin that occurs with some long-term drug therapies, as well as Hartnup's disease—a genetic disease that affects tryptophan absorption—may also lead to a niacin deficiency. In all of these cases, supplemental niacin brings marked improvements in symptoms, if not an outright cure.

Niacin and High Cholesterol

Although extremely effective at bringing down elevated blood cholesterol levels, megadoses of niacin also cause serious side effects. "Niacin flush" is the common name for the red head and neck one gets about 15 to 30 minutes after taking nicotinic acid. The flushing effect can go on for half an hour or longer before wearing off. Other side effects include itching skin, stomach upset, and occasional **hyperglycemia** (high blood sugar levels). These effects are reversed if the dose of nicotinic acid is reduced or discontinued, and tolerance can be built up by gradually taking larger doses.

Sustained-release, or time-release, nicotinic acid was developed to provide the benefits of niacin without causing niacin flush. It worked well, but unfortunately was later discovered to cause its own set of side effects, including upset stomach, fatigue, and liver damage or liver failure, perhaps due to its chemical structure. Therefore, time-release niacin supplements are no longer recommended. The best way to prevent niacin side effects may be to take the vitamin in the form of inositol hexaniacinate (IHN), available only recently in the United States, although doctors in Europe have prescribed IHN for years. It's just as effective at reducing high cholesterol levels as nicotinic acid, but eliminates the flushing and risk of liver damage. IHN doses higher than 2,000 milligrams per day may also have a blood-thinning effect.

Niacin and Cardiovascular Risk

Homocysteine, an amino acid–like substance, has been found to be a risk factor for heart disease when present in high levels in the blood. Results of the Cholesterol Lowering Atherosclerosis Study, published in 1991, showed an increase in blood homocysteine levels in study participants who received niacin and another cholesterol-lowering agent compared with the placebo group. Taking this study one step further to determine if niacin alone would increase homocysteine levels, the one-year long Arterial Disease Multiple Intervention Trial was recently conducted with over 450 participants. All participants received 1,000 milligrams of niacin daily for the first four weeks, and an 18 percent increase in average homocysteine levels was noted. Some participants were then assigned to a treatment group and received increasing amounts of niacin—up to 3,000 milligrams per day. The remaining participants received a placebo. In the treatment group homocysteine levels increased a total of 55 percent, while the placebo group experienced declining homocysteine levels. The increase in homocysteine with niacin appeared to be dose related—that is, the more niacin taken, the higher the homocysteine levels.

Although it is not known whether the beneficial effects of niacin on cholesterol levels offset the negative effect it has on homocysteine, the risks of taking large amounts of niacin should be considered when evaluating the usefulness of the vitamin for heart disease patients. One animal study showed that combining niacin and vitamin B$_6$ supplements normalizes homocysteine levels without diminishing the cholesterol-lowering ability of niacin.

What to Know about Taking Niacin Supplements

- Niacin is sold in tablet and capsule forms. Multivitamins contain about 25 milligrams of niacinamide (or sometimes nicotinic acid); B-complex supplements contain 50 to 100 milligrams of niacinamide; and a single niacin supplement usually contains 500 milligrams.

Niacin in Food

Niacin is widely distributed in both plant and animal foods. Good sources include yeast, meats, fortified breakfast cereals, legumes, and seeds. Green leafy vegetables, fish, coffee, and tea also contain some niacin, as do grains, but it's only about 30 percent available (see "Food Sources of Niacin"). Since we need relatively little niacin, it's not difficult to consume the recommended amount through a normal diet.

Since niacin is a water-soluble vitamin, some of it will be lost if foods are cooked in liquid. To preserve as much niacin as possible, try to cook high-niacin foods in a minimum of liquid, or steam them.

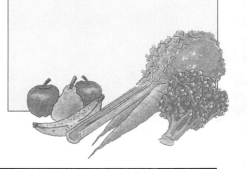

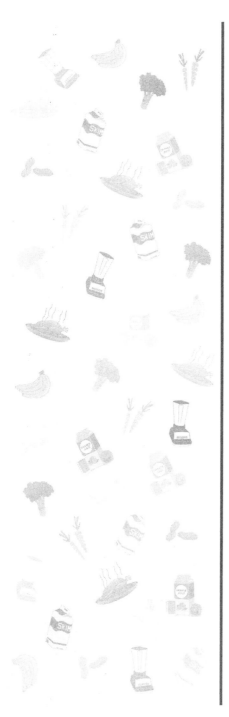

- Niacin taken in large (and even not-so-large) doses is considered a drug. If you're considering taking niacin in amounts greater than those found in multivitamins, talk to your doctor first.
- If you want to take niacin or IHN to lower cholesterol, see your doctor for the recommended dosage. Continued medical supervision is necessary in order to monitor effectiveness and safety when taking these supplements.
- For circulatory problems, 500 milligrams of IHN is suggested. See your doctor before beginning supplements to make sure this dosage is appropriate for you.
- If, for any reason, you're taking niacin daily for long periods, see your doctor for periodic monitoring of liver function.
- Inadequate iron, riboflavin, or vitamin B_6 status decreases the conversion of tryptophan to niacin, but it's currently unknown how much this affects the niacin requirement. Therefore, increasing niacin intake to compensate for this decrease isn't recommended at this time.
- Since dietary supplements (or claims for them) are not reviewed by the Food and Drug Administration, quality control and potency problems may exist with niacin supplements.

FOOD SOURCES OF NIACIN

FOOD SOURCES	SERVING SIZE	NIACIN (MG)*
Ground beef, broiled	3½ ounces	6.0
Oatmeal, instant	1 packet, prepared	5.5
Chicken, fried	1 drumstick	3.0
Bread, white	1 slice	1.0
Fish stick	1 stick	0.6
Popcorn, air-popped	3½ cups	0.5

Source: *Pennington, Bowes & Church's Food Values of Portions Commonly Used,* 17th Ed., Revised by Jean Pennington, Ph.D., R.D., 1998.
*mg = milligrams.

RECOMMENDED DIETARY ALLOWANCES (RDA)* FOR NIACIN

SEX/AGE	NIACIN (MG NE)**
Males	
9–13 years	12
14–18+ years	16
Females	
9–13 years	12
14–18+ years	14
Pregnant women	18
Lactating women	17

Reprinted with permission of The National Academy of Sciences, 1998. Courtesy of the National Academy Press, Washington D.C.
*There is no RDA for infants due to insufficient information.
**One niacin equivalent (NE) = 1 milligram preformed niacin = 60 milligrams tryptophan.

TOLERABLE UPPER INTAKE LEVEL (UL)[a] FOR NIACIN[b]

AGE	NIACIN (MG)*
0–½ year	ND[c]
½–1 year	ND
1–3 years	10
4–8 years	15
9–13 years	20
14–18 years	30
19+ years	35
Pregnancy	
≤18 years	30
19–50 years	35
Lactation	
≤18 years	30
19–50 years	35

Source: National Academy of Sciences, 1998
[a] = The maximum level of daily nutrient intake that is likely to pose no risk of adverse effects.
[b] = The UL for niacin applies to forms obtained from supplements, fortified foods, or a combination of the two.
*mg = milligrams.
[c] = Not determinable due to lack of data of adverse effects in this age group and concern with regard to lack of ability to handle excess amounts. Source of intake should be from food only to prevent high levels of intake.

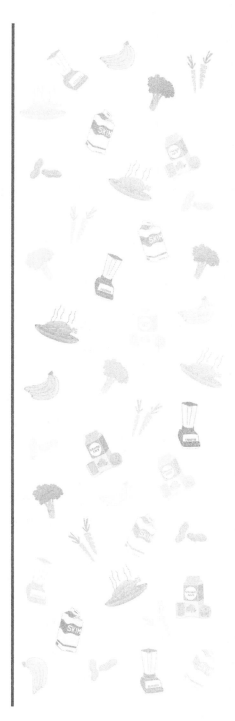

Pantothenic Acid

Pantothenic acid (pronounced PAN-to-THEN-ic) is a B vitamin that is essential for human and animal growth, reproduction, and normal physiological functions.

Pantothenic acid's main function is its role as a component of coenzyme A, which is involved with the metabolism of carbohydrates and fat. Coenzyme A also plays a role in the production of cholesterol, **phospholipids**, steroid hormones, and red blood cells.

Pantothenic Acid in Food

Pantothenic acid is found in all plant and animal tissue. Excellent sources include egg yolk, kidney, liver, and yeast; fair sources include broccoli, lean beef, milk, sweet potatoes, and molasses (see "Food Sources of Pantothenic Acid"). Quite a bit of pantothenic acid is lost in meat during thawing, and as much as 33 percent is lost in cooking. Roughly 50 percent is lost in the milling of flour. Pantothenic acid loss during processing is significant since it is stable in neutral conditions, but readily destroyed by heat in either alkaline or acidic conditions.

Pantothenic acid is a water soluble vitamin, so when you boil a food containing this nutrient, much will be lost into the water. Try to steam vegetables in as little water as possible, and avoid overcooking foods.

When to Supplement with Pantothenic Acid

Pantothenic acid deficiency is rare; in fact, the average American diet provides 2–3 milligrams of pantothenic acid per 1,000 calories—which puts daily totals near the suggested intake of 5 milligrams for adult men and women (see "Adequate Intakes of Pantothenic Acid"). Children do not need pantothenic acid supplements.

Reported symptoms of pantothenic acid deficiency include depression, fatigue, abdominal pain, sleep disturbances, cardiac instability, and neurological disorders such as numbness, paresthesia ("burning feet" syndrome), muscle weakness, and cramps. Biochemical changes include lowered blood cholesterol, decreased potassium in the blood, and **insulin** sensitivity.

Caution!

- Since deficiencies are rare, diet and a multivitamin should provide most people with the pantothenic acid they need each day.
- If you have a medical condition or are pregnant or lactating, talk to your doctor before taking any supplement.

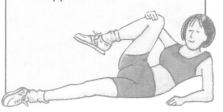

FOOD SOURCES OF PANTOTHENIC ACID

FOOD SOURCES	SERVING SIZE	PANTOTHENIC ACID (MG)*
Liver, beef	3 ounces	3.89
Salmon, baked	3 ounces	1.25
Yogurt, low fat, with fruit	1 cup	1.20
Chicken, white meat, baked	3 ounces	0.79
Milk, 2% fat	1 cup	0.78
Corn, cooked	½ cup	0.72
Dates	10	0.65
Oatmeal, cooked	1 cup	0.47
Strawberries	½ cup	0.25
Bread, whole wheat	1 slice	0.16

Source: USDA Nutrient Database for Standard Reference, Release 13, 1999.
*mg = milligrams.

ADEQUATE INTAKES (AI) OF PANTOTHENIC ACID*

AGE/SEX	PANTOTHENIC ACID (MG)**
Males	
9–13 years	4
14+ years	5
Females	
9–13 years	4
14+ years	5
Pregnant women	6
Lactating women	7

Reprinted with permission of The National Academy of Sciences, 1998. Courtesy of the National Academy Press, Washington D.C.
*There are no RDAs for pantothenic acid due to insufficient information.
**mg = milligrams.

Riboflavin (B₂)

Riboflavin (pronounced RIBE-o-flay-vin), also known as vitamin B_2, is a yellow, fluorescent compound. Like all B vitamins, riboflavin is water-soluble, but it's more heat-stable than most. Vitamin B_2 in the body is found in the form of the coenzymes, flavin mononucleotide (FMN) and flavin-adenine dinucleotide (FAD). FAD, the predominant form of riboflavin, is an essential component of energy production and helps to metabolize carbohydrates, protein, and fat.

What to Know about Taking Pantothenic Acid Supplements

- Pantothenic acid is often sold in 250- to 500-milligram capsules.
- Although no serious toxic effects are known, supplemental intakes above 10 to 20 grams per day may cause diarrhea.
- Since dietary supplements (or claims for them) are not reviewed by the Food and Drug Administration, quality control and potency problems may exist with pantothenic acid supplements.

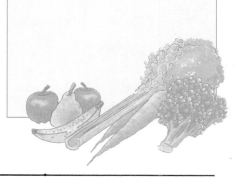

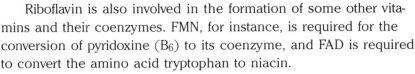

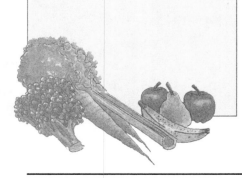

Riboflavin is also involved in the formation of some other vitamins and their coenzymes. FMN, for instance, is required for the conversion of pyridoxine (B_6) to its coenzyme, and FAD is required to convert the amino acid tryptophan to niacin.

Although this important nutrient is found in small amounts in the liver and kidneys, it is not stored to any great extent in the body. Therefore, riboflavin must be supplied in the diet and any excess is eliminated through the urine.

The Benefits of Riboflavin

Riboflavin and Migraine Headaches

Preliminary research indicates that taking a high dose of riboflavin (400 milligrams) every day may help prevent **migraine headaches**. In one study, people who took riboflavin supplements for three months had 37 percent fewer migraines than those taking a placebo. Although studies to date have used high doses of riboflavin, further research will investigate the effects of lower doses.

Researchers caution that the riboflavin treatment isn't for everyone. First, you need to make sure that your headaches are true migraines, and second, the treatment is only recommended for people who have migraines at least twice a month.

For those with diagnosed migraines, supplementing with riboflavin might be worth a try. Most riboflavin supplements contain no more than 100 milligrams per tablet, so you'll need a prescription to get one that contains 400 milligrams. Talk to your doctor before treating your migraines with riboflavin supplements.

Riboflavin in Food

Most plant and animal tissues contain some riboflavin. However, the foods that contribute the most riboflavin to the U.S. diet are milk and milk drinks, followed by bread products and fortified cereals (see "Food Sources of Riboflavin"). National food surveys show that the median daily intake of riboflavin in the United States is about 2 milligrams for men and roughly 1.5 milligrams for women, well above the recommended levels of 1.3 milligrams and 1.1 milligrams, respectively.

When to Supplement with Riboflavin

Although a true riboflavin deficiency (called ariboflavinosis) is uncommon in the United States, certain groups of people are at a greater risk, including individuals with kidney disease who are being treated with dialysis; individuals with absorption problems; women who are pregnant with more than one fetus; and women who are breastfeeding more than one infant.

Ariboflavinosis can also result from diverse causes, including the use of certain drugs, inadequate dietary intake, rare genetic defects, and hormonal disorders. In addition, chronic diseases such as cancer, heart disease, and diabetes mellitus are known to trigger or exacerbate riboflavin deficiency.

Symptoms of ariboflavinosis include weakness, sore throat, **edema** (fluid retention) of the mucous membranes in the mouth and throat, cheilosis (dermatitis around the nose and lips), stomatitis (cracking of the corners of the mouth), photophobia (hypersensitivity to light, reddening of cornea), and anemia.

FOOD SOURCES OF RIBOFLAVIN

FOOD SOURCES	SERVING SIZE	RIBOFLAVIN (MG)*
Liver, beef	3 ounces	3.49
Yogurt, fruit flavored, low fat	1 cup	0.44
Milk, 2% fat	1 cup	0.40
Trout, baked	3 ounces	0.36
Ice milk, soft serve	1 cup	0.31
Custard, baked	½ cup	0.29
Pork, roast loin	3 ounces	0.26
Egg	1 medium	0.25
Cheese, feta	1 ounce	0.24
Spinach, fresh, cooked	½ cup	0.22
Cheese, cottage, 2% fat	½ cup	0.21
Chicken, dark meat	3 ounces	0.17
Rice, brown, cooked	1 cup	0.05
Orange	1 medium	0.05

Source: USDA Nutrient Database for Standard Reference, Release 13, 1999.
*mg = milligrams.

Caution!

- Since deficiency is uncommon, a well balanced diet and a multivitamin, or B-complex supplement, should provide most people with the riboflavin they need.
- If you have a medical condition or are pregnant or lactating, talk to your doctor before taking any supplement.

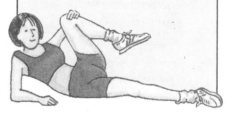

- Riboflavin is sold in tablet and capsule forms. Multivitamins contain about 1.7 milligrams of riboflavin, and B-complex and single riboflavin supplements can provide 100 milligrams.

- Although there is no known toxicity with riboflavin supplements (one study showed no short-term side effects in people who took 400 milligrams of riboflavin per day for at least three months), if you're considering taking a supplement, it's probably wise to stay under 100 milligrams per day. Additionally, humans have a limited ability to absorb riboflavin—the extra is excreted in urine.

- Since dietary supplements (or claims for them) are not reviewed by the FDA, quality control and potency problems may exist with riboflavin supplements.

ADEQUATE INTAKES (AI) FOR RIBOFLAVIN*

AGE/SEX	RIBOFLAVIN (MG)**
Infants	
0–½ year	0.3
½–1 year	0.4

*There is no RDA for infants due to insufficient information.
**mg = milligrams.

RECOMMENDED DIETARY ALLOWANCES (RDA) FOR RIBOFLAVIN

AGE/SEX	RIBOFLAVIN (MG)*
Children	
1–3 years	0.5
4–8 years	0.6
Males	
9–13 years	0.9
14+ years	1.3
Females	
9–13 years	0.9
14–18 years	1.0
19+ years	1.1
Pregnant women	1.4
Lactating women	1.6

Reprinted with permission of The National Academy of Sciences, 1998. Courtesy of the National Academy Press, Washington D.C.
*mg = milligrams.

Thiamin (B₁)

Thiamin (pronounced THIGH-uh-min), also known as vitamin B_1, is a water-soluble vitamin. The first B vitamin to be identified, it is found in skeletal muscle, the heart, liver, kidney, and brain.

Thiamin diphosphate (ThDP) is the active form of thiamin and acts as a coenzyme (a small molecule that works with an enzyme to promote the enzyme's activity) in the metabolism of carbohydrate and protein. It is also involved in the synthesis of DNA. As a result, thiamin is also used in a negative way, for tumor growth. In fact, limiting thiamin can slow tumor cell production.

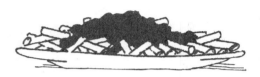

Thiamin in Food

Although pork and sunflower seeds are the richest sources of thiamin, Americans get most of this vitamin from enriched, fortified, or whole grain products such as bread and bread products, mixed foods whose main ingredient is a grain, and ready-to-eat cereals (see "Food Sources of Thiamin"). The USDA Continuing Survey of Food Intakes by Individuals 1994–96 showed an average intake of 1.9 milligrams of thiamin for males aged 20 and older, and 1.33 milligrams for females aged 20 and older. The recommended intake for thiamin is 1.2 milligrams and 1.1 milligrams per day for adult males and females, respectively (see "Recommended Dietary Allowances for Thiamin").

If you can't get enough of sushi, you might want to think twice. Raw fish contains thiaminase—an enzyme that deactivates thiamin. Cooking fish will make the enzyme inactive.

FOOD SOURCES OF THIAMIN

FOOD SOURCES	SERVING SIZE	THIAMIN (MG)*
Yeast, brewer's	1 tablespoon	1.25
Sunflower seeds, shelled	¼ cup	0.83
Pork chop, lean	3 ounces	0.76
Malt-o-Meal	1 cup	0.48
Wheat germ, raw	¼ cup	0.47
Beans, baked	1 cup	0.39
Corn flakes	1 cup	0.36
Pasta, cooked	1 cup	0.30
Rice, white, enriched, cooked	1 cup	0.26
Orange juice	1 cup	0.22
Bread, white	1 slice	0.10

Source: USDA Nutrient Database for Standard Reference, Release 13, 1999.
* mg = milligrams.

What to Know about Taking Thiamin Supplements

- Thiamin is sold in tablet and capsule forms. Multivitamins contain about 1.5 milligrams of thiamin; B-complex supplements contain about 15 milligrams of thiamin; and a single thiamin supplement may provide as much as 100 milligrams.

- Thiamin supplements can be taken with a meal or on an empty stomach.

- Although there is no known toxicity with thiamin supplements (there are a few reports of allergic reactions from intravenous thiamin), if you are considering taking an individual thiamin supplement, it's probably wise to stay under 50 milligrams per day.

- Since dietary supplements (or claims for them) are not reviewed by the FDA, quality control and potency problems may exist with thiamin supplements.

When to Supplement with Thiamin

Because the biological half-life of thiamin in the body is about 15 days, deficiency symptoms can be seen in people on a thiamin-deficient diet in as little as 18 days. Although a true thiamin deficiency (called **beriberi**) is uncommon in the United States, certain groups of people are at a greater risk, including individuals with kidney disease being treated with dialysis; individuals with malabsorption syndrome or genetic metabolic disorders; women who are pregnant with more than one fetus; seniors; chronic dieters; elite athletes; and alcoholics.

Signs of beriberi primarily involve the nervous and cardiovascular systems and include dementia (mental confusion), **Wernicke–Korsakoff syndrome** (muscle wasting, or "dry" beriberi), edema (wet beriberi), peripheral paralysis, high blood pressure, and an enlarged heart. The "dry" form of beriberi is associated with a low calorie intake and inactivity, with a loss of function or paralysis of the lower limbs. The "wet" form of the deficiency disease, resulting from a high carbohydrate intake and strenuous physical exertion, is associated with edema, or fluid retention, due to heart failure. Beriberi in infants, although rare, is caused by feeding babies thiamin-free formula. The effect can be sudden and rapid, ending in heart failure. Most infant formula in the United States is fortified with thiamin.

In industrialized countries, thiamin deficiency is most often due to a high alcohol intake combined with reduced food consumption. Alcohol can impair the absorption and storage of thiamin, resulting in alcohol-related thiamin deficiency (or Wernicke–Korsakoff syndrome)— the third most common form of dementia in the United States.

Treatment of thiamin deficiency often involves 50 to 100 milligram of thiamin/day (given intramuscularly or **intravenously**) for 7 to 14 days, followed by oral therapy. This treatment can quickly reverse many of the acute symptoms, but often leaves residual neurologic signs such as memory loss (called the chronic phase of Wernicke–Korsakoff syndrome). Recent studies suggest that thiamin deficiency may be related to Alzheimer's disease, although much more research is needed.

ADEQUATE INTAKES (AI)* FOR THIAMIN

AGE/SEX	THIAMIN (MG)**
Infants	
0–0.5 year	0.2
0.5–1 year	0.3

*There is no RDA for infants due to insufficient information.
**mg = milligrams.

RECOMMENDED DIETARY ALLOWANCES (RDA) FOR THIAMIN

AGE/SEX	THIAMIN (MG)*
Children	
1–3 years	0.5
4–8 years	0.6
Males	
9–13 years	0.9
14+ years	1.2
Females	
9–13 years	0.9
14–18 years	1.0
19+ years	1.1
Pregnant women	1.4
Lactating women	1.5

Reprinted with permission of The National Academy of Sciences, 1998. Courtesy of the National Academy Press, Washington D.C.
*mg = milligrams.

Caution!

- Since thiamin is one of the vitamins most commonly fortified in foods, most people get the amount they need. Supplementing with extra thiamin (other than what is contained in a B-complex or multivitamin) is not necessary.
- If you have a medical condition or are pregnant or lactating, talk to your doctor before taking any supplement.

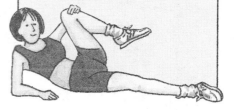

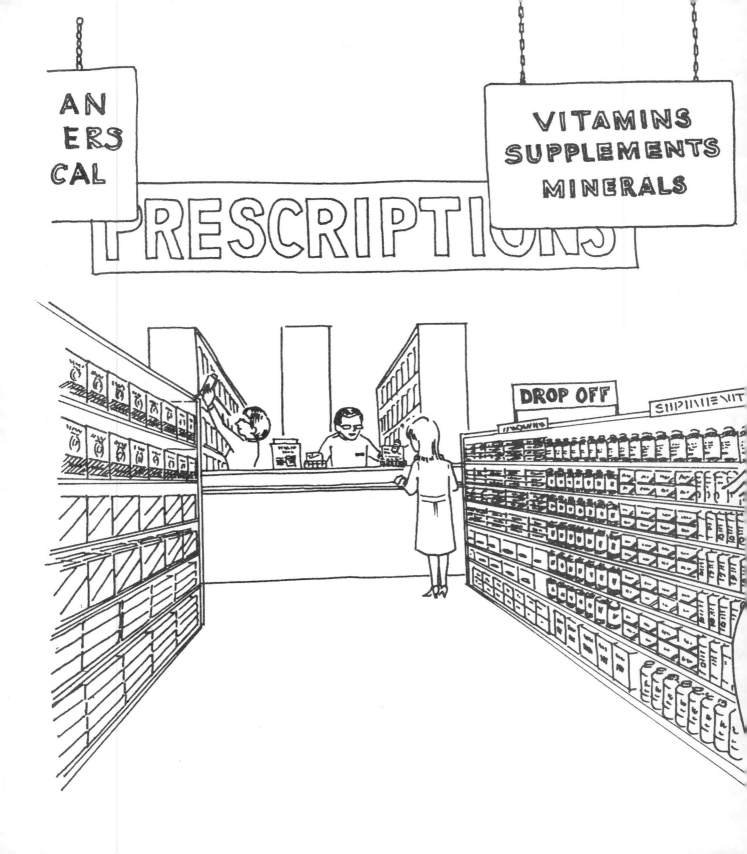

CHAPTER 3:

Minerals:
Elements of Good Health

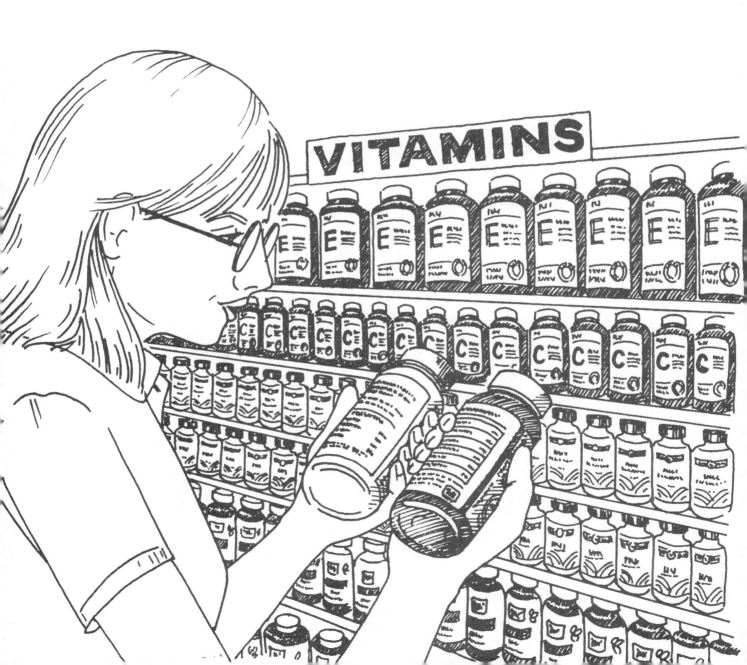

Most of us know arsenic as a deadly poison, but it was identified as an essential trace element mineral in the mid-1970s. Although arsenic's functions as a nutrient aren't yet well defined, it's believed to affect the body's utilization of the amino acids methionine, taurine, cysteine, and arginine. It's also involved in certain enzyme reactions in the body. In humans, decreased blood arsenic concentrations have been correlated with central nervous system problems, cancer, and other diseases. Although there is no recommended intake for arsenic, the estimated requirement for humans is 12–25 micrograms per day. Worldwide, the average daily arsenic intake is 12–40 micrograms, with most of it coming from fish, grains, and cereal products. Too much arsenic (greater than 250 micrograms per day) can cause hair loss, skin disorders, liver damage, lack of appetite, weight loss, and death.

There are about 60 minerals in the human body, making up about 4 percent of total body weight. Unlike vitamins, minerals don't contain the element carbon in their chemical structures, so they are inorganic elements (the word "organic" in chemistry means "carbon-containing"). These elements are found in the crust of the earth. Soil, water, oceans, plants, animals, and humans all contain minerals in varying amounts.

Getting the proper amount of minerals—not too much, but not too little—is important not only for preventing deficiency disease and symptoms, but also because the body depends on minerals for nearly every bodily process. For example, minerals are required for transporting oxygen to body cells, regulating heartbeat and blood pressure, and producing hormones (chemicals produced by glands that influence growth and other body processes) and enzymes (proteins that speed up chemical reactions in the body) that are crucial to many body processes.

Major Minerals

The minerals that we need in the largest quantity (hundreds of milligrams per day) are called "major" minerals or "macro" minerals. Calcium, phosphorus, and magnesium are three of the six major minerals. Each of the major minerals has been scientifically studied for years, and there is a lot of information available about how they function in the body to keep us healthy. The major minerals each have their own section in this chapter.

Trace Minerals

Those that are required in much smaller amounts are called "trace" or "micro" minerals. The **trace minerals** include iron, zinc, iodine, copper, manganese, fluoride, chromium, selenium, molybdenum, boron, nickel, and silicon. Lithium, tin, cobalt, and vanadium are probably also essential, but only in very tiny amounts. Strangely, arsenic, which is a deadly poison, is an essential mineral, but obviously supplements aren't necessary!

Lesser-Known Trace Minerals

The biochemical functions of a number of trace minerals, including nickel, silicon, and vanadium, have not been completely identified. Nevertheless, scientists have determined that these minerals are essential for life. How? By observing that when people (and/or animals) ingest diets low in these minerals, various negative effects occur and these negative effects are reversed when the mineral content of the diets is returned to normal. The essentiality of the remaining minerals, including lithium, cobalt, cadmium, aluminum, lead, mercury, and tin, is debatable because there simply isn't enough scientific information available.

What do we know about the lesser-known trace minerals—nickel, silicon, and vanadium? Much of the research has been conducted on animals and may or may not apply to humans. However, here is a synopsis of what's known:

Nickel. Not considered essential until the 1970s, nickel is known to be involved in a number of enzymatic reactions. Too little nickel affects the functioning of other nutrients, including calcium, iron, zinc, and vitamin B_{12}. The effects of too much nickel are not well documented, but in animals excess nickel worsens symptoms of iron and copper deficiencies. Americans typically get 69–162 micrograms of nickel per day, mostly from chocolate, nuts, beans, peas, and grains. This amount is considered sufficient intake.

Silicon. Silicon is required for collagen and **cartilage** formation, but its major roles appear to be bone-related. Deficiencies of the mineral in animals cause bone abnormalities, including poorly formed joints and irregular bone growth. The human requirement for silicon is estimated to be 2–5 milligrams per day. Silicon is nontoxic when taken orally. In fact, magnesium trisilicate, an over-the-counter antacid (which contains a form of silicon), has been used by people for more than 40 years without obvious negative effects. Silicon is also found in some food additives. The richest food sources of silicon are unrefined grains, cereal products, and root vegetables.

Vanadium. Considered essential only since 1987, vanadium is involved in a huge number of complex biochemical reactions—so

Major and Trace Minerals

Major Minerals
- Calcium
- Chloride
- Magnesium
- Phosphorus
- Potassium
- Sodium

Trace Minerals
- Boron
- Chromium
- Cobalt
- Copper
- Fluoride
- Iodine
- Iron
- Manganese
- Molybdenum
- Nickel
- Selenium
- Vanadium
- Zinc

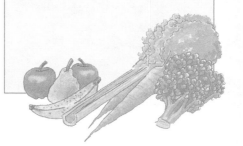

A Word about Colloidal Minerals

Colloidal mineral supplements, available in either liquid or capsule form, are combinations of many minerals—some that are essential for health, and some that aren't. Colloidal mineral supplements are frequently marketed as being necessary to make up for mineral deficiencies in the soil, or as being more easily absorbed than other supplements or minerals in food because they are smaller particles. There is no scientific backing to these claims. Colloidal minerals are not better absorbed. Mineral absorption is more a reflection of the body's needs than of the mineral's size. What's more, the amount of minerals that colloidal supplements contain has nothing to do with human requirements—they often contain few of the minerals we need more of (calcium and magnesium, for example) and more of the minerals we don't need. Finally, poor quality control, along with frequent contamination problems, makes these supplements a risky way to get your minerals.

many that it's difficult to narrow down the mineral's major role. It's estimated that a daily intake of 10 micrograms of vanadium is sufficient. Deficiency in animals caused decreased growth and decreased thyroid function, among other things, while too much vanadium causes gastrointestinal upset, lack of appetite, and death. Foods rich in vanadium include shellfish, mushrooms, and some spices, including dill seed, parsley, and black pepper.

Mineral Deficiencies and Toxicities

The body is good at regulating its mineral balance. In many cases, excesses are excreted in the urine. And, when the body stores of a mineral are running low, more of that mineral will be absorbed from food. However, some people are genetically predisposed to retain excessive amounts of certain minerals, such as sodium or iron, which can lead to health problems.

In general, mineral deficiencies are rare in the United States, with the exception of iron and calcium, and sometimes magnesium. Trace mineral deficiencies are very unlikely because these minerals are found in a wide variety of foods and also in water. For the minerals phosphorus and sodium, the concern is usually about getting too much, not too little.

There's also the question of whether or not getting more of a mineral will improve your health—beyond just preventing deficiency. Some experts think that the Recommended Dietary Allowance or Adequate Intake levels are set too low for some nutrients, and in fact, the RDAs have recently been revised and are now higher for some minerals, such as calcium. However, in many cases there simply isn't enough evidence yet to recommend consuming minerals (especially trace minerals) in amounts above the RDA and AI levels.

Although taking extra calcium in the form of a supplement is a common practice these days—and one that's frequently recommended for certain population groups—it pays to exercise great caution when considering whether to take other mineral supplements. Getting too much of many minerals can be extremely dangerous, and in some cases it doesn't take a lot to do damage. When possible, try to get your minerals—especially trace minerals—from food instead of supplements.

Boron

Boron is a trace mineral that, before 1980, was considered essential only for plants. Since then, evidence has been accumulating that boron is indeed an essential nutrient for animals—including humans—although no official requirement has yet been set. Boron's functions, although not completely known, include assisting in calcium metabolism, cell membrane functioning, energy utilization, and the development and maintenance of bone.

The Benefits of Boron

Preliminary research suggests that boron's beneficial role in calcium metabolism may translate to a benefit for bone health—especially for postmenopausal women. A U.S. Department of Agriculture study published in 1987 showed that supplementing a low-boron diet with 3 milligrams of boron per day helped prevent calcium loss and bone demineralization. However, this area of research is in its infancy, and no researchers recommend boron supplementation for bone maintenance or osteoporosis prevention at this time.

When to Supplement with Boron

The human requirement for boron is estimated to be between 0.3 and 1 milligram per day—an amount easily consumed through a normal diet. Nutritional surveys indicate that daily intakes of boron range from 0.5 to 3.1 milligrams, but the average intake for both men and women is about 1 milligram per day, with vegetarians consuming slightly higher amounts. It is not recommended that children take boron supplements.

No boron deficiencies have been documented in free-living populations. However, in study subjects living in special supervised settings, reducing the amount of dietary boron has been found to cause changes in blood glucose (and the body's use of fat) similar to those seen in boron-deficient animals. Very low intakes of boron may also aggravate the symptoms of arthritis.

For all practical purposes, getting too much boron through a normal diet is impossible. The body tightly regulates the amount of

Boron in Food

Boron is found in a variety of foods. Rich sources of boron include noncitrus fruits, leafy vegetables, nuts, and legumes. Wine, cider, and beer are also high in boron. Other sources of boron include: apples/applesauce, dried beans, broccoli, grapes/grape juice, lentils, nuts/peanut butter, peaches, pears, raisins, and spinach.

Despite the fact that coffee and milk are low in boron, they make up 12 percent of the average American daily dietary intake because of the volume consumed.

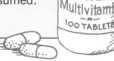

boron it contains by excreting nearly all that it obtains through food. However, this control process can be overwhelmed by very high boron intakes, which are generally achieved only through excessive supplementation or the ingestion of borax or other boron-containing compounds. Signs of boron toxicity include poor appetite, nausea, vomiting, diarrhea, weight loss, and lethargy. The minimum lethal amount of boron for humans isn't known, although single doses of 18 to 20 grams have been fatal for adults. However, taking a supplement that contains up to 3 milligrams of boron—such as some multivitamin and mineral supplements—is considered to be safe.

What to Know about Taking Boron Supplements

- Boron is sold in capsule and tablet form, usually as a combined mineral supplement, or as part of a multivitamin supplement. The amount of boron per serving is typically 3 milligrams or less.
- Since dietary supplements (or claims for them) are not reviewed by the Food and Drug Administration, quality control and potency problems may exist with boron supplements.

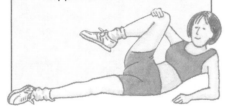

Caution!

- Taking more than 3 milligrams of boron per day is not recommended.
- If you have or are at risk for breast cancer or prostate cancer, talk to your doctor before taking a supplement containing boron, as this mineral can affect hormone levels.
- If you have a medical condition or are pregnant or lactating, talk to your doctor before taking any supplement.

TOLERABLE UPPER INTAKE LEVEL (UL)[a] FOR BORON

AGE	BORON (MG)*
9–13 years	11
14–18 years	17
19+ years	20
Pregnancy	
14–18 years	17
19+ years	20
Lactation	
14–18 years	17
19+ years	20

Source: National Academy of Sciences, 2001

*mg = milligram

[a] = The maximum level of daily nutrient intake that is likely to pose the risk of adverse effects.

Calcium

Calcium is the most abundant mineral in the human body. Over 99 percent of the body's calcium is found in bones and teeth. The remainder is found in blood, bodily fluids, muscle, and other tissues where it plays a role in blood vessel contraction and dilation, muscle contraction, nerve transmission, and glandular secretion. Calcium is probably most recognized for its important role in maintaining bone health. The skeleton not only provides structural support for muscles, it protects vital organs and serves as a storage site for calcium.

The Benefits of Calcium

Calcium and Osteoporosis

Osteoporosis is a debilitating disease affecting more than 25 million Americans—80 percent of whom are women. Osteoporosis, or porous bone, is caused by low bone mass and the structural deterioration of bone tissue, leading to bone fragility and an increased susceptibility to fractures of the hip, spine, and wrist. Fifty percent of all women over age 50 will have an osteoporosis-related fracture in their lifetime. A Caucasian woman's risk of hip fracture is equal to her risk of breast, uterine, and ovarian cancers combined. The incidence of osteoporosis in men is rising. In fact, 20 to 25 percent of all hip fractures in the United States occur in men, and as in women, the chance of occurrence increases dramatically with age. Because of the aging population, the incidence of hip fractures is expected to triple by the year 2040.

In the United States, approximately 21 percent of post-menopausal Caucasian and Asian women, 16 percent of Hispanic women, and 10 percent of African-American women have osteoporosis. An additional 38 percent of American women over the age of 50 years have osteopenia (the beginning stages of osteoporosis.)

Why are so many women at risk for osteoporosis? A decreased **estrogen** level beginning at menopause is associated with accelerated bone loss, especially from the lumbar spine, for about five years. During this period a woman may lose an average of 3 percent

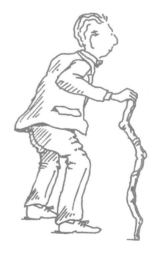

of her skeletal mass per year! Additionally, lower estrogen levels may decrease calcium absorption and increase rates of bone turnover.

Bone is an active tissue that is constantly undergoing "remodeling" that involves resorption (old bone is removed) and formation (new bone is formed). The rate of remodeling in children can be as high as 50 percent per year compared to about 5 percent in adults. Until the age of 30 or so, we build and store bone efficiently. Then, as part of the aging process, bones begin to break down faster than new bone can be formed. If bone calcium stores are not sufficient, as the aging process takes over, the risk of osteoporosis increases.

Moreover, since bone serves as a "bank" for calcium and other minerals, as blood levels of calcium fall, the mineral is pulled out of the bone via resorption. When blood calcium levels rise, the mineral can be redeposited into the bones in the formation phase. If more calcium is pulled out of the bone than is put into bone, osteoporosis can occur.

In addition to calcium, magnesium and vitamin D are also needed to prevent osteoporosis. According to experts, calcium increases bone density, but magnesium is involved in the construction of the matrix, a flexible scaffold into which bone tissue is deposited. The matrix allows the skeleton to absorb bone-fracturing shocks. Vitamin D plays an important role in the body's absorption and use of calcium.

Calcium and Blood Pressure

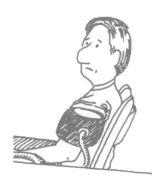

In a review of 22 studies, calcium supplementation was found to reduce blood pressure modestly in adults with **hypertension**, or high blood pressure, but had little effect on people with normal blood pressure. Findings from the recent DASH study (Dietary Approaches to Stop Hypertension) suggest that a diet high in calcium, magnesium, and potassium, and lower in sodium and fat, can lower high blood pressure significantly.

Calcium and Pre-eclampsia

Calcium is now recognized as a treatment for pre-eclampsia, or pregnancy-induced hypertension. In a review of 14 studies, pregnant women who supplemented with 1,500 to 2,000 milligrams of calcium per day had a significant lowering of both their **systolic** (the top number in a blood pressure reading) and **diastolic** (the lower number) **blood pressure**. In another study of 82 pregnant women, those who consumed more than 900 milligrams of calcium (the amount found in three glasses of milk) had lower blood pressure than those who consumed less calcium.

Getting adequate amounts of calcium when pregnant can also save your baby's bones. A study at the University of Tennessee showed that women who consumed fewer than 600 milligrams of the mineral per day during pregnancy had babies with 15 percent less bone density than babies born to women who consumed up to 2,000 milligrams of calcium per day.

Calcium and Colon Cancer

Colon cancer is one of the most common cancers in the Western world. Research has shown that colon cancer incidence rates are inversely proportional to calcium intake—as intakes go up, cancer rates go down. One study indicates that most cases of colon cancer may be prevented with regular calcium intake for men and women around 1,800 milligrams and 1,000 milligrams per 1,000 calories per day, respectively, along with 800 IUs of vitamin D per day.

New findings indicate that calcium may help reduce the recurrence of colon polyps (benign tumors that often turn cancerous). Researchers studied 930 people who had previously had colon polyps surgically removed. Half of the group took 1,200 milligrams of calcium carbonate per day, and the other half received a placebo. After four years, 7 percent fewer people in the calcium group developed at least one new polyp compared to those taking the placebo. Researchers suspect that calcium may prevent polyp formation by binding to **carcinogens** and thereby inhibiting abnormal cell growth.

Calcium and Premenstrual Syndrome (PMS)

In a study of 466 premenopausal women, ages 18 to 45, who suffered from recurring premenstrual syndrome (PMS), supplementing with calcium carbonate lessened the symptoms. Researchers gave each woman either 600 milligrams of calcium carbonate or a

Risk Factors for Osteoporosis

- Being female
- Being Caucasian or Asian, although African-Americans and Hispanic Americans are at significant risk as well
- Thin and/or small frame
- Advanced age
- A family history of osteoporosis
- Postmenopause, including surgically induced menopause (i.e., hysterectomy)
- Abnormal absence of menstrual periods
- Anorexia nervosa or bulimia
- A diet low in calcium
- Use of certain medications such as glucocorticoids, used to treat asthma or arthritis
- Low testosterone levels in men
- Smoking
- Excessive use of alcohol
- An inactive lifestyle

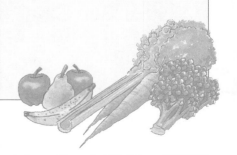

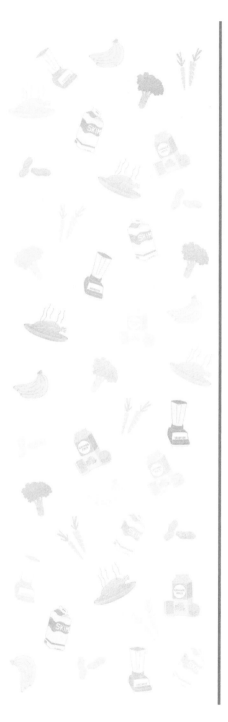

placebo twice a day for three menstrual cycles. By the third treatment cycle, those taking the calcium supplements reported a 48 percent reduction in overall symptoms during the two weeks prior to their menstrual cycle. Those taking the placebo, however, reported only a 30 percent reduction. The symptoms that improved included depression, mood swings, anxiety, water retention, breast tenderness, cramps, food cravings, and headaches. Insomnia and fatigue did not improve in either group. More research is needed to determine if other forms and/or doses of calcium would provide the same effect.

Calcium in Food

Calcium is found in a variety of foods (see "Food Sources of Calcium"), including dairy products and dark leafy vegetables such as kale, collards, turnip greens, and broccoli, as well as clams, oysters, and salmon with bones. According to 1994 data, 73 percent of the calcium in the U.S. food supply comes from milk products, 9 percent comes from fruits and vegetables, 5 percent is from grain products, and the remaining 12 percent from other sources. Although grains are not particularly high in calcium, because they are consumed in such great quantities, they account for a substantial proportion of the calcium intake. Corn tortillas, for instance, are the second best source of calcium (after milk) among Mexican American adults, and white bread is the second most important source among Puerto Rican adults.

Not all calcium sources are alike. Calcium may be poorly absorbed from foods high in **oxalic acid** (spinach, sweet potatoes, beans, or rhubarb) and phytic acid (unleavened bread, nuts, seeds, raw beans, grains, and soy isolates—isolated soy protein made from defatted and dehulled soybeans, at least 90 percent protein by weight).

When to Supplement with Calcium

Most Americans do not get the calcium they need. According to a recent statement from the National Institutes of Health, only about 25 percent of boys and 10 percent of girls meet the recommended daily levels of calcium consumption. The USDA Continuing

Survey of Food Intakes by Individuals 1994–96 showed an average daily intake of 925 milligrams of calcium for males aged 9 and older, and 657 milligrams for females aged 9 and older. The National Academy of Sciences recently increased the recommended intake of calcium for adults, both male and female, to 1,000 to 1,300 milligrams per day (see "Adequate Intakes for Calcium").

Some argue that these new levels are not high enough. Experts at the 1994 NIH Consensus Development Conference on Optimal Calcium Intake recommended that women over the age of 50 who are not on estrogen, and all women over the age of 65, should consume 1,500 milligrams of calcium per day. And the American Academy of Pediatrics has recommended that children ages 9 to 18 should also get as much as 1,500 milligrams of calcium per day.

Moreover, certain groups of the population are at greater risk for calcium deficiency, including menopausal women; young women who lose their periods due to anorexia nervosa and/or exercise-induced anorexia; individuals with **lactose intolerance**; strict vegetarians; and other individuals with poor calcium intakes. Many chronic illnesses that affect children also affect calcium metabolism and bone formation, including rheumatologic conditions, renal disease, liver failure, and insulin-dependent diabetes mellitus.

Although lack of calcium is much more common than too much calcium, toxicity can occur with calcium supplementation. Too much calcium can cause kidney stone formation and kidney failure, and it can interfere with the absorption of other nutrients such as zinc, iron, phosphorus, and magnesium.

Calcium and Magnesium

Although calcium and magnesium often work together, they can also compete against one another. Calcium helps muscles contract, while magnesium helps them to relax. However, too much magnesium can inhibit bone hardening, or calcification, while too much calcium can lessen the amount of magnesium absorbed by the body. Therefore, it is essential to maintain a balance between these two minerals. Experts recommend a two-to-one ratio of calcium to magnesium. If you regularly supplement with extra calcium, be sure to increase your magnesium intake, too.

Calcium in Soy Milk

Although soy beverages are growing in popularity, you may have to drink more than you bargained for to get the calcium you need. The calcium in soy milk is typically 25 percent less absorbed than calcium in cow's milk. According to one study, an extra 500 milligrams of calcium should be added to most soy beverages to equal cow's milk.

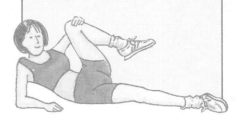

What to Know about Taking Calcium Supplements

- Calcium supplements come in many different forms (see "Choosing a Calcium Supplement"), but avoid bone meal, dolomite (a naturally occurring calcium-magnesium combination), and oyster shell, as they are not scrutinized and may contain lead or other dangerous heavy metals.

- Research shows that calcium is best absorbed in doses of 500 milligrams or less. If you're taking higher doses, be sure to divide them up throughout the day. Also, breakfast is often a calcium-rich meal. If you eat a bowl of cereal and milk (about 300 to 500 milligrams of calcium), along with calcium-fortified orange juice (about 300 to 350 milligrams of calcium), hold off until later in the day to take a calcium supplement.

(continued on next page)

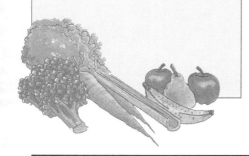

Calcium and Iron

Calcium and iron fight one another for absorption, and calcium can reduce absorption of **nonheme iron** (the form found in plants, fortified foods, and supplements) when eaten together. On average, though, research has shown that the two nutrients balance out in the long run. For instance, if you eat a bowl of iron-fortified cereal with a cup of milk, you may not absorb all of the iron. On the other hand, vitamin C aids iron absorption, so adding a glass of orange juice can actually increase the amount of iron absorbed from the cereal. The exception is when iron supplements are taken for anemia. In this case, do not take iron supplements at the same time as calcium supplements.

Calcium and Sodium

Calcium also interacts with sodium. An increase in sodium intake can cause increased sodium *and* calcium losses in the urine. However, there has been no research to date on the effects of a high sodium diet on bone loss.

Calcium and Caffeine

According to some experts, caffeine has a moderate impact on calcium retention in the body and has been associated with increased hip fractures in women. However, this association has been seen primarily in postmenopausal women with low calcium intakes (less than 800 milligrams per day) who drank the equivalent of two or more cups of coffee per day. Caffeine causes a short-term increase in calcium excretion in the urine, and may slightly decrease calcium absorption. Simply increasing calcium intake can decrease any impact from caffeine.

Choosing a Calcium Supplement

Calcium comes in a variety of forms, including carbonate, citrate, citrate malate, gluconate, phosphate, lactate, and microcrystalline hydroxyapatite. Calcium is also available in fortified foods such as juice, chocolates, yogurt, and cereal. Some calcium sources are better than others, and some are cheaper.

- *Calcium carbonate* is generally the cheapest form of calcium because it's the most concentrated and therefore, fewer supplements are necessary. It should be taken with meals to increase absorption.
- *Calcium citrate malate (CCM)* is available in tablet form and in fortified juice. The low calcium content requires a greater number of tablets per day (2–5 tablets) and it's more expensive. However, studies have shown that this particular form of calcium is the best absorbed. Typically, people absorb 35 percent of the calcium in this form, versus 30 percent of the calcium in calcium carbonate and other supplements. The citrate portion may also help reduce the risk of kidney stones.
- *Calcium citrate and calcium lactate* can be taken between meals.
- If you're not a pill-taker, juice fortified with CCM or other calcium forms may be your best bet.

FOOD SOURCES OF CALCIUM

FOOD SOURCES	SERVING SIZE	CALCIUM (MG)*
Yogurt, low fat, with fruit	1 cup	372
Milk, nonfat	1 cup	302
Milk, 2% fat	1 cup	297
Cheese, Gruyere	1 ounce	287
Ice milk, soft serve	1 cup	225
Salmon, canned, with bones	3½ ounces	211
Tofu, firm	½ cup	204
Cheese, cheddar	1 ounce	204
Rhubarb, cooked	½ cup	174
Ice cream, vanilla	1 cup	173
Spinach, frozen, cooked	½ cup	122
Almonds	1 ounce	69
Baked beans	½ cup	64
Mustard greens, cooked	½ cup	52
Broccoli, cooked	½ cup	36
Cheese, cream	2 tablespoons	23
Cream, half and half	1 tablespoon	16

Source: USDA Nutrient Database for Standard Reference, Release 13, 1999.
*mg = milligrams.

What to Know about Taking Calcium Supplements

(continued from previous page)

- Multivitamin and mineral supplements provide calcium, but only in small amounts. If you want more than about 20 percent of the RDA, you'll probably have to buy a separate calcium supplement.
- The National Academy of Sciences recommends no more than 2,500 milligrams of supplemental calcium per day. No cases of calcium toxicity have ever been reported from food sources.
- Since dietary supplements (or claims for them) are not reviewed by the FDA, quality control and potency problems may exist with calcium supplements.

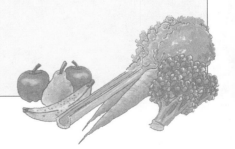

TOLERABLE UPPER INTAKE LEVEL (UL)[a] FOR CALCIUM

AGE	CALCIUM (MG)*
0–1 year	ND[b]
1+ years	2,500
Pregnancy	2,500
Lactation	2,500

Reprinted with permission of The National Academy of Sciences, 1997. Courtesy of the National Academy Press, Washington D.C.

*mg = milligrams.

[a] = The maximum level of daily nutrient intake that is likely to pose no risk of adverse effects. Unless otherwise specified, the UL represents total intake from food, water, and supplements.

[b] = Not determinable because of lack of data or adverse effects in this age group and concern with regard to lack of ability to handle excess amounts. Source of intake should be from food only to prevent high levels of intake.

ADEQUATE INTAKES (AI) FOR CALCIUM*

AGE/SEX	CALCIUM (MG)**
Infants	
0–½ year	210
½–1 year	270
Children	
1–3 years	500
4–8 years	800
Males	
9–18 years	1,300
19–50 years	1,000
51+ years	1,200
Females	
9–18 years	1,300
19–50 years	1,000
51+ years	1,200
Pregnant women	
≤18 years	1,300
19–50 years	1,000
Lactating women	
≤18 years	1,300
19–50 years	1,000

Reprinted with permission of The National Academy of Sciences, 1997. Courtesy of the National Academy Press, Washington D.C.

*There is no RDA due to insufficient information.

**mg = milligrams.

Caution!

- Individuals prone to kidney stones or those with kidney disease should consult with their physician before supplementing with calcium.
- If you have a medical condition or are pregnant or lactating, talk to your doctor before taking any supplement.
- Calcium supplementation is a good idea for anyone who is not currently meeting his or her calcium needs through diet alone.

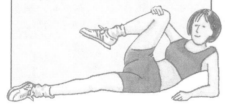

Chloride

Chloride is a mineral that's generally consumed as sodium chloride, or table salt. Because sodium and chloride are so strongly linked in the diet, it's rare that levels of one or the other would vary independently. In other words, it's hard to get a lot of chloride without also getting lots of sodium in the diet.

Chloride usually receives very little attention because getting too much or too little of it is not a common problem. However, chloride does have important functions in the body.

The Benefits of Chloride

Chloride is an **electrolyte**—an electrically charged mineral that dissolves in water. Chloride has a negative charge, while sodium and potassium have positive charges. As a result, electrolytes can easily move back and forth across the body's cell membranes. This is essential because as they move in and out of cells, they carry things with them, such as nutrients, water, and waste products.

The functions of electrolytes in the body include maintaining the body's water balance, carrying nerve impulses, and helping muscles contract and relax. Electrolytes also keep the body from becoming too acidic or alkaline. Although chloride's main function is fluid balance, it's also used to make stomach acid that's necessary for digestion.

Chloride in Food

Table salt is the primary source of chloride in the diet, and most everyone gets plenty of this mineral (as well as sodium) via the foods we eat and the added salt we use.

When to Supplement with Chloride

Chloride is not something that people need to add to their diets via supplements, so it's not added to multivitamin and mineral formulas, nor is it found as a single supplement. Chloride deficiency is rarely seen, since the body conserves chloride when

Chloride and Babies

Infants who are breastfed receive chloride from human milk. Although at one time infant formulas were deficient in chloride, they are now required to contain 55 to 65 milligrams per 100 calories in order to prevent chloride deficiency in babies who are formula fed.

intake is low. However, a deficiency of chloride only—that is, without an accompanying sodium deficiency—can occur in a number of circumstances. These situations include frequent vomiting (such as with prolonged illness or the eating disorder bulimia) and Bartter's syndrome, a genetic condition in which chronic diarrhea is accompanied by inadequate chloride reabsorption by the kidneys.

Losses of both chloride and sodium occur with kidney disorders (the kidneys regulate how much chloride is eliminated from the body), cystic fibrosis, excessive sweating, Addison's disease (which affects chloride and sodium reabsorption), and use of **diuretics**.

ESTIMATED CHLORIDE MINIMUM REQUIREMENTS OF HEALTHY PERSONS[a]

AGE	WEIGHT (KG)[*]	CHLORIDE (MG)[b,**]
0–5 months	4.5	180
6–11 months	8.9	300
1 year	11.0	350
2–5 years	16.0	500
6–9 years	25.0	600
10–18 years	50.0	750
>18 years	70.0[c]	750[c]

Reprinted with permission of The National Academy of Sciences, 1989. Courtesy of the National Academy Press, Washington D.C.

*kg = kilograms (1 kilogram = 2.2 pounds)

**mg = milligrams.

[a] = No allowance has been included for large, prolonged losses from the skin through sweat.

[b] = There is no evidence that higher intakes confer any health benefit.

[c] = No allowance included for growth. Values for those below 18 years assume a growth rate at the 50th percentile reported by the National Center for Health Statistics and averaged for males and females.

Caution!

- People with Bartter's syndrome and those who vomit frequently may need chloride supplements (see "When to Supplement with Chloride"). Everyone else gets enough through food sources.

Chromium

Chromium (pronounced CROW-me-um) is a trace mineral that's essential for maintaining normal blood sugar levels by helping insulin (a hormone that transfers blood sugar to the body's cells) do its job. It also helps the body break down fats and carbohydrates. There are three forms of chromium used in supplements: chromium picolinate, chromium polynicotinate, and chromium chloride.

The Benefits of Chromium

Chromium and Glucose Intolerance/Insulin Resistance

Insulin resistance (sometimes called glucose intolerance) is a condition in which the body's cells don't respond adequately to insulin. Because of this, glucose (blood sugar) doesn't get cleared from the blood as easily, leading to higher circulating blood sugar levels. The pancreas, sensing the need for more insulin, increases its production of the hormone. Eventually, insulin resistance can lead to diabetes.

In several studies conducted by the U.S. Department of Agriculture's Beltsville Human Nutrition Research Center, glucose-intolerant people who took 200 micrograms of chromium a day were better able to clear excess glucose from their blood after meals than those who took a placebo. However, the declines in blood sugar levels that were observed, although positive, weren't enough to bring the levels down to normal range. What's more, the results were more striking in those people who consumed a low chromium diet—not those who consumed a normal, varied diet.

In people with insulin resistance, the beneficial effect of chromium supplements is related to the severity of the intolerance. That is, chromium only seems to work for people who are insulin resistant; people with good glucose tolerance do not respond to supplemental chromium.

Chromium and Diabetes

People with diabetes have a higher requirement for chromium since they have impaired mechanisms to convert chromium to a usable form in the body. Although 200 micrograms might be helpful with glucose intolerance, it isn't enough to produce a positive effect with Type 2 diabetes.

A number of research studies with diabetics have yielded positive results with chromium supplements of 400 to 1,000 micrograms per day. In these people, insulin sensitivity and action was increased, and blood sugar control was better. And, although chromium picolinate appeared to be more effective than chromium chloride supplements in

Chromium in Food

Animal products are generally low in chromium, with a few exceptions, and although fruits, vegetables, whole grains, and seeds are a better source, they vary widely in content of the mineral. Other food sources of chromium are: beef, whole wheat bread, brewer's yeast, broccoli, whole-grain or fortified cereals, American cheese, chicken, calf's liver, oysters, and wheat germ.

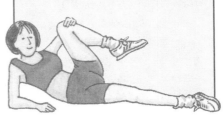

What to Know about Taking Chromium Supplements

- Chromium supplements are available in 200-microgram capsules, tablets, or softgels.
- Chromium supplements usually contain chromium picolinate, chromium polynicotinate, or chromium chloride. There's no evidence that one type of chromium is more effective than any other. However, for safety reasons, avoid chromium picolinate.
- Chromium is better absorbed when taken with foods high in vitamin C, or with a vitamin C supplement.
- Calcium carbonate supplements or antacids can reduce chromium absorption.
- Since dietary supplements are not reviewed by the FDA, quality control and potency problems may exist.
- Rumor has it that taking chromium supplements can extend life. If only it were so! Only one study has been done on this topic—and it was performed with rats. What's more, it wasn't apparent that the life-prolonging effects were due to the chromium at all.

some studies, this has not been shown across the board. Diabetics should discuss chromium supplementation with their doctors.

Chromium and Other Potential Benefits

There are a number of other claims made for chromium supplements. Two of the most popular claims—and the ones that probably lure the most consumers to the supplements—are that chromium picolinate causes fat loss and weight loss, and that it increases muscle mass. In truth, these claims are largely unsupported. Only a few small studies were conducted—all by one researcher—and he used a scientifically unreliable measuring tool (testing body fat levels with calipers). Follow-up studies using a more reliable measurement of fat and muscle (underwater weighing) have shown no effect of chromium supplementation on muscle, fat, or weight. In fact, in November of 1996, the Federal Trade Commission ordered one chromium picolinate supplement manufacturer to stop making unsubstantiated weight loss and health claims for their supplement.

In a few animal studies, chromium has been shown to lower blood cholesterol levels; however, in people, the results are inconclusive. Chromium has also been proposed as a treatment for migraine headaches. More research is needed to determine if chromium supplements provide any of these benefits in humans.

When to Supplement with Chromium

Although there's no RDA for chromium (it's unknown exactly how much the body needs), it's widely agreed that most people probably don't get enough from their diets. Some estimates put typical consumption between 25 and 35 micrograms per day—short of the Adequate Intake level for some groups. For most people, a varied diet along with a chromium-containing multivitamin should be sufficient. It is not recommended that children take chromium supplements.

Although side effects from chromium appear to be rare, there have been some reports of skin reactions from chromium picolinate supplements. It's also possible that chromium supplements will induce anemia in women who take them for more than a few months.

A recent research report linking chromium picolinate supplements to cancer in animals garnered plenty of media attention. Apparently, the picolinate part of the supplement is the problem—not the chromium part. Of course, negative findings such as this are always cause for some concern. However, this was only one study, and therefore its conclusions should not be accepted as a final answer on chromium safety (just as one study on a chromium benefit shouldn't be accepted as the whole story). If you're determined to use a chromium supplement, don't choose one with picolinate. Or, use supplemental brewer's yeast, which has chromium but no picolinate.

ADEQUATE INTAKES (AI) FOR CHROMIUM[a,b]

AGE/SEX	CHROMIUM (MCG)*
Males	
9–13 years	25
14–50 years	35
51+ years	30
Females	
9–13 years	21
14–18 years	24
19–50 years	25
51+ years	20
Pregnancy	
14–18 years	29
19+ years	30
Lactation	
14–18 years	44
19+ years	45

Source: The National Academy of Sciences, 2001.
[a] = Because there is less information on which to base allowances, these figures are not given in the main table of RDA.
[b] = Since the toxic levels for many trace elements may be only several times usual intakes, the upper levels for the trace elements given should not be habitually exceeded.
*mcg = microgram

Caution!

- Healthy people don't need chromium supplements. They may provide some benefit to people with diabetes and insulin resistance. Keep in mind, this research is preliminary.
- If you have diabetes, talk to your doctor before taking chromium. It may alter your dosage for insulin or other medications.
- Specific foods may negatively affect body chromium status. Not only are foods high in simple carbohydrates (such as refined grain products and sweets) usually low in chromium, they also enhance chromium losses.
- If you have a medical condition or are pregnant or lactating, talk to your doctor before taking any supplement.

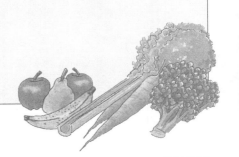

Copper

Copper is a trace element that is essential for humans. Like some other trace minerals, copper's main role is assisting with the proper functioning of enzymes (proteins that accelerate chemical reactions in the body). The enzymes that depend on copper have many functions including energy production; the protection of cells from free radical damage; the strengthening of connective tissues, bones, and blood vessels; the formation of skin and hair pigments; the production of **neurotransmitters** and other hormones; and the absorption, storage, and metabolism of iron.

The Benefits of Copper

Copper and Osteoporosis

Copper's role in preserving bone health is not yet well understood. However, preliminary research suggests that getting the Adequate Intake level of copper may be helpful in preventing osteoporosis. Unfortunately, there aren't enough studies from which to draw any real conclusions, and most of those that do exist study a combination of trace minerals—not just copper.

Copper and Heart Disease

According to one researcher, copper deficiencies increase the risk of high cholesterol (**hypercholesterolemia**) and heart disease. Although other scientists have also found that hypercholesterolemia occurs with inadequate copper status, there is little evidence at this time to conclude that heart disease always follows. In fact, a clinical trial of copper supplements showed that they had no effect on heart disease risk. Nevertheless, this is a promising area of research that warrants additional study.

When to Supplement with Copper

The Recommended Dietary Allowance (RDA) for copper is 900 micrograms for adults aged 19 years and over (it is not recommended for children). Compared to some other minerals, copper is relatively easily absorbed by the body. We absorb about 30 to 40 percent of the copper in our diets, although high intakes of some other nutrients, such as vitamin C and the minerals zinc, iron, manganese, and molybdenum, can decrease copper absorption and the body's level of copper.

Estimates of actual adult copper intake vary widely, but average about 1 milligram per day—less than estimated requirements. Yet, despite low intakes, copper deficiency within the United States is rare, leading some researchers to theorize that copper absorption adapts somewhat to copper intake. That is, copper absorption may become more efficient when copper intake is reduced, and vice versa, in order to keep the body's copper balance stable.

A true copper deficiency usually only occurs in individuals with the inherited condition called **Menkes disease** (sometimes known as "kinky" or "steely" hair disease), in which copper absorption in the intestine is inhibited. However, taking excessive vitamin C, iron, or zinc supplements can also interfere with copper absorption and trigger deficiency symptoms. The most common symptoms of copper deficiency include anemia, heart problems such as blood vessel and heart rupture, abnormal heart rhythms, a low number of white blood cells, and elevated triglycerides, cholesterol, and glucose levels. A lifetime of marginal dietary copper intake may lead to heart disease.

Toxicity from dietary copper is rare, but consuming supplements that provide more than 3 milligrams of copper per day for an extended period of time can be dangerous. Doses of 10 milligrams per day over several weeks can lead to toxic symptoms such as weakness and nausea. With very high intakes there is injury to the digestive tract, kidneys, liver, brain, and other organs. **Wilson's disease**, a genetic disease in which copper accumulates in the body, can lead to severe liver damage and neurological problems. Individuals with Wilson's disease should *not* take copper supplements.

What to Know about Taking Copper Supplements

- Copper is found in multivitamin and mineral formulas, or combined with zinc (because copper decreases zinc absorption and vice versa) in varying dosages.
- Although sometimes it's suggested that zinc and copper be taken separately because of their antagonism toward each other, this is not necessary when taking a multivitamin/ mineral supplement because the zinc level is not high.
- Copper supplements are available in tablets or capsules as copper aspartate, copper citrate, copper gluconate, or copper picolinate. There is no evidence that one form is better than another.
- Avoid *excessive* iron, manganese, molybdenum, zinc, and vitamin C supplements, which can decrease copper absorption. Amounts in a typical diet or in a regular supplement don't cause problems. Ask your doctor if extra copper is necessary.
- Since dietary supplements are not reviewed by the FDA, quality control and potency problems may exist.

FOOD SOURCES OF COPPER

FOOD SOURCES	SERVING SIZE	COPPER (MG)*
Liver, beef	3 ounces	3.8
Sunflower seeds, kernels	1/4 cup	0.6
Walnuts	1 ounce	0.5
Tofu, firm	1/2 cup	0.3
Chocolate chips, semisweet	1/4 cup	0.3
Milk chocolate	1 ounce	0.1

Source: USDA Nutrient Database for Standard Reference, Release 13, 1999.
*mg = milligrams.

ADEQUATE INTAKES (AI)[a] FOR COPPER

AGE	COPPER (MCG)*
Infants	
0–1/2 year	200
1/2–1 year	220

[a] = The AI levels for the first six months of life reflect the average iron intake of infants principally fed human milk, with an added increment for food in infants 6 months and older.
*mcg = micrograms.

RECOMMENDED DIETARY ALLOWANCES (RDA) FOR COPPER

AGE	COPPER (MCG)*
Children	
1–3 years	340
4–8 years	440
9–13 years	700
Adults	
19+ years	900
Pregnancy	
14+ years	1,000
Lactation	
14+ years	1,300

Source: The National Academy of Sciences, 1989.
*mcg = micrograms.

Copper in Food

Copper is found in a variety of foods. Good sources include oysters and other shellfish, nuts, grains, seeds, and legumes. In seeds and grains, the **bran** and germ parts of the grain contain most of the copper. Therefore, refined flour, which has these parts removed, isn't a great source of copper (see "Food Sources of Copper").

Sometimes drinking water is listed as a source of dietary copper if it travels through copper pipes. However, since only minute amounts of copper normally leach into the water, it's not a good source of the mineral.

TOLERABLE UPPER INTAKE LEVEL (UL)[a] FOR COPPER

AGE	COPPER (MCG)*
0–1 years	ND[b]
1–3 years	1,000
4–8 years	3,000
9–13 years	5,000
14–18 years	8,000
19+ years	10,000
Pregnancy	
14–18 years	8,000
19+ years	10,000
Lactation	
14–18 years	8,000
19+ years	10,000

Source: National Academy of Sciences, 2001.
a = The maximum level of daily nutrient intake that is likely to pose no risk of adverse effects.
b = Not determinable due to lack of data of adverse effects in this age group. Source of intake should be from food and formula only.
*mcg = micrograms.

Fluoride

Fluoride is a form of the trace element fluorine. About 99 percent of the fluoride in humans is found in bone and teeth. It is best known for its ability to protect against and reverse the development and progression of dental **caries** (cavities). Dental caries are caused by bacteria. When we eat food, bacteria in the mouth multiply (forming plaque), producing organic acids. Loss of tooth enamel occurs as long as the pH of plaque is acidic. Fluoride can stop this process by reducing the acids on the teeth.

The Benefits of Fluoride

Fluoride and Teeth

Consuming fluoride is essential throughout life. In infancy, during the period of tooth formation—before the teeth penetrate the gum—

Caution!

- If you have a medical condition or are pregnant or lactating, talk to your doctor before taking any supplement.
- A combined daily copper intake (from food sources and supplements) of up to 3 milligrams—no more— is considered to be safe and adequate.

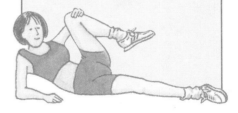

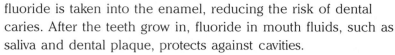

Fluoride in Food and Drink

Fluoride is found in fluoridated water, beverages, infant formulas that are made with fluoridated water, teas, and some marine fish. Brewed tea contains roughly 1 to 6 milligrams/liter of fluoride, depending on the amount of tea used, the water fluoride concentration, and brewing time. Interestingly, decaffeinated teas contain twice as much fluoride as caffeinated teas.

The average daily intake of fluoride in fluoridated areas has remained constant since 1980 at about 0.05 milligrams/kilogram/day from infancy to early childhood. In communities without fluoridated water, average intakes are about 50 percent lower.

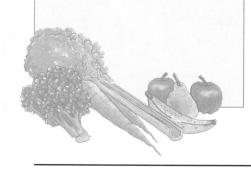

fluoride is taken into the enamel, reducing the risk of dental caries. After the teeth grow in, fluoride in mouth fluids, such as saliva and dental plaque, protects against cavities.

Fluoride balance in the body changes with age. In young children, for instance, as much as 80 percent of the fluoride consumed goes into skeleton and teeth for growth, with only 20 percent excreted in the urine. On the other hand, young or middle-aged adults who are healthy lose as much as 50 percent via urine. Although there are no data for the elderly, experts believe that older persons excrete even more fluoride in urine.

Fluoride and Bone Health

In a recent study, researchers compared a low-fluoride control group of perimenopausal women (those nearing menopause) with other perimenopausal women who had consumed fluoridated water for 10 years or more. Vertebral bone mineral density was slightly increased in the women who had been using fluoridated water. Previous research has shown that fluoride may stimulate new bone growth, prompting its use as an experimental treatment in osteoporosis. For optimal results, some experts recommend combining fluoride (1 milligram/kilogram body weight/day) with calcium and low-dose (400 International Units) vitamin D supplementation. Keep in mind, however, that long-term supplementation of fluoride has not been fully studied. Consult with your doctor before supplementing with fluoride for the prevention of osteoporosis.

Fluoride and Crohn's Disease

People who suffer from Crohn's disease, chronic inflammation of the small and/or large intestine, are at an increased risk of decreased bone density and osteoporosis. Earlier studies have shown that supplementing with calcium and vitamin D can prevent further bone loss. A new study found that adding sodium fluoride, in combination with calcium and vitamin D, is even more effective in increasing bone density of the spine.

When to Supplement with Fluoride

A lack of fluoride at any age will increase the risk of cavities. Research shows that the earlier children are exposed to fluoridated water or supplements, the greater the reduction in dental caries in both baby and permanent teeth.

Fluoride supplements are available only by prescription and are intended for use by children (they're rarely prescribed for adults) living in areas with low fluoride concentrations (see "Dietary Fluoride Supplement Dosage Schedule for Children"). The purpose is to bring the fluoride intakes in these children up to the levels of children living in areas with fluoridated water (about 1.0 milligram/liter).

Although too little fluoride is definitely a problem, more is not necessarily better. Too much fluoride before the age of eight can result in **fluorosis**—chronic fluoride "poisoning" or overconsumption. Mild fluorosis, or mottled tooth enamel (white horizontal lines on the teeth), develops on permanent teeth while they're still forming. Although fluorosis may be aesthetically objectionable, it has no effect on tooth function.

However, in extreme cases of chronic fluoride consumption, fluorosis can also affect the skeleton in three different stages. Stage 1 symptoms include occasional stiffness or joint pain. Stages 2 and 3 can result in dose-related calcification (or hardening) of ligaments, muscle loss, and neurological defects due to hypercalcification of vertebra. Most studies indicate that an intake of at least 10 milligrams per day for 10 years or more is needed to produce the milder forms of this condition.

Although fluorosis of bones may be uncommon, fluorosis of teeth is not. Fluoridated dental products (i.e., toothpaste, mouthwash) are one of the biggest culprits. Fluoride consumption from these products can equal or exceed intake from the diet, especially in young children. Kids can swallow about 0.3 milligrams of fluoride each time they brush, averaging about 0.6 milligrams of fluoride per day—especially if they don't rinse well.

Believe it or not, baby food can also be a culprit. Ready-to-eat foods with chicken may provide quite a bit of fluoride, possibly

Does Your Bottled Water Pass the Fluoride Test?

If you and your family prefer bottled water over tap water, you may want to take note. In a recent survey in Cleveland, only 5 percent of the bottled water purchased fell within the required fluoride range recommended by the state of Ohio, compared with 100 percent of the tap water samples. The tap water also met the optimal fluoride level of 1.0 milligram/liter, which maximizes the reduction in cavities, while minimizing the risk of fluorosis.

The Environmental Protection Agency (EPA) requires community water systems to regularly report to the public the quality (and fluoride content) of local tap water. Currently, there are no similar requirements for bottled water manufacturers. To find out whether your bottled water provides fluoride, contact the International Bottled Water Association at 800/WATER-11 to receive a list of brands that contain this important nutrient.

because of the way they're made. The mechanical deboning process may leave some skin and residual bone particles in the food. Since fluoride is stored mostly in bones, higher concentrations are found in chicken-containing products.

Some experts argue that there is no longer a need for fluoride supplements in the United States. According to researchers at the University of Michigan, because there are alternative forms of fluoride (i.e., drinking water, toothpaste, gels, rinses, processed foods, and beverages) the risk of using supplements in small children outweighs the benefits.

ADEQUATE INTAKES (AI) FOR FLUORIDE*

AGE/SEX	FLUORIDE (MG)**
Infants	
0–1/2 year	0.01
1/2–1 year	0.5
Children	
1–3 years	0.7
4–8 years	1
Males	
9–13 years	2
14–18 years	3
19+ years	4
Females	
9–13 years	2
14+ years	3
Pregnant women	3
Lactating women	3

Reprinted with permission of The National Academy of Sciences, 1997. Courtesy of the National Academy Press, Washington D.C.
*There are no RDAs for fluoride due to insufficient information.
**mg = milligrams.

Caution!

Before giving your child fluoride supplements, talk to your dentist and do some checking. Consider how much fluoride your child is getting in the water supply, toothpaste, and baby food.

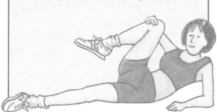

DIETARY FLUORIDE SUPPLEMENT DOSAGE SCHEDULE FOR CHILDREN:
Recommended Supplemental Amount for Various Levels of Fluoride in Drinking Water Drinking Based on Water Fluoride Concentration (MG/LITER)*

AGE OF CHILD	<0.3	0.3–0.6	>0.6
6 months to 3 years	0.25[a]	0	0
3 to 6 years	0.50	0.25	0
6 to 16 years	1.00	0.50	0

Reprinted with permission of The National Academy of Sciences, 1997. Courtesy of the National Academy Press, Washington D.C.

*mg = milligrams.

[a] = Fluoride supplement values are given in milligrams of fluoride per day (2.2 milligrams sodium fluoride = 1.0 milligram fluoride). Depending on the amount of fluoride in your water, (<0.3–>0.6), your child may or may not need fluoride supplements.

TOLERABLE UPPER INTAKE LEVEL (UL)[a] FOR FLUORIDE

AGE	FLUORIDE (MG)*
0–$\frac{1}{2}$ year	0.7–2.2
9+ years	10.0
Pregnancy	10.0
Lactation	10.0

Source: The National Academy of Sciences, 1997.

*mg = milligrams.

[a] = The maximum level of daily nutrient intake that is likely to pose no risk of adverse effects. Unless otherwise specified, the UL represents total intake from food, water, and supplements.

Iodine

When most people think of iodine, they recall the antiseptic their parents used to put on cuts. However, this mineral plays a much more important role in the body. Roughly 75 to 80 percent of the iodine in the body is found in the butterfly-shaped **thyroid gland** in the neck.

The Benefits of Iodine

Iodine is an essential part of the thyroid hormones, thyroxin and triiodothyronine. These hormones are necessary for maintaining normal metabolism and are critical for normal growth and development of a healthy fetus and infant. The biggest benefit of dietary

Iodine in Food

The iodine content of food and water depends on the amount of iodine in the soil. Areas that are mountainous or experience heavy rainfalls are likely to be low in iodine, placing humans and animal populations at risk. Fortunately, since the 1920s, iodine has been added to salt in the United States, enabling Americans to get the iodine they need. Foods typically high in iodine include iodized table salt, seafood, sea vegetables, such as kelp, and cheese (see "Food Sources of Iodine").

If you're not buying iodized salt because you prefer sea salt or eat a lot of salty snack foods, you might want to reconsider. Sea salt loses its iodine during processing, and most popular snack foods are not made with iodized salt.

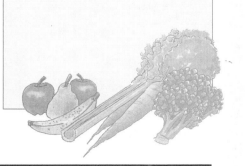

Iodine Supplementation Helps Millions Worldwide

In 1990, iodine deficiency affected almost one-third of the world's population and was the most common preventable cause of brain damage and mental retardation. That same year, following a resolution adopted by the World Summit for Children, major iodine supplementation programs were implemented by the governments of the affected countries with the aid of major donors. Iodization of salt was the method of choice, and nine years later, in 1999, 75 percent of the affected countries had legislation on salt iodization and 68 percent of the affected populations had access to iodized salt. The prevalence of iodine deficiency disorders decreased dramatically in most countries, and disappeared completely in some areas, such as Peru.

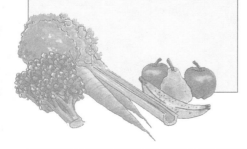

iodine may be the prevention of iodine deficiency disorders (IDD), the result of insufficient iodine.

Iodine and Goiter

Goiter is the classic iodine deficiency disease. When the iodine level in the blood is low, the cells of the thyroid gland enlarge in an attempt to trap as many particles of iodine as possible. If the gland enlarges until it's visible at the neck, it is called simple goiter.

Another form of goiter is called toxic goiter. This occurs as a result of eating too many plants from the cabbage family and others (cabbage, Brussels sprouts, legumes, and cassava) that contain an antithyroid substance that interferes with iodine absorption. As with a simple goiter, the thyroid gland enlarges until it's visible at the neck. However, this is only a problem when these foods are eaten in large quantities and dietary iodine intake is also low.

Iodine and Birth Defects

Iodine deficiency can impair growth and neurological development, which can damage the brain. Depending on its severity and the stage of development at which deficiency occurs, a lack of iodine can lead to a number of health problems ranging from mild intellectual impairment to severe mental retardation (**cretinism**), growth stunting, apathy, and impaired speech, hearing, or movement. Individuals suffering from cretinism can have an IQ as low as 20 and an abnormal face and body.

Although cretinism is rare, the more "mild" deficiency symptoms are all too common in undeveloped areas of the world. Fortunately, universal salt iodization provides the most effective and affordable way to prevent IDD. Currently, more than 90 countries iodize their salt (see "Iodine Supplementation Helps Millions Worldwide"). Other avenues for providing iodine include water, grain, and dairy products. In remote areas of the world where the use of iodized salt is not feasible, iodized oil supplements are sometimes used.

Iodine and Breast Cancer

There is some suggestive evidence linking iodine to a reduced risk of breast cancer. Japanese women, for instance, have a low rate of benign and malignant breast disease. They also tend to eat quite a bit of seaweed, which is a rich source of iodine. In both animal and human studies, iodine has been shown to cause regression of benign breast tissue. However, these findings are preliminary, and researchers caution that much more research is needed.

FOOD SOURCES OF IODINE

FOOD SOURCES	SERVING SIZE	IODINE (MCG)*
Salt, iodized	1 teaspoon	400
Haddock	3 ounces	104–145
Bread, made with regular process	1 slice	35
Cheese, cottage, 2% fat	½ cup	26–71
Shrimp	3 ounces	21–37
Egg	1 medium	18–26
Cheese, cheddar	1 ounce	5–23
Ground beef	3 ounces	8

Source: *Krause's Food, Nutrition, and Diet Therapy*, Revised by L.K. Mahan, R.D., C.D., M.S., and M.T. Arlin, R.D., M.S., 8th Ed., 1992.
*mcg = micrograms.

ADEQUATE INTAKES (AI) FOR IODINE

AGE/SEX	IODINE (MCG)*
Infants	
0–1/2 year	110
1/2–1 year	130

*mcg = micrograms.

Caution!

- Since the introduction of iodized salt, iodine supplements are unnecessary and *not* recommended for most people. Consumption of iodized salt *is* recommended.
- High doses of iodine (several milligrams per day) can interfere with normal thyroid function and should not be taken without consulting a doctor first.
- Children and individuals with thyroid problems should not take iodine supplements.
- If you have a medical condition or are pregnant or lactating, talk to your doctor before taking any supplement.

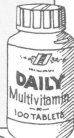

What to Know about Taking Iodine Supplements

- Iodine supplements are available in tablet, capsule, and liquid forms in varying doses. Iodine is often combined with potassium.
- Strict vegetarians who avoid salt and sea vegetables, such as kelp, may wish to supplement with 150 micrograms or less of iodine per day.
- Supplementing at levels greater than 3 milligrams (3,000 micrograms) per day can result in goiter, similar to that seen with iodine deficiency. And, there are no proven benefits from taking this much iodine.
- Since dietary supplements are not reviewed by the FDA, quality control and potency problems may exist.

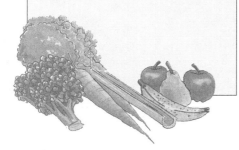

RECOMMENDED DIETARY ALLOWANCES (RDA) FOR IODINE

AGE/SEX	IODINE (MCG)*
Children	
1–8 years	90
Males	
9–13 years	120
14+ years	150
Females	
9–13 years	120
14+ years	150
Pregnant women	220
Lactating women	290

Source: National Academy of Sciences, 2000.
*mcg = micrograms.

TOLERABLE UPPER INTAKE LEVEL (UL)[a] FOR IODINE

AGE	IODINE (MCG)*
0–1 year	Not possible to establish; intake should be from food and formula only
1–3 years	200
4–8 years	300
9–13 years	600
14–18 years	900
19+ years	1,100
Pregnancy	
14–18 years	900
19+ years	1,100
Lactation	
14–18 years	900
19+ years	1,100

Source: The National Academy of Sciences, 2000.
[a] = The maximum level of daily nutrient intake that is likely to pose no risk of adverse effects. Unless otherwise specified, the UL represents total intake from food, water, and supplements.
*mcg = micrograms.

Iron

The most studied and best understood mineral, iron was identified as a component of blood back in the 18th century. About three-fourths of the body's iron is found in **hemoglobin**, a key component of red blood cells. Hemoglobin's job is to deliver oxygen to the body's cells and carry carbon dioxide—a waste product—away from the cells to the lungs. Exhaling rids the body of the carbon dioxide. The rest of the body's iron is found in enzymes and myoglobin (temporary iron storage in the muscles and heart) with longer-term storage in the liver, spleen, and bone marrow.

The Benefits of Iron

Iron and Anemia

Iron deficiency anemia is characterized by low iron stores and depressed hemoglobin production. Anemia decreases the amount of oxygen delivered to the body tissues. The body compensates for this by extracting more oxygen from hemoglobin, redistributing blood flow to vital organs at the expense of other tissues, and making the heart work harder to circulate the blood. These compensatory measures put stress on the body, and when combined with other disease states or medical problems, extreme illness can result.

Symptoms of anemia come on gradually and include pale skin, weakness, lack of energy, breathlessness, inability to maintain body temperature, increased susceptibility to infections, and irregular heartbeat. During pregnancy, anemia increases the risk of having a premature and low birth weight baby. In young children, iron deficiency is associated with learning disabilities and behavioral problems such as reduced attention span, as well as increased absorption of lead. In fact, in the United States, children who have iron deficiency have a three to four times higher prevalence of lead poisoning than children who aren't iron deficient.

Interestingly, research indicates that some of the symptoms that people normally associate with iron deficiency anemia, such as fatigue and impaired muscular function (which frequently shows up as difficulty walking), are probably not due to the anemia, but are

Iron in Food

Iron is found in many common foods (see "Food Sources of Iron"). When present in animal products it's called **heme iron**; in plant foods it's called nonheme iron. Heme iron is much more readily absorbed than **nonheme iron**, which is why the body absorbs about 20 percent of the iron in meat, a little less from dairy products, and only 3 to 5 percent of iron in vegetables.

The iron content of breast-milk is similar to that of cow's milk, but about 50 percent of the iron in breast-milk is absorbed, making it a great source of the mineral for infants (as is iron-fortified infant formula).

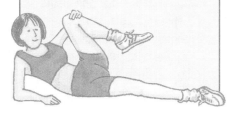

likely caused by the effects of the deficiency on iron-containing enzymes in the body.

Iron supplementation is highly effective at reversing anemia, producing results after about one month of treatment. (If there is no correction after a month, further medical evaluation is necessary—there may be other causes for the anemia.) In children, research in many countries shows that iron therapy can help reverse the learning problems associated with anemia, but it may not be 100 percent effective in this regard. Some studies suggest that children who experienced iron deficiency at a young age and over a long time never catch up to their peers intellectually.

When to Supplement with Iron

In the United States, where meat consumption is generally high, most people have little difficulty meeting the Recommended Dietary Allowance for iron—the exception to this is girls and women who are menstruating. The USDA Continuing Survey of Food Intakes by Individuals in 1996 revealed that the average iron intake for females aged 20 and over was 13 milligrams (5 milligrams less than the RDA); for males it was 19 milligrams. Only supplement children with iron if prescribed by a physician.

Additional data from this survey, which averaged food intake over two days, showed that the RDA for iron was met by only 20 percent of women aged 40 to 49, 27 percent of females aged 12 to 29, and only 32 percent of those aged 30 to 39. This "snapshot" look at iron intake does not reveal how many of these females had iron deficiency. In addition, had the survey been conducted on different days, the results could very well have shown adequate iron consumption. Nevertheless, surveys such as this are some of the best tools we have to indicate probable areas where nutrient intakes don't match up with needs.

Iron Deficiency

Iron deficiency is the most common nutritional deficiency in the United States and worldwide, affecting mainly older infants, young children, and females of childbearing age. In developing countries it's estimated that 30 to 40 percent of young children and pre-menopausal women are deficient in iron. In the United States, the third National Health and Nutrition Examination Survey, conducted in 1991, showed that about 5 percent of children aged 1 to 2 had iron deficiency, and about half of those were anemic as well.

Iron deficiency most commonly occurs as a result of increased needs during periods of growth—pregnancy, infancy, early childhood, and puberty, for example. Breastfed infants can be at risk if they aren't receiving supplemental iron or aren't eating iron-fortified foods. Women in the childbearing years require about twice the iron of men in order to cover menstrual blood losses. Adolescent females are particularly at risk for deficiency because they're growing *and* they're losing blood. Individuals who have suffered blood loss (i.e., from an accident) are also at risk for iron deficiency.

A person who is iron deficient isn't automatically anemic; iron deficiency progresses in three stages. First, iron stores in the bone marrow, liver, and spleen are depleted. Next, red blood cell production is reduced, and finally, hemoglobin production falls, resulting in anemia. Blood tests can diagnose iron deficiency in any of these stages.

The body has an interesting way to fight against iron deficiency. As is the case with many nutrients, when the body is low on iron, it adapts to absorb more. However, the body goes one step further in the case of iron. Studies show that when the diet is high in nonheme iron (from plant foods) but contains little heme iron (from animal products), the body increases its ability to absorb nonheme iron. This enables people who derive their iron primarily from vegetable sources to better maintain their body stores. The diet does not need to contain animal products for proper iron intake. Iron is also contained in iron-fortified products such as cereals and breads, so vegetarians don't have to consume animal products. (This adaptation does not appear to work in reverse. In other words, the body does not begin to absorb less iron when a high heme iron diet is consumed.)

Iron deficiency is effectively treated with iron supplements, which have been used since 1832. They efficiently reverse iron deficiency and can correct iron-deficiency anemia. However, they

Iron Facts

- Because iron isn't generally well absorbed, the dietary requirement for iron is about 10 times higher than our biological needs.
- Pagophagia, an abnormal desire to eat large amounts of ice, is linked to iron deficiency. Once the body's iron stores reach normal levels, the cravings disappear.
- For more information about iron, contact the Iron Disorders Institute (864/241–0111) at *www.irondisorders.org.*

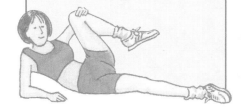

frequently produce gastrointestinal side effects, the most common of which are nausea and constipation. The risk of side effects is directly proportional to the iron dose. According to experts, doses larger than 120 milligrams are the most likely to cause unpleasant symptoms. Such large doses are not necessary in most cases.

Iron Toxicity

Too much iron is just as serious a problem as too little. Excessive iron intake can result in a number of health problems in both the short term and the long term.

Iron poisoning, or toxicity, can result from an excessive dose of iron from supplements. This mainly happens in children who swallow iron supplements intended for their mothers or other women in the household. Vomiting and bloody diarrhea—the first signs of iron poisoning—can lead to gastrointestinal tract damage.

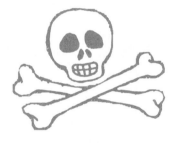

WARNING: Children and Iron Poisoning

According to the Food and Drug Administration, iron-containing supplements are the leading cause of pediatric poisoning deaths for children under age six in the United States. Between June 1992 and January 1993, five toddlers died after eating iron supplements, according to the national Centers for Disease Control and Prevention.

Iron poisoning in children causes problems within minutes or hours after ingestion. Early symptoms include nausea, vomiting, diarrhea, and gastrointestinal bleeding, developing into shock, coma, seizures, and death. Even if no symptoms appear, or if the child seems to be recovering, medical treatment is necessary. A child who survives iron poisoning can experience health problems (gastrointestinal obstruction and liver damage) up to a month after the incident.

Iron is always included in prenatal vitamins prescribed for pregnant women, and is often included in multivitamin formulas for children and adults. Children's chewable supplements often taste just like candy, leading kids to want more than the recommended dose. Iron supplements (as a single nutrient and not part of a multivitamin) are usually available without a prescription and can be found in many supermarkets, drugstores, and health food stores in a wide variety of potencies. For a small child, as little as 600 milligrams of iron can be fatal. Depending on the dosage, this amount can be found in as few as four tablets.

Iron supplements are tempting to children because they frequently look like candy. They're round and often red in color, and some have a sweet-tasting coating to cover up the bad-tasting iron. In 1993, the Nonprescription Drug Manufacturers Association, which includes companies that manufacture about 95 percent of the nonprescription medicines available today, adopted a policy that called for the elimination of sweet coatings on iron-containing supplements that provided 30 milligrams or more iron per dose. They also agreed to new voluntary warning labels for these products. In 1997, FDA required "unit-dose" packaging for iron-containing products with 30 milligrams or more of iron per dose. This packaging features individual "bubbles" from which a paper or foil covering must be peeled before the supplement will come out. It's believed that this packaging will discourage children from taking the supplements, or at least limit the number of tablets a child would swallow. This requirement is in addition to existing U.S. Consumer Product Safety Commission regulations, which require child-resistant packaging for most iron-containing products.

If you suspect a child has overdosed on an iron-containing supplement, call the nearest poison control center or the child's physician first, then follow their instructions. Of course, taking steps to avoid an iron-poisoning situation first is the best plan:

- Always close a supplement container completely as soon as you've finished using it.
- Properly secure the child-resistant packaging, and put it away immediately in a place where children can't see or reach it.
- Keep supplements in their original containers.
- Never keep supplements on a countertop or bedside table.
- If you spill some of the supplements, immediately pick them up. Do not dispose of them in a place where a child could get them.
- Never refer to vitamins as candy.

Iron Deficiency

Iron deficiency primarily affects:

- Children
- Adolescent girls
- Pregnant women
- Females who have very heavy menstrual periods
- People who have medical conditions that cause loss of blood (i.e., wounds, bleeding ulcers)
- People who have recently undergone surgery
- Women who regularly donate blood (blood donations do not appear to significantly affect the body iron stores of men)
- Strict vegetarians (vegans)
- Female athletes or women who regularly engage in strenuous exercise (especially premenopausal women and adolescents)
- People who take cholesterol-lowering medications

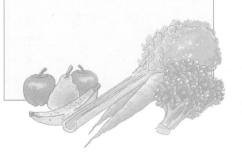

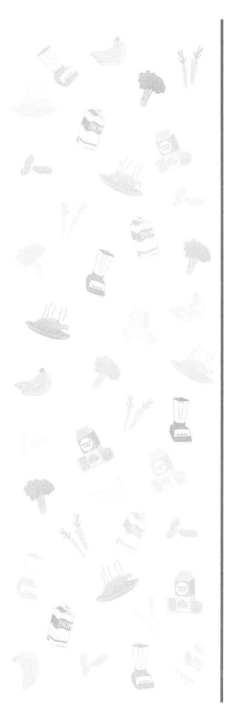

Hemochromatosis

Overloading the body's iron stores by chronically taking too much supplemental iron (or sometimes by blood transfusions) can damage various organs by causing excessive iron storage. The best known, and probably the most common, form of chronic iron overload is hereditary **hemochromatosis**. Of course, people diagnosed with the disease should not take iron supplements.

In population groups with European ancestry, approximately three in 1,000 have hemochromatosis, a genetic abnormality that causes a greater than normal absorption of iron. The organs most affected are the liver, heart, pancreas, and pituitary gland; the joints are also impacted. When total body iron accumulates to 20 to 40 grams (about 10 percent more than normal), signs of the abnormality—including arthritis, diabetes, **cirrhosis** of the liver, sexual dysfunction, and heart failure—begin to show. Although it can vary, symptoms of hemochromatosis don't usually surface until later in life, when bodily needs for iron have decreased—that's why many people with this disorder don't even know they have it. In men symptoms typically appear around age 30 to 50; in women, it's after menopause.

Even if you have no symptoms, it's not difficult to be screened for hemochromatosis. A simple blood test will reveal if your **transferrin** (protein in the blood that carries iron) is saturated with iron. The main treatment for the disease is phlebotomy, or removal of blood from the body. When phlebotomy is started before clinical signs of the disease appear, organ damage can be prevented. However, the treatment will not reverse organ damage that has already occurred. For this reason, screening is recommended for people who may be at risk for hemochromatosis—even if they show no symptoms.

Some research has linked high iron levels with cancer, increased rates of tumor growth, and **coronary heart disease**. With the exception of an increased risk of liver cancer among people with hemochromatosis (due to chronic injury of the liver from high levels of iron stored there), further study has not supported these associations.

Dietary Factors That Affect Nonheme (Plant-Derived) Iron Absorption

Absorption is increased by:

- The presence of meat, fish, poultry, shellfish, or meat products at the same meal
- Vitamin C*
- Cooking in iron cookware, such as a cast-iron skillet

Absorption is hindered by:

- Calcium**
- Soy protein
- Wheat bran and other dietary fiber (phytic acids bind the iron)
- Tea (**tannin** is the component in tea that can decrease iron absorption) and coffee
- Egg yolks

The latest research shows that vitamin C's effect is not as great as previously thought.
**Recent research shows that long-term calcium supplementation does not adversely affect the body's iron stores.

FOOD SOURCES OF IRON

FOOD SOURCES	SERVING SIZE	IRON (MG)*
Clams	3 ounces	24
Cereal, fortified	1 cup	1–15
Liver, beef	3 ounces	5.7
Beans and franks, canned	1 cup	4.4
Chicken leg	1	1.5
Rice, white, enriched	1 cup	1.9
Beef, ground	3 ounces	1.7
Cashews	1 ounce	1.4
Bread, whole wheat	1 slice	0.9
Egg	1	0.7
Milk, 2% fat	1 cup	0.1

Source: USDA Nutrient Database for Standard Reference, Release 13, 1999.
*mg = milligrams.

Caution!

- Self-treatment with iron supplements can be dangerous. Do not take iron supplements unless advised to do so by a doctor.
- Keep all supplements containing iron out of reach of children. Relatively small amounts of iron can be fatal to children.
- Iron supplements can interfere with the absorption and utilization of antibiotics and some other medications.
- Premature infants who receive iron-fortified formula or oral iron supplements should also take vitamin E to prevent oxidative damage from the iron.
- Iron supplements can be dangerous, *especially* for adult men, post-menopausal women, and people diagnosed with hemochromatosis. For children, adolescent females, and women who have not reached menopause, a multivitamin containing the RDA for iron is considered safe, but may not be necessary. When in doubt, ask your doctor to check your iron status before taking any iron-containing supplements.

ADEQUATE INTAKE (AI)[a] FOR IRON

AGE	IRON (MG)*
Infants	
0–1/2 year	0.27

a = The AI levels for the first six months of life reflect the average iron intake of infants principally fed human milk.
*mg = milligrams.

RECOMMENDED DIETARY ALLOWANCES (RDA) FOR IRON

AGE/SEX	IRON (MG)*
Infants	
1/2–1 year	11
Children	
1–3 years	7
4–8 years	10
Males	
9–13 years	8
14–18 years	11
19+ years	8
Females	
9–13 years	8
14–18 years	15[a]
19–50 years	18[a]
51+ years	8
Pregnancy	
14+ years	27
Lactation	
14–18 years	10
19+ years	9

Source: The National Academy of Sciences, 2001.
a = Because the use of oral contraceptives decreases menstrual blood loss and therefore lowers iron needs, the RDAs for those taking oral contraceptives are lowered to 11.4 and 10.9 for adolescent girls and premenopausal women, respectively.
*mg = milligrams.

TOLERABLE UPPER INTAKE LEVEL (UL)[a,b] FOR IRON

AGE	IRON (MG)*
0–13 years	40
14+ years	45
Pregnancy	
14+ years	45
Lactation	
14+ years	45

Source: The National Academy of Sciences, 2001.
[a] = The maximum level of daily nutrient intake that is likely to pose no risk of adverse effects.
[b] = Individuals with conditions that make them susceptible to the adverse effects of excess iron intake may not be protected by the UL.
*mg = milligrams.

INCREASING THE IRON CONTENT OF FOOD BY USING IRON COOKWARE

FOOD SOURCES	IRON IN MG PER 3½ OUNCES RAW FOOD	NON-IRON COOKWARE	IRON COOKWARE
Baked corn bread	0.67	0.83	0.86
Beef vegetable stew	0.66	0.81	3.40
Fried egg	1.92	1.84	3.48
Pancakes	0.63	0.81	1.31
Spanish rice	0.87	0.83	2.25
Spaghetti sauce	0.61	0.69	5.77
Stir-fried green beans	0.64	0.69	1.18
Unsweetened applesauce	0.35	0.28	7.38
White rice	0.67	0.86	1.97

Copyright ©The American Dietetic Association. Reprinted by the permission of the *Journal of the American Dietetic Association*, 1986; Vol. 86, pp. 897–901.

Magnesium

Magnesium (pronounced mag-KNEE-see-um) is an essential mineral, and like calcium, it is stored largely in the bones. In fact, as much as 60 percent of the body's store of magnesium is in bones; the other 40 percent is found in muscle and soft tissues. The kidneys regulate magnesium balance in the body, ensuring that there will be enough magnesium on hand for a number of important bodily

What to Know about Taking Magnesium Supplements

- Magnesium supplements come in the form of sulfate, lactate, hydroxide, oxide, chloride, and glycerophosphate. Any of these forms are fine, but *avoid* dolomite as it may contain lead.

- Multivitamin and mineral supplements provide magnesium, but rarely contain a day's recommended dose because the 300 to 400 milligrams necessary would never fit into a small pill. If you want more than about 25 percent of the RDA, you'll probably have to buy a separate magnesium supplement.

- Magnesium is prescribed in divided doses 3 to 4 times per day to avoid diarrhea.

- The National Academy of Sciences recommends no more than 350 milligrams of supplemental magnesium per day. No cases of magnesium toxicity have ever been reported from food sources.

- Since dietary supplements are not reviewed by the FDA, quality control and potency problems may exist.

functions. For example, magnesium activates more than 300 enzymes that keep our cells and organs functioning properly.

Magnesium is also necessary for releasing energy that is stored in muscles, manufacturing proteins, repairing cell damage, and regulating body temperature. Together with calcium, magnesium helps to maintain normal muscle and nerve function, keeps heart rhythm steady and bones strong, and promotes resistance to tooth decay by holding calcium in tooth enamel.

The Benefits of Magnesium

Magnesium and Heart Disease

For years researchers have observed that people who live in areas with "hard" drinking water (which contains more minerals, including magnesium, than "soft" water) have lower rates of heart disease and stroke. Although the amount of magnesium in a cup of water is only a fraction of an individual's daily food intake, the possible link to decreasing the risk of heart disease has prompted researchers to take a closer look.

A deficiency of magnesium can cause metabolic changes that may contribute to heart attacks and strokes. There is some evidence that low body stores of magnesium can increase the risk of abnormal heart rhythms, which in turn may increase the risk of complications associated with a heart attack. Higher blood levels of magnesium have been associated with lower risk of coronary heart disease, and higher magnesium intakes have been linked to a lower risk of stroke.

Magnesium and Blood Pressure

Studies show that magnesium may also play an important role in regulating blood pressure. When the muscles lining the major blood vessels contract, blood pressure rises. Many theorize that since magnesium helps muscles relax, it can reduce blood pressure.

In a study with 30,000 U.S. male health professionals, researchers found that those who ate more magnesium had lower blood pressure than those who had lower magnesium intakes. Similar findings were seen in a study with 40,000 female nurses. The recent DASH study

Magnesium in Food

Magnesium is found in a variety of foods (see "Food Sources of Magnesium"), including dark leafy greens, nuts, whole grain cereals, cocoa, and legumes. The magnesium content of refined foods is usually low. For example, whole wheat bread provides twice as much magnesium as white bread because the mineral is removed when white flour is processed. Hard water and mineral water can also be good sources of this important mineral.

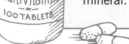

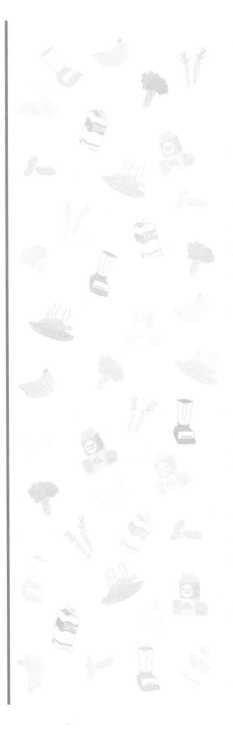

(Dietary Approaches to Stop Hypertension) suggested that a diet high in calcium, magnesium, and potassium, and lower in sodium and fat, could lower high blood pressure significantly.

The evidence to date is strong enough that the Joint National Committee on Prevention, Detection, Evaluation and Treatment of High Blood Pressure recommends maintaining an adequate magnesium intake to prevent and manage high blood pressure.

Magnesium and Osteoporosis

Magnesium is important in vitamin D and calcium metabolism, and can affect the hormone that regulates calcium in the body. As a result, magnesium may play a key role in preventing post-menopausal osteoporosis. A number of studies have suggested that supplementing with magnesium may improve bone density, but more research is needed. Interestingly, while calcium gives bones strength, magnesium makes them flexible, helping the skeleton to withstand trauma.

Magnesium and Diabetes

Diabetes mellitus is thought to be the most common disorder associated with magnesium deficiency. Without magnesium, the pancreas won't secrete enough insulin to control glucose (blood sugar) levels. And without insulin, magnesium cannot be transported from the blood into cells where it does most of its work.

Two large population studies have found that people with low magnesium intakes have a greater risk of developing Type 2, or adult-onset, diabetes. In a study of 65,000 female nurses, those who consumed roughly 220 milligrams of magnesium per day were 33 percent more likely to develop diabetes over the next six years than those who consumed about 340 milligrams per day. Similar findings were also seen in a study of 43,000 male health professionals.

What about magnesium's effect on someone who already has diabetes? Elevated blood glucose levels increase the amount of magnesium that is excreted (lost) in the urine, which can cause low blood levels of magnesium, or hypomagnesemia. In fact, many people with poorly controlled diabetes have hypomagnesemia, but it's not clear which came first, the diabetes or the deficiency. And, researchers aren't sure whether or not magnesium supplements can help diabetics, although they may help improve insulin sensitivity, which in turn would improve diabetes control, and decrease the risk of a heart attack or stroke.

Magnesium and Other Potential Benefits

There are a number of alleged benefits of magnesium supplements, but the evidence to support such claims is very preliminary. One example is the possible use of magnesium to treat migraine headaches. It seems that people who suffer from migraine headaches may also be magnesium deficient. In one study, migraine patients who took 600 milligrams of magnesium per day for 12 weeks went from three attacks per month down to two. Migraine patients who were given the placebo noticed no change in the number of headaches.

Researchers are also looking at a potential role of magnesium in the treatment of premenstrual syndrome (PMS). A deficiency in magnesium has been associated with PMS alone, or in combination with low levels of zinc, linolenic acid, the B vitamin pyridoxine, and high calcium intake. Several studies have shown an improvement in PMS symptoms with magnesium supplementation, but more research is needed.

When to Supplement with Magnesium

Most Americans do not get all of the magnesium they need. The USDA Continuing Survey of Food Intakes by Individuals 1994–96 showed an average intake of 323 milligrams of magnesium for males aged 9 and older, and 228 milligrams for females aged 9 and older (magnesium supplements are not recommended for children). The recommended intake for magnesium for adult males is 410 to 420 milligrams per day, and 310 to 320 milligrams for adult females (see "Recommended Dietary Allowances for Magnesium").

Moreover, certain groups of the population are at greater risk for magnesium deficiency. The elderly, for instance, often have low magnesium intakes, possibly due to poor appetite, loss of taste and

Caution!

- Individuals with kidney disease should consult with their physician before supplementing with magnesium.
- Before adding magnesium supplements (other than a multivitamin), check with your doctor to see if it's necessary. A simple blood test will let you know if your magnesium stores are depleted.
- If you have a medical condition or are pregnant or lactating, talk to your doctor before taking any supplement.

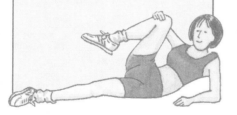

smell, poorly fitting dentures, and difficulty in shopping and preparing meals. Add to this the fact that magnesium absorption decreases with age (most adults only absorb about 50 percent of the magnesium in the diet) and urinary losses increase.

Cancer patients receiving chemotherapy, cisplatin, or individuals on diuretics or various antibiotics such as gentamicin, amphotericin, and cyclosporin may excrete more magnesium in the urine. Others at risk for magnesium deficiency are those who suffer from medical conditions such as chronic malabsorption and diarrhea, poorly controlled diabetes, and alcoholism.

People with chronically low blood levels of potassium and calcium may actually have a magnesium deficiency. Adding magnesium supplements to their diets may make calcium and potassium supplementation more effective. In fact, doctors routinely evaluate magnesium status when calcium and potassium blood levels are abnormal. Also, phosphate binds with magnesium, so people on high phosphate diets often have decreased magnesium absorption.

Symptoms of magnesium deficiency include confusion, loss of appetite, muscle cramps, tingling, numbness, high blood pressure, arrhythmias (or abnormal heart rhythms), coronary spasms, and seizures. When blood levels are mildly low, increasing dietary intake of magnesium can help restore the levels to normal. On the other hand, if magnesium blood levels are very low, an intravenous drip may be needed to return levels to normal. Magnesium tablets may be prescribed, but some forms, especially magnesium salts, can cause diarrhea.

Keep in mind that too much magnesium can be too much of a good thing. While dietary magnesium has never been a problem (it's difficult to consume too much through food), adding too much in supplement form can be. High doses of magnesium supplements, which may be added to laxatives, can promote diarrhea. And very large doses of laxatives have been associated with magnesium toxicity (hypermagnesemia). The elderly are at risk for magnesium toxicity, for example, because they are more likely to take magnesium-containing laxatives and antacids. And kidney function declines with age, thereby reducing the kidney's ability to remove excess magnesium from the body. Magnesium toxicity can produce signs similar

Calcium and Magnesium

Although calcium and magnesium often work together, they can also compete against one another. Calcium, for instance, helps muscles contract, while magnesium helps them to relax. Too much magnesium can inhibit bone hardening, or calcification, while too much calcium can lessen the amount of magnesium absorbed by the body. For this reason, it is essential to maintain a balance between these two minerals. Experts recommend a two-to-one ratio of calcium to magnesium. If you regularly supplement with extra calcium, be sure to increase your magnesium intake, too.

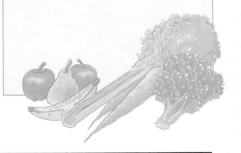

to magnesium deficiency, including mental status changes, nausea, diarrhea, muscle weakness, difficulty breathing, very low blood pressure, and irregular heartbeat.

FOOD SOURCES OF MAGNESIUM

FOOD SOURCES	SERVING SIZE	MAGNESIUM (MG)*
Wheat bran, crude	1 ounce	177
Wheat germ, toasted	1 ounce	91
Almonds	1 ounce	77
Spinach, cooked	½ cup	78
Seeds, pumpkin	½ ounce	75
Cashews, dry roasted	1 ounce	73
Cereal, shredded wheat	2 rectangular biscuits	54
Chocolate bar	1.45 ounces	45
Vegetarian baked beans	½ cup	40
Potato, baked with skin	1 medium	39
Avocado	½ medium	39
Banana, raw	1 medium	34
Shrimp, raw	3 ounces (12 large)	29
Tahini	2 tablespoons	28
Bread, whole wheat	1 slice	24
Broccoli, chopped, boiled	½ cup	19

Source: USDA Nutrient Database for Standard Reference, Release 13, 1999.
*mg = milligrams.

TOLERABLE UPPER INTAKE LEVEL (UL)[a] FOR MAGNESIUM

AGE	MAGNESIUM (MG)[b],*
9+ years	350
Pregnancy	350
Lactation	350

Reprinted with permission of The National Academy of Sciences, 1997. Courtesy of the National Academy Press, Washington D.C.
*mg = milligrams.
[a] = The maximum level of daily nutrient intake that is likely to pose no risk of adverse effects. Unless otherwise specified, the UL represents total intake from food, water, and supplements.
[b] = The ULs for magnesium do not include intake from food and water.

RECOMMENDED DIETARY ALLOWANCES (RDA) FOR MAGNESIUM (IN MG)

AGE	MAGNESIUM (MG)*
Males	
9–13 years	240
14–18 years	410
19–30 years	400
31+ years	420
Females	
9–13 years	240
14–18 years	360
19–30 years	310
31+ years	320
Pregnant women	
≤18 years	400
19–30 years	350
31–50 years	360
Lactating women	
≤18 years	360
19–30 years	310
31–50 years	320

Reprinted with permission of The National Academy of Sciences, 1997. Courtesy of the National Academy Press, Washington D.C.
*mg = milligrams.

Manganese

Manganese (pronounced MAN-ga-neez) is an element that has been recognized since the Roman Empire. Its name is derived from the Greek word for "magic," which is suitable given its wide range of metabolic functions. Manganese was proven to be an essential mineral in 1931, when it was discovered that low intake resulted in poor growth and impaired reproduction in animals. Like copper, molybdenum, and various other minerals, manganese is a required component for several enzymes. Some of these enzymes help break down fats and carbohydrates, strengthen bone, and form cartilage. Manganese also helps to activate numerous other enzymes.

Manganese in Food

Manganese is present in a wide variety of foods (see "Foods That Contain Manganese"). In general, sugary and refined foods as well as proteins (such as meat, dairy products, poultry, and fish) contain little manganese; vegetables contain a moderate amount; and nuts, cereals, and dried fruit are considered some of the best food sources of this mineral.

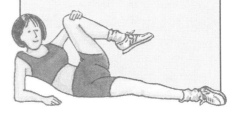

What to Know about Taking Manganese Supplements

- Manganese supplements are available in tablet form, and typically contain 2.5 to 5 milligrams of the mineral as a chloride, chelate, or carbonate complex. Manganese is also frequently found in multivitamins in varying amounts.
- A number of dietary components can decrease manganese absorption and retention, including iron, calcium, phosphorus, phytates, and fiber.
- Excessive amounts of manganese can interfere with the body's ability to absorb iron.
- Since dietary supplements (or claims for them) are not reviewed by the Food and Drug Administration, quality control and potency problems may exist with manganese supplements.

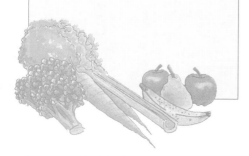

The Benefits of Manganese

Manganese and Bone Health

The effects of manganese deficiency on bone development show that inadequate intake of this mineral results in shortened and thickened limbs, curvature of the spine, and swollen and enlarged joints. In animals, too little manganese reduces bone cell activity. This is particularly relevant since researchers have found that women with osteoporosis tend to have low blood levels of manganese. Some researchers have examined whether manganese supplements—either alone or in combination with other trace minerals—help prevent bone loss in animals. In one study, a manganese supplement was found to be effective at inhibiting loss of bone mass in rats. Manganese deficiency has also been suggested as a potential factor in the development of joint disease and hip abnormalities—a promising area of continuing research.

Manganese and Heart Disease

Although research in this area is in its infancy, it's been found that animals deficient in manganese produce a substance called glycosaminoglycan—an important component of the connective tissue found in arteries. Researchers believe that this may encourage LDL ("bad" cholesterol) to stick to artery walls, thereby increasing risk of coronary artery disease.

When to Supplement with Manganese

Altough there are no Recommended Dietary Allowances for manganese, the Adequate Intake for adults 19 and over is 2.3 and 1.8 milligrams per day for males and females, respectively. Usual dietary intakes in the United States are about 2.2 and 2.7 for adult women and men, respectively. It is not recommended that children take manganese supplements. Results from the Food and Drug Administration's Total Diet Study (1982–1986) showed that adolescent and adult females had manganese intakes that were slightly lower than the Adequate Intake levels (2 to 5 milligrams per day). However, much higher intakes (up to 18 milligrams) can be found in vegetarian diets and those based on whole-grain products.

Deficiencies in manganese are not common, since it is so widely available in foods. Manganese toxicity, though very serious, is also quite rare and is usually seen in people exposed to high levels of manganese in industrial environments, such as mines, or in people who drink water containing high levels of the mineral. However, isolated cases of manganese toxicity from dietary exposure (from supplements, not typical diets) have been reported in the scientific literature.

In its most severe forms, manganese toxicity can result in a collection of psychiatric symptoms, including hallucinations, violence, hyperirritability, and schizophrenia. Toxicity can also cause nervous disorders resembling signs of **Parkinson's disease**. Subtle signs of manganese toxicity include delayed reaction time, impaired coordination, and memory problems. In general, the lack of toxicity seen in the population as a whole—as well as the fact that reliable methods of assessing body manganese status are still being developed—indicates that perhaps the low end of the AI range for adults is too conservative.

For those tempted to use manganese supplements to head off osteoporosis, be aware that although the research is promising, a lack of this mineral is not seen as a major underlying factor in the disease because manganese deficiency in humans is not common.

With an increasing proportion of the population adopting a vegetarian eating style, there is a concern that among vegetarians, body levels of manganese could cause problems over time. Why? First, vegetarians have a higher manganese intake due to their dietary choices, and second, iron deficiency (not uncommon among vegetarians) tends to increase manganese absorption. Currently there is no evidence that vegetarians as a whole are at an increased risk for manganese toxicity, but U.S. Department of Agriculture researchers believe that more human toxicity studies with longer time frames and more sensitive analysis methods are needed. Until more research is done, vegetarians might do well to choose a multivitamin with a low level of manganese, or not take manganese supplements at all.

Manganese in Food

Some foods that contain manganese are: pecans, peanuts, pineapple/juice, oatmeal, wheat bran cereals, legumes, rice, spinach, sweet potatoes, and whole wheat bread.

ADEQUATE INTAKE (AI)[a] FOR MANGANESE

AGE	MANGANESE (MG)[b],*
Infants	
0–½ year	0.003
½–1 year	0.6
Children	
1–3 years	1.2
4–8 years	1.5
Males	
9–13 years	1.9
14–18 years	2.2
19+ years	2.3
Females	
9–18 years	1.6
19+ years	1.8
Pregnancy	
14+ years	2
Lactation	
14+ years	2.6

Source: The National Academy of Sciences, 2001.

a = The maximum level of daily nutrient intake that is likely to pose no adverse effects.

b = Since the toxic levels for many trace elements may be only several times higher than usual intakes, the upper levels for the trace elements given in this table should not be habitually exceeded.

*mg = milligrams.

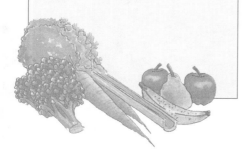

TOLERABLE UPPER INTAKE LEVEL (UL)[a] FOR MANGANESE

AGE	MANGANESE (MG)*
0–1 year	Not possible to establish
1–3 years	2
4–8 years	3
9–13 years	6
14–18 years	9
19+ years	11
Pregnancy	
14–18 years	9
19+ years	11
Lactation	
14–18 years	9
19+ years	11

Source: National Academy of Sciences, 2001.
a = The maximum level of daily nutrient intake that is likely to pose no risk of adverse effects.
*mg = milligrams.

Molybdenum

Molybdenum (pronounced mo-LIB-duh-num) is an essential trace mineral that functions as an enzyme cofactor. In other words, a number of enzymes (proteins that help speed up chemical reactions in the body) depend on the presence of molybdenum in order to become activated.

The Benefits of Molybdenum

Since humans get all the molybdenum necessary through the diet, there is a lack of information regarding benefits associated with supplements. However, molybdenum is important because it helps to activate enzymes. Some of the enzymatic reactions in which molybdenum plays a role include the breakdown of certain amino acids and the utilization of iron.

What to Know about Taking Molybdenum Supplements

- Molybdenum is available combined with other trace minerals in tablet or capsule forms, usually in a 300 microgram dosage, which poses no health problem.
- Since dietary supplements (or claims for them) are not reviewed by the Food and Drug Administration, quality control and potency problems may exist with molybdenum supplements.

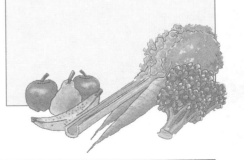

Molybdenum in Food

Molybdenum is found in milk and milk products, dried legumes, organ meats (liver and kidney), cereal products, baked goods, and leafy green vegetables. Poor sources include fruits, oils, sugar, fats, and fish. The molybdenum content of the soil greatly affects the amount of the mineral found in food. Molybdenum is also found in water, and most public water supplies are estimated to contribute between 2 and 8 micrograms of the mineral per day.

When to Supplement with Molybdenum

The Recommended Dietary Allowance (RDA) for molybdenum is 45 micrograms for people aged 19 years and older (it is not recommended for children). One study shows that average dietary intake of molybdenum in the United States is 180 micrograms per day, while the Food and Drug Administration's 1984 Total Diet Study estimates intake at 76 to 109 micrograms per day for adult females and males, respectively. The National Academy of Sciences does not recommend molybdenum supplements, since most diets should meet the requirements.

Molybdenum deficiency is extremely rare, in part because the human requirement is very small and because molybdenum absorption is very efficient. Symptoms of deficiency include irritability, amino acid intolerance, and eventually, coma. Some people have a rare genetic metabolic defect that results in their inability to make three molybdenum-containing enzymes. There is no treatment for this rare disease, which results in seizures and other neurological symptoms in infants and children, and death in early childhood.

Molybdenum is relatively nontoxic because the body is good at regulating its content of the mineral through excretion in the urine. In fact, large oral doses (generally only achieved through excessive supplementation) are necessary to overcome these control mechanisms. Nevertheless, molybdenum toxicity is much more likely than deficiency. In general, 10 to 15 milligrams of molybdenum per day is considered excessive and may result in goutlike symptoms (acute arthritic joint pain), anemia, and growth problems. Excess molybdenum can also interfere with the body's absorption of copper.

Caution!

- Molybdenum supplements aren't necessary, carry no known benefits, and can be dangerous, so supplements are not recommended. However, taking a multivitamin that contains the AI level of molybdenum—or less—is considered safe.
- If you have a medical condition or are pregnant or lactating, talk to your doctor before taking any supplement.

One study found that a molybdenum intake of just 0.54 milligrams per day was associated with loss of copper in the urine.

Recently, the first known case of molybdenum poisoning from an individual molybdenum supplement was reported in the scientific literature. The subject, a male in his late thirties, consumed 300 to 800 micrograms of molybdenum (up to three times the AI amount) daily for 18 days. The subject suffered a series of seizures, visual and auditory hallucinations, and brain damage. One year later he was still having problems such as learning disabilities, major depression, and post-traumatic stress disorder.

ADEQUATE INTAKE (AI)[a] FOR MOLYBDENUM

AGE	MOLYBDENUM (MCG)*
0–½ year	2
½–1 year	3

[a] = The AI levels for infants reflect the average molybdenum intake of infants principally fed human milk, with an added increment for foods from ½–1 year old infants.
*mcg = micrograms.

RECOMMENDED DIETARY ALLOWANCES (RDA) FOR MOLYBDENUM

AGE	MOLYBDENUM (MCG)*
1–3 years	17
4–8 years	22
9–13 years	34
14–18 years	43
19+ years	45
Pregnancy	
14+ years	50
Lactation	
14+ years	50

Source: The National Academy of Sciences, 2001.
*mcg = micrograms.

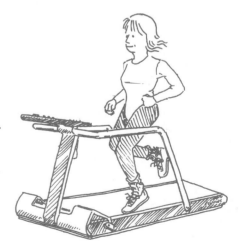

Phosphorus

Phosphorus (pronounced FOS-for-us) is one of the most essential minerals, ranking second only to calcium in abundance in human tissues. Eighty-five percent of phosphorus is located in bones and teeth, combined with calcium, and 15 percent is in muscle and other soft tissues. It is commonly found in the form of phosphate and has a number of important functions in the body.

The Benefits of Phosphorus

Phosphorus is necessary for healthy bones and teeth, and is an essential part of the nucleic acids, DNA and RNA. Phosphorus is also a part of phospholipids (fatty-like substances), which are key components in the structure of cell membranes. This important mineral helps to convert protein, carbohydrate, and fat into energy. And, it acts as a cofactor (an essential component of an enzyme) for a variety of enzymes, and helps to maintain normal pH in the body.

When to Supplement with Phosphorus

Most Americans get more than enough phosphorus in their diets. The USDA Continuing Survey of Food Intakes by Individuals 1994–96 showed an average intake of 1,495 milligrams of phosphorus for males aged nine and older, and 1,024 milligrams for females aged nine and older (it is not recomended for children). The recommended daily intake for phosphorus for adults is 700 milligrams (see "Recommended Dietary Allowances for Phosphorus").

In the past 20 years, both the use of phosphate salts as additives and the amount per serving have increased substantially. These salts are used in processed foods for moisture retention, smoothness, and binding. As a result, people who eat a lot of processed foods may have higher phosphorus intakes than the averages listed here. In fact, many of us are consuming as much as 10–15 percent more phosphorus now than we were 20 years ago.

In addition, colas and other soft drinks provide a lot of this mineral. A 12-ounce beverage contains about 50 milligrams of phos-

What to Know about Taking Phosphorus Supplements

- Phosphorus supplements come in capsule, tablet, liquid, and powder forms.
- The National Academy of Sciences recommends no more than 4,000 milligrams of supplemental phosphorus up to age 70, and then 3,000 milligrams for those older than 70 years of age. No cases of phosphorus toxicity have ever been reported from food sources.
- For years, experts believed that increased phosphorus in the diet would lead to decreased calcium levels in bone, but studies have shown little or no evidence to support this. A bigger issue is the fact that many people have replaced milk with soda, thereby decreasing their calcium intake.
- Since dietary supplements are not reviewed by the FDA, quality control and potency problems may exist.

phorus, which is only 5 percent of the typical intake of an adult female. However, if five or more sodas are consumed in a day, these beverages can contribute a large portion to our phosphorus intake.

Although inadequate phosphorus, or hypophosphatemia, is very rare, it can occur with various diseases or conditions, such as gastrointestinal malabsorption, diabetes mellitus, kidney disease, antacid abuse, and premature birth. Symptoms include anorexia, anemia, muscle weakness, bone pain, rickets (abnormally shaped bones in children) and osteomalacia (adult form of rickets), increased susceptibility to infection, ataxia (poor muscular coordination), confusion, and even death.

Too much phosphorus, or hyperphosphatemia, is also rare; in fact, it generally occurs as a result of nondietary reasons. For instance, it is often seen in people with kidney failure since their bodies are unable to excrete enough excess phosphorus in the urine.

FOOD SOURCES OF PHOSPHORUS

FOOD SOURCES	SERVING SIZE	PHOSPHORUS (MG)*
Grilled cheese sandwich	1	531
Macaroni and cheese	1 cup	250
Split pea soup	1 cup	250
Sole, baked	3 ounces	246
Tofu, firm	½ cup	239
Milk, 2% fat	1 cup	232
Ham	3 ounces	224
Milkshake, vanilla	10 ounces	212
Oatmeal	1 cup	178
Tostada with beans and beef	1	173
Cheese, Swiss, processed	1 ounce	171
Cashews, dry roasted	1 ounce	137
Pistachios	1 ounce	136
Shrimp, boiled	3 ounces (12 large)	116
Egg	1	89
Bread, whole wheat	1 slice	64
Lettuce, romaine	1 cup	25

Source: USDA Nutrient Database for Standard Reference, Release 13, 1999.
*mg = milligrams.

Phosphorus in Food

Phosphorus is found widely distributed in the food supply (see "Food Sources of Phosphorus"). The average contributions of food groups to phosphorus intake are 60 percent from milk, meat, poultry, fish, and eggs; 20 percent from cereals and legumes; 10 percent from fruits and fruit juices; 4 percent from alcoholic beverages; and 3 percent from soft drinks and other beverages.

If you regularly consume antacids and soft drinks with aluminum hydroxide, you may want to reconsider. Too much aluminum hydroxide may interfere with phosphorus absorption.

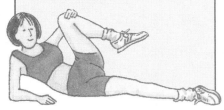

RECOMMENDED DIETARY ALLOWANCES (RDA)* FOR PHOSPHORUS

AGE	PHOSPHORUS (MG)**
Males	
9–18 years	1,250
19+ years	700
Females	
9–18 years	1,250
19+ years	700
Pregnant women	
≤18 years	1,250
19+ years	700
Lactating women	
≤18 years	1,250
19+ years	700

Reprinted with permission of The National Academy of Sciences, 1997. Courtesy of the National Academy Press, Washington D.C.
*There is no RDA for infants due to insufficient information.
**mg = milligrams.

TOLERABLE UPPER INTAKE LEVEL (UL)[a] FOR PHOSPHORUS

AGE	PHOSPHORUS (MG)*
9–70 years	4,000
>70 years	3,000
Pregnancy	3,500
Lactation	4,000

Reprinted with permission of The National Academy of Sciences, 1997. Courtesy of the National Academy Press, Washington D.C.
*mg = milligrams.
[a] = The maximum level of daily nutrient intake that is likely to pose no risk of adverse effects. Unless otherwise specified, the UL represents total intake from food, water, and supplements.

Potassium

Like sodium and chloride, potassium is an electrolyte—an electrically charged mineral that dissolves in water—and is critical for proper fluid regulation in the body. As electrolytes, potassium and sodium carry positive charges, while chloride has a negative charge, thus enabling them to easily move back and forth across the body's cell membranes. This is essential because as they move in and out of

Caution!

- Individuals with kidney disease should consult their physician before supplementing with phosphorus.
- Since the typical American diet provides more than enough phosphorus, supplementing is not necessary for most people. Before adding phosphorus supplements to your diet (other than a multivitamin), check with your doctor to see if it's necessary.
- If you have a medical condition or are pregnant or lactating, talk to your doctor before taking any supplement.

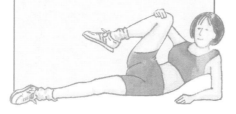

cells, they carry things with them, such as nutrients, water, and waste products. The functions of electrolytes in the body include maintaining the body's water balance, carrying nerve impulses, and helping muscles contract and relax. Electrolytes also keep the body from becoming too acidic or alkaline.

Potassium is the most essential cation (or positively charged mineral) in cells. It is found primarily in muscle tissue and is related to muscle mass. Therefore, when building muscle, sufficient potassium is essential. This important mineral is also critical to maintaining a heartbeat. In fact, sudden deaths that occur from severe diarrhea or in children with malnutrition are often due to heart failure caused by potassium loss.

The Benefits of Potassium

Potassium and Blood Pressure

The recent multicenter study called Dietary Approaches to Stop Hypertension (DASH) involved more than 450 adults with mild hypertension (high blood pressure). The participants were divided into groups, and each group followed a specific dietary plan for eight weeks. The most effective diet was one that was low in fat and cholesterol and rich in foods containing potassium, magnesium, and calcium—such as fruits, vegetables, legumes, and dairy foods. The diet reduced systolic blood pressure (the top number) by an average of six points, and the diastolic blood pressure (bottom number) by three points. The results were even more significant for those with higher blood pressure.

Potassium and Stroke

Studies have also shown that potassium may reduce the risk of stroke. Researchers at Harvard looked at the relationship between potassium (and other nutrients) and the risk of stroke in 43,738 men, 40–75 years old, without diagnosed diabetes or cardiovascular disease. The results of the study showed that diets rich in potassium, magnesium, and cereal fiber can reduce the risk of stroke, especially in men with high blood pressure. In a similar study in middle-aged women, researchers concluded that diets low in calcium and potassium may contribute to an increased risk of stroke.

What to Know about Taking Potassium Supplements

- Potassium supplements come in capsule, tablet, or liquid forms as potassium gluconate, aspartate, citrate or hydrochloride.
- Because of the dangers of too much potassium, the FDA allows no more than 99 milligrams of potassium per supplement dose. Higher dosages are available only by prescription.
- Some people who take potassium supplements experience gastric irritation and other side effects.
- Diuretics can deplete the body of potassium. If you're taking any kind of diuretic, talk to your doctor about your potassium needs.
- Since dietary supplements are not reviewed by the FDA, quality control and potency problems may exist.

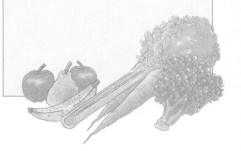

Although it's true that exercise can cause losses of potassium and sodium (up to 180 milligrams of potassium and 1,000 milligrams of sodium during a two-hour workout), the truth is that unless you exercise for an extended period of time—such as when running a marathon—you are unlikely to deplete your body's stores of these minerals. The main function of sports drinks is to replace fluid, not electrolytes. In fact, the purpose of adding electrolytes to sports drinks at all is to enhance the body's absorption of the water they contain. Although they won't hurt you, the electrolytes contained in sports drinks certainly won't come close to "replacing" those lost during exercise. For most of us, staying hydrated (getting enough fluid) is more important than worrying about electrolytes—try to drink about 1 cup of water or other fluid every 20 minutes of exercise.

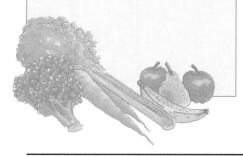

Potassium in Food

Potassium is found in most foods. The best sources are vegetables; fruits and fruit juices, such as figs, orange juice, and bananas; and potatoes.

FOOD SOURCES OF POTASSIUM

FOOD SOURCES	SERVING SIZE	POTASSIUM (MG)*
Figs	10	1,353
Lentils	1 cup	731
Kidney beans	1 cup	713
Black beans	1 cup	611
Potato, baked with skin	1 medium	610
Avocado	½ medium	601
Orange juice	8 ounces	496
Cantaloupe	1 cup	494
Banana	1 medium	467
Spinach, cooked	½ cup	419
Tomato juice	6 ounces	400
Sweet potato	1 medium	397
Milk, 2% fat	8 ounces	377
Pistachios	1 ounce	289
Orange	1 medium	237
Hazelnuts	1 ounce	190
Beef, ground	3 ounces	190

Source: USDA Nutrient Database for Standard Reference, Release 13, 1999.
*mg = milligrams.

When to Supplement with Potassium

Most Americans get more than enough potassium in their diets. The average intake for adults is about 4,000 milligrams per day, while the recommended level is 2,000 milligrams (see "Estimated Potassium Minimum Requirements of Healthy Persons"). Potassium supplements are not recommended for children.

Potassium deficiency from low dietary intake is rare—except for starvation. **Hypokalemia** (low blood levels of potassium) is the result of excessive losses of potassium in the urine, usually due to the use of diuretics, or "water pills," to treat hypertension (high blood pressure). Too little potassium can result in cardiac failure.

Too much potassium is also a problem. Although the body usually maintains a balance by excreting excess potassium in the urine, individuals who use liberal amounts of potassium-containing salt substitutes may be getting more potassium than they need—especially those with impaired cardiovascular or kidney function who also take diuretics. Too much of this nutrient in the body can cause cardiac arrest.

ESTIMATED POTASSIUM MINIMUM REQUIREMENTS OF HEALTHY PERSONS

AGE	WEIGHT (KG)[a],*	POTASSIUM (MG)[b],**
0–½	4.5	500
½–1	8.9	700
1	11.0	1,000
2–5	16.0	1,400
6–9	25.0	1,600
10–18	50.0	2,000
>18	70.0[c]	2,000[c]

Reprinted with permission of The National Academy of Sciences, 1989. Courtesy of the National Academy Press, Washington D.C.
*kg = kilograms (1 kilogram = 2.2 pounds).
**mg = milligrams.
[a] = No allowance has been included for large, prolonged losses from the skin through sweat.
[b] = Desirable intakes of potassium may considerably exceed these values (3,500 milligrams for adults).
[c] = No allowance included for growth. Values for those below 18 years assume a growth rate at the 50th percentile reported by the National Center for Health Statistics and averaged for males and females.

Selenium

Selenium (pronounced se-LEN-ee-um) is a trace mineral and part of an antioxidant enzyme called glutathione peroxidase. As an antioxidant, selenium works closely with vitamin E, protecting body tissues against oxidative damage from free radicals. It is present in every cell in the body, especially in the kidneys, liver, spleen, pancreas, and testes. Selenium is also necessary for thyroid health, as well as normal development, growth, and metabolism.

Ironically, the potential benefits of selenium have traditionally been ignored, primarily because deficiencies are rare and toxicity is a risk. In fact, it wasn't until the 1950s that selenium was even considered an essential nutrient. However, in recent years this important mineral has moved into the spotlight as a potential disease fighter.

Caution!

- Individuals with heart or kidney disease should consult with their physicians before supplementing with potassium.
- Since the typical American diet provides more than enough potassium, and too much (more than 18,000 milligrams) can be deadly, supplementing is not recommended for most people. Before adding potassium supplements (other than a multivitamin), check with your doctor.
- If you have a medical condition or are pregnant or lactating, talk to your doctor before taking any supplement.

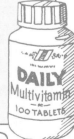

Selenium in Food

Selenium is found in animal tissues and in grains and seeds, although the amount can vary in plant foods depending on the selenium content of the soil. Generally, beef, pork, bread, chicken, and eggs account for nearly half of the selenium content in the American diet. The most concentrated source of selenium is in Brazil nuts—just one nut provides more than the RDA for men and women (see "Food Sources of Selenium").

On average, American adults consume about 80 to 100 micrograms of selenium per day. The recommended intake is 70 micrograms per day for men, and 55 micrograms of selenium for women.

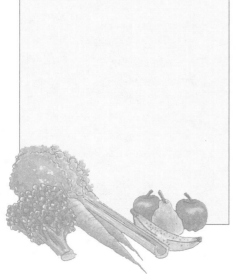

The Benefits of Selenium

Selenium and Cancer

The first signs of selenium as a potential cancer fighter came from animal studies conducted about 30 years ago. Human studies began more than a decade ago, when researchers set out to test selenium's effect on skin cancer in 1,312 people in a 10-year clinical trial. Study participants were given 200 micrograms of selenium (as high-selenium yeast) or a placebo per day. Although supplementation with selenium had no effect on skin cancer, the researchers were amazed to find that the people taking selenium supplements had much lower rates of colon, prostate, and lung cancers than those taking the placebo. Moreover, the selenium supplement group also had a decrease in total cancer incidence and total cancer death. The findings were so dramatic that the study was halted early for ethical reasons.

Although the data is very promising, there are some limitations with the study. For instance, it was done in the Southeast, where many people don't get much selenium from their food because it's grown in selenium-poor soil. Researchers question whether the effect would be as dramatic in parts of the country where people get more selenium from their food. In the meantime, research is underway to explore the findings further.

A more recent study from the Health Professionals Follow-up Study at Harvard University supports selenium's role in cutting the risk of prostate cancer. Researchers found that among 33,737 men, those with the lowest selenium levels in toenail clippings (see "Testing for Selenium") had twice the risk of prostate cancer compared to men with the highest levels.

Although selenium's antioxidant properties may play a beneficial role in fighting cancer, there may be other anticancer processes involved. Researchers believe that one way our bodies are able to fight off cancer is through apoptosis—cell suicide. The body literally encourages cancer cells to self-destruct. If apoptosis is suppressed through genetics or environmental factors, including diet, cancer can develop. On the other hand, certain substances, such as selenium, may promote apoptosis of cancer cells, thereby reducing the risk of cancer.

Selenium and Heart Disease

Low blood levels of selenium have also been associated with heart attacks and an increased number of deaths from cardiovascular disease. In addition, selenium deficiency can result in a buildup of fatty acid deposits in the heart, leading to an increased risk of blood clot formation, which can cause a heart attack.

Selenium and Kidney Disease

Low selenium levels in the blood have been seen in patients with chronic renal failure and those undergoing hemodialysis. Although a selenium deficiency per se is not believed to be the cause of renal disease, it may exacerbate other conditions in people with kidney disease. Studies show that selenium supplementation can be effective in improving the selenium status and immune function of these individuals.

Selenium and Other Potential Benefits

Selenium may help infertile couples. Preliminary research indicates that infertile men supplemented with selenium and vitamin E show improvements in sperm motility, vitality, and morphology.

This important antioxidant may also have a positive effect on people with HIV. Some studies have shown that HIV patients have lower selenium levels and suggest that selenium supplementation may be beneficial in the treatment of HIV. Studies are currently underway to test this theory. Finally, as part of a potent antioxidant "system," selenium may help reduce the risk of cataracts.

When to Supplement with Selenium

Selenium deficiency is rare in humans (supplementing with selenium is not recommended for children), although there are two diseases that occur in areas where the soil is low in selenium. Keshan disease is a cardiomyopathy (a disease of the heart muscle) that mainly affects children and was first seen in the Keshan province of China in 1979. It can be prevented with selenium supplementation. Keshan–Beck disease occurs in preadolescent and adolescent

Testing for Selenium

Because food can vary in its selenium content, depending on the soil it was grown in, the most accurate way to determine selenium intake is by testing selenium concentrations in blood and toenails. Selenium in toenails reflects intake from the previous 6 to 12 months. If selenium intake is low, a limited amount of the mineral is deposited into the nails because most of it will be used by the body. At higher intakes, the body's demands are met and the excess selenium accumulates in the nails. Interestingly, testing hair is not recommended because of possible selenium contamination by widely used selenium-containing anti-dandruff shampoos.

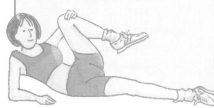

What to Know about Taking Selenium Supplements

- The form of selenium is important. Much of the research has used high-selenium yeast. However, most supplements on the market, including vitamin/mineral supplements, use inorganic forms of selenium (sodium selenite or selenate), which may not be utilized as well in the body. Additionally, some high-selenium yeast supplements on the market are often made by spraying yeast with inorganic sodium selenite, and may therefore not be much of an improvement over inorganic forms.
- Selenium is sold in capsule and tablet form.
- If you are considering taking a selenium supplement, make sure that your total intake does not exceed 800 micrograms per day.
- Since dietary supplements are not reviewed by the FDA, quality control and potency problems may exist.

children and involves stiffness, swelling, and joint pain, followed by osteoarthritis.

Selenium toxicity is actually more of a concern than deficiency. Because the toxicity threshold for selenium is rather low, it's important not to oversupplement. In the 13th century, Marco Polo first observed the effects of selenium toxicity in the mountainous region of western China. The soil was very rich in selenium, and when his horses ate the selenium-rich vegetation some became so ill that their hooves literally fell off. This was also observed in animals the late 19th and early 20th centuries in Nebraska, the Dakotas, and other Western territories.

Classic toxicity symptoms in humans occur at levels of about 900 to 1,000 micrograms and include skin changes (red, blistered, and swollen) and hair and nail damage (brittle, discolored, and eventual loss), anorexia, abdominal pain, and diarrhea. The most severe changes occur in the nervous system and can result in convulsions, paralysis, and motor disturbance—even death.

FOOD SOURCES OF SELENIUM

FOOD SOURCES	SERVING SIZE	SELENIUM (MCG)*
Brazil nuts (unshelled)	½ ounce (4 nuts)	436
Tuna, light, canned in water	3½ ounces	80
Beef, liver, cooked	3½ ounces	55
Pork, leg (ham) cooked	3½ ounces	45
Egg noodles, cooked	1 cup	35
Pink salmon, canned	3½ ounces	33
Spaghetti/macaroni, cooked	1 cup	30
Chicken, roasted	3½ ounces	24
Oatmeal, cooked	1 cup	19
Egg	1 large	15
Puffed wheat cereal	1 cup	15
Rice, white, long grain, cooked	1 cup	12
Beans, Great Northern, canned	1 cup	11
Bread, whole wheat	1 slice	10
Yogurt, plain, low fat	1 cup	8

Source: USDA Nutrient Database for Standard Reference, Release 13, 1999.
*mcg = micrograms.

RECOMMENDED DIETARY ALLOWANCES (RDA)* FOR SELENIUM

AGE	SELENIUM (MCG)**
Males	
9–13 years	40
14+ years	55
Females	
9–13 years	40
14+ years	55
Pregnant women	60
Lactating women	70

Reprinted with permission of The National Academy of Sciences, 2000. Courtesy of the National Academy Press, Wassington D.C.

*There is no RDA for infants due to insufficient information.

**mcg = micrograms.

TOLERABLE UPPER INTAKE LEVEL (UL)[a] FOR SELENIUM

AGE	SELENIUM (MCG)*
0–½ year	45
½–1 year	60
1–3 years	90
4–8 years	150
9–13 years	280
14+ years	400
Pregnancy	400
Lactation	400

Reprinted with permission of The National Academy of Sciences, 2000. Courtesy of the National Academy Press, Washington D.C.

*mcg = micrograms.

[a] = The maximum level of daily nutrient intake that is likely to pose no risk of adverse effects. Unless otherwise specified, the UL represents total intake from food, water, and supplements.

Caution!

- Many experts believe that more research is needed before suggesting that people supplement with selenium. However, most agree that a multivitamin or selenium supplement that provides no more than 200 micrograms of the mineral is safe.
- If you have a medical condition or are pregnant or lactating, talk to your doctor before taking any supplement.

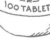

Sodium

Sodium is an essential mineral that's generally consumed as sodium chloride, or table salt. Sodium and chloride are so strongly linked in the diet that it's rare that levels of one or the other would vary independently.

In the past couple of decades, sodium has received plenty of attention for its role in blood pressure regulation and hypertension. Although sodium supplements, or "salt pills," are not necessary for anyone, this chapter will discuss the functions of sodium in the body in order to provide background on hypertension (high blood pressure)—a condition for which other mineral supplements may be justified.

The Benefits of Sodium

Sodium is an electrolyte—an electrically charged mineral that dissolves in water. These charges (either positive or negative) allow electrolytes to easily move back and forth across the body's cell membranes. This is essential because as they move in and out of cells, they carry things with them, such as nutrients, water, and waste products.

The functions of electrolytes in the body include maintaining the body's water balance, carrying nerve impulses, and helping muscles contract and relax. Electrolytes also keep the body from becoming too acidic or alkaline. Although sodium's major role in the body is fluid balance (as is chloride's), it's also involved in the control of blood volume, the absorption of glucose (blood sugar), and the transport of other nutrients within the body.

Sodium and Pregnancy

Until recently, pregnant women were advised to decrease their salt intake in order to reduce edema (swelling) of the face, legs, and feet. It is now believed that pregnancy increases the need for sodium because of increased blood volume. However, this requirement is relatively small, and the vast majority of pregnant women already consume enough sodium in their diets to meet this extra need.

Caution!

- People with kidney disease must avoid sodium and potassium, and should follow their doctors' orders regarding how much to consume.
- Cutting back on sodium may help your blood pressure medications work better, allowing you to eventually decrease the dosage. However, you should never stop taking medications, or change your dosage without consulting your doctor first.
- Certainly, none of us needs to add more sodium to our diets, and some of us could benefit from less. Since the experts have not reached an agreement on the importance of sodium in hypertension, in the meantime the DASH diet appears to be the way to go.

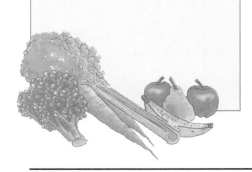

When to Supplement with Sodium

There are no Recommended Dietary Allowances for sodium, although the National Academy of Sciences estimates that the minimum requirement for sodium ranges from 120 milligrams per day for infants to 500 milligrams (a little less than a teaspoon of salt) per day for adults and children over age 10. In the United States, sodium consumption averages 3,500 milligrams per day—much more than our bodies really need—so getting too much sodium is frequently more of a problem than getting enough. The National Institutes of Health (NIH) recommends limiting sodium consumption to 2,400 milligrams per day or less, while the American Heart Association is a little more liberal, suggesting Americans get no more than 3,000 milligrams of sodium each day.

Sodium Deficiency

Sodium supplements, or "salt pills," used to be more widely available and were sometimes advised for people who spent long periods of time working or exercising outdoors in the sun in order to prevent excessive sodium loss through perspiration. Now, however, sports drinks are the popular way to replenish electrolyte losses. In reality, even sports drinks are rarely necessary because the normal diet provides more sodium (and other electrolytes) than we generally need, and sodium deficiency is practically unheard of.

It is, however, possible to lose a lot of sodium through extremely heavy, prolonged sweating; chronic or severe diarrhea; and the use of diuretics (drugs that cause the kidneys to remove more water and salt from the body). In addition, some people may have medical problems that cause the kidneys to be unable to reabsorb sodium when it's needed. In these instances sodium and potassium depletion is a possibility and can lead to a fall in blood pressure (caused by decreased blood volume) and shock.

Sodium Toxicity

Consuming a large amount of sodium at one time can cause edema and hypertension as water is pulled from cells. As long as water needs are met, the kidneys can rid the body of excess

Sodium in Food

Natural sodium is found in fresh foods from animal sources and, to a lesser extent, plant sources. The amount of sodium found in foods naturally, however, accounts for only about 10 percent of the sodium we consume. Roughly 75 percent of our sodium intake comes from food processing and preparation (including restaurant foods), while 15 percent is "discretionary" salt—added to food at the table and in home cooking. Sodium is also found in drinking water and many medications.

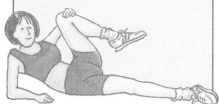

sodium, so sodium is generally considered nontoxic for healthy adults. In infants, excessive consumption can lead to death due to the limited function of immature kidneys.

The Sodium–Blood Pressure Controversy

The relationship between sodium and high blood pressure has been an area of intense research and controversy for years—and it shows no signs of letting up. The two schools of thought on the issue are basically this: (1) excessive sodium intakes are primarily responsible for high blood pressure (hypertension) and its potentially fatal consequences, including heart and kidney disease and stroke; and (2) sodium intake is just one factor to be considered in the high blood pressure equation—and it is really only significant when the intake of other minerals is inadequate.

Sodium's role in this controversy hinges on the balance of water and sodium in the body. The body constantly adjusts to maintain a relatively stable sodium–water ratio. When sodium intake is high, the thirst mechanism is triggered, so the body gets more water in order to dilute the sodium. The kidneys also play an important role. When sodium levels in the body get too high, the kidneys dump it out via urine; when the body needs sodium, the kidneys return it to the blood.

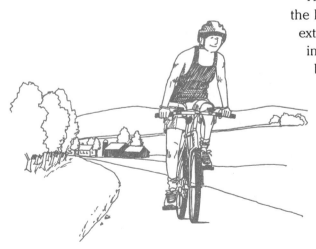

High blood pressure develops when, for some reason, the kidneys fail to rid the body of enough sodium. The extra sodium attracts water and causes blood volume to increase. At the same time, the blood vessels can become waterlogged and contract. Since more blood now has to pass through the narrower vessels, the blood pressure increases.

According to the NIH, a strong positive relationship between sodium intake and blood pressure has been long established for some people. In other words, when sodium intake increases, so does blood pressure and risk of hypertension. This is why for years, experts and health authorities around the world, including the U.S. Surgeon General, the American Heart

Association, and the World Health Organization (WHO), have recommended that people limit their sodium intake. However, there is just as strong evidence to show that universal salt restriction may not be necessary.

Experts estimate that only about 30 to 35 percent of the general population (50 percent of hypertensive people) is sodium sensitive. That is, for these people, when sodium intake increases, so does blood pressure and risk of stroke. This is especially so for certain population segments such as African-Americans, people with a family history of hypertension, and older individuals. A recent study suggests that increased sodium consumption may also affect the health of overweight people more than those who aren't overweight. In a study of approximately 2,700 overweight and 6,800 nonoverweight people, who were followed for 19 years, sodium intake had no effect on stroke, heart disease, or mortality for normal weight people. However, for overweight people a high sodium intake increased the risk of stroke and mortality from heart disease (and all other causes) by as much as 89 percent.

For the majority of Americans, though, research shows that sodium restriction has no effect on blood pressure. So how do you know if you're sodium sensitive? Currently there's no easy way to tell—that's why most health authorities are taking the "better safe than sorry" approach and standing by their universal sodium restriction advice. However, a study published in 2001 discusses research on a new testing method to predict sodium sensitivity. The test, which is conducted over three days, offers the first real method for determining who is sodium-sensitive and to what degree.

Another compelling reason the experts are divided on the issue of sodium restriction is that other nutrients may be just as important as sodium when it comes to controlling blood pressure. A multicenter study called the Dietary Approaches to Stop Hypertension (DASH) trial involved more than 450 adults with mild hypertension. The participants were divided into groups, and each group followed a specific type of dietary plan for eight weeks. Although the study wasn't designed to identify *which* nutrients effectively reduced blood pressure, the results showed that mineral consumption was very

More on Blood Pressure

There are two numbers involved with blood pressure, or the pressure exerted by the blood on any vessel wall, such as a vein or artery.

Systolic (the top number) is the pressure that occurs when the heart contracts—usually between 100 and 140.

Diastolic (the bottom number) is the pressure that occurs between heartbeats when the heart muscle relaxes—usually around 60–90.

Some lifestyle changes that can help decrease high blood pressure are:

- Lose weight
- Get regular aerobic exercise
- Reduce sodium intake
- Consume a diet that's low in fat and cholesterol and contains lots of fruits, vegetables, legumes, nuts, and low-fat dairy products
- Have your blood pressure checked every year or two

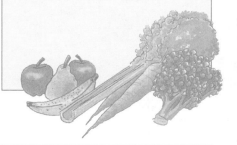

important in this regard. In fact, the most effective diet was the one that was low in fat and cholesterol, contained plenty of fruits and vegetables, and contained excellent food sources of potassium, magnesium, and calcium. This diet reduced systolic blood pressure (the top number in a blood pressure reading) by an average of six points, and diastolic blood pressure (the bottom number) by three points. The results were even more significant for those with higher blood pressure.

What's really interesting about the DASH study is that all three diets contained the same amount of sodium—about 3,000 milligrams per day. This indicates that the effects of sodium on blood pressure are tempered when adequate calcium, potassium, and magnesium are also consumed. In this respect the DASH findings reinforced previous findings that showed that when adults meet or exceed the Recommended Dietary Allowances for these minerals, the simultaneous consumption of a diet high in sodium is not associated with increased blood pressure.

Calculating Sodium Content

- 1 gram of salt contains 0.4 grams sodium

- 1 teaspoon salt contains 2.1 grams (2,100 milligrams) sodium

- 2.5 grams salt contains 1 gram sodium

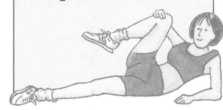

ESTIMATED SODIUM MINIMUM REQUIREMENTS OF HEALTHY PERSONS[a]

AGE	WEIGHT (KG)[a],*	SODIUM (MG)[b],**
Months		
0–5	4.5	120
5–11	8.9	200
Years		
1	11.0	225
2–5	16.0	300
6–9	25.0	400
10–18	50.0	500
>18	70.0[c]	500[c]

Reprinted with permission of The National Academy of Sciences, 1989. Courtesy of the National Academy Press, Washington D.C.

*kg = kilograms (1 kilogram equals 2.2 pounds).

** mg = milligrams

[a] = No allowance has been included for large, prolonged losses from the skin through sweat.

[b] = There is no evidence that higher intakes confer any health benefit.

[c] = No allowance included for growth. Values for those below 18 years assume a growth rate at the 50th percentile reported by the National Center for Health Statistics and averaged for males and females.

Zinc

Although zinc has been known to be an essential mineral for more than 50 years, for much of that time it was considered a relatively unimportant nutrient. However, the past few years have seen interest in zinc increase dramatically—not only in nutrition and health circles, but among consumers as well. Why the sudden interest? Numerous new studies about zinc's many functions show it to be of crucial importance to human health. Zinc is a component of more than 200 enzymes, which are necessary for many bodily processes. Zinc is also essential for growth, immune system function, taste and smell sensation, reproductive health, wound healing, and more.

The Benefits of Zinc

Zinc and Immunity

Even moderate degrees of zinc deficiency can compromise the immune system. T-cell lymphocytes, the white blood cells that help fight infection, don't function well when zinc stores are low. Therefore, people who are zinc-deficient have a more difficult time resisting infections. Research has shown that when zinc supplements are given to individuals with low zinc levels, the numbers of T-cell lymphocytes circulating in the blood increase, and the ability of these cells to fight infection improves. Limited data also suggest that the incidence of certain respiratory infections and malaria may also be reduced by zinc supplements.

Zinc and the Common Cold

There is much debate about whether zinc lozenges help make colds more bearable. A study of more than 100 employees of the Cleveland Clinic suggested that sucking on zinc lozenges decreased the duration of colds by one-half—or about three days—and lessened the severity of colds as well. This study has been criticized by some researchers, since zinc lozenges are known for their unappealing taste—a factor that could make it obvious to study participants whether they were taking the zinc or the placebo lozenges,

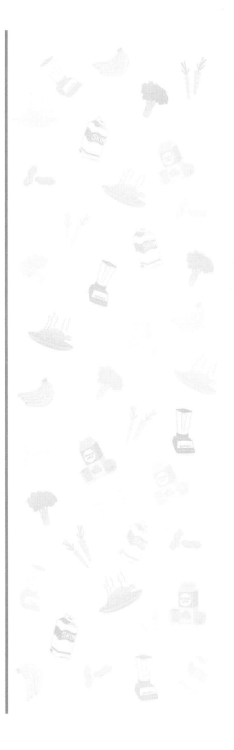

thereby skewing the study results. Other studies have found no effect from zinc lozenges.

It's important to note that the lozenges used in these studies contained zinc gluconate. Other forms of zinc, such as zinc acetate, zinc aspartate, and zinc citrate, which are found in some "cold season" products, have *no* published studies to back up their claims for alleviating cold symptoms.

If you decide to take zinc gluconate lozenges for a cold, begin taking them every few hours as soon as your symptoms show up. Don't exceed the recommended dosage, and don't take the lozenges for more than a week. Taking zinc supplements (tablets, capsules, etc.) won't work for colds because the form used to make the lozenges, zinc gluconate, is generally not available in capsule form. This is the best form for treating colds.

Zinc and Diarrhea

Inadequate zinc intakes are prevalent in developing countries. Studies of zinc-deficient children in India, Africa, South America, and Southeast Asia have found that zinc supplements help decrease the incidence of diarrhea, as well as lessen the severity and duration of the condition. A study during which zinc supplements were provided for two weeks resulted in preventive effects against diarrhea for three months afterward. Diarrhea is of particular concern since it both causes zinc losses and results from severe zinc deficiency, creating a dangerous cycle.

Zinc and Wound Healing

Zinc supplements have been shown to increase rates of wound healing, including burns. Skin irritations and bedsores are helped by zinc supplements (not lozenges), but only if the person is zinc-deficient in the first place. In other words, when zinc levels are normal, taking zinc supplements to help a wound heal doesn't work.

Zinc and Other Potential Benefits

There are many other purported benefits of zinc supplements, but the scientific research to support such uses of the mineral is preliminary, contradictory, or significantly lacking at this time. Some of these uses for zinc include the treatment of rheumatoid arthritis and lupus, which involve the immune system. Zinc is necessary to make testosterone and other hormones, so it may be useful for enhancing fertility in both women and men. Zinc may also slow vision loss in people with macular degeneration, a common cause of blindness in those over age 50. Osteoporosis, hemorrhoids, inflammatory bowel disease, prostatic hypertrophy (enlarged prostate gland), and ulcers are other health problems for which zinc may eventually prove beneficial.

Zinc in Food

Zinc is found in protein foods. Beef, pork, organ meats, poultry (especially dark meat), eggs, and seafood (especially oysters) are the best sources. Other sources include beans, nuts, seeds, and wheat germ. According to experts, people eating a typical Western diet get about half of their dietary zinc from meat, fish, and poultry. Another 20 percent comes from dairy products, some comes from grains, and a small amount from beans, nuts, and soy products (see "Food Sources of Zinc").

Humans absorb only about 33 percent of the total zinc in our diets. Zinc from animal foods is better absorbed than zinc from plant foods (because of the fiber and phytic acid contained in plants). This can be a problem for strict vegetarians (vegans) whose diets contain lots of high-fiber foods. Also, infants absorb less zinc when fed soy-based formula, which contains phytate, than when fed a milk-based formula.

What to Know about Taking Zinc Supplements

- Zinc supplements are available in tablet, capsule, lozenge, and liquid forms—all in varying dosages.
- Zinc picolinate, acetate, citrate, glycerate, or monomethionine are all equally well absorbed, although zinc sulfate can cause an upset stomach.
- Zinc supplements can interfere with copper absorption. If you regularly take extra zinc, you may also need to take a little extra copper. Check with your doctor.
- Be aware that calcium and iron supplements can decrease absorption of zinc.
- Since dietary supplements (or claims for them) are not reviewed by the Food and Drug Administration, quality control and potency problems may exist with zinc supplements.

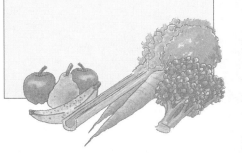

FOOD SOURCES OF ZINC

FOOD SOURCES	SERVING SIZE	ZINC (MG)*
Oysters, Pacific	6	50
Oysters, Eastern	6	27
Liver, beef	3 ounces	5
Wheat germ, toasted	1 ounce	4.7
Beef, ground, lean	3 ounces	4.6
Chicken leg, cooked	1	3
Pecans	1 ounce	1
Rice, wild, cooked	½ cup	1
Cheese, Edam	1 ounce	1
Milk, 2% fat	1 cup	1
Salmon	3 ounces	0.8
Egg	1	0.5

Source: USDA Nutrient Database for Standard Reference, Release 13, 1999.
*mg = milligrams.

When to Supplement with Zinc

Extra zinc is needed during periods of rapid growth, pregnancy, and lactation. However, according to two national surveys, the National Health and Nutrition Examination Survey (1988–1991) and the USDA Continuing Survey of Food Intakes of Individuals 1994–96, pregnant and breastfeeding women (as well as people aged 51 and older) don't get the recommended amounts of zinc. Additional surveys also revealed that young children, aged one to six years, adolescents, and low-income adults also consume less than the recommended amounts. However, consult your pediatrician before giving children zinc supplements.

The body works hard to maintain the proper level of zinc by increasing its absorption efficiency when intake of the mineral is low. However, chronic low intake can cause a zinc deficiency. Increased losses of zinc from the body or an increased need for zinc can also cause deficiency. Chronically decreased food intake, which frequently is a concern in older people, low-income population groups, or those who suffer from alcoholism, is a risk factor for zinc deficiency. Other circumstances during which zinc intake may be less than optimal include regular fasting (going without food completely) and consuming a vegetarian diet that's low in legumes and nuts. The body's requirement for zinc increases during pregnancy and lactation, times of infection, and during recovery from surgery, but frequently intake doesn't keep pace. People with AIDS and those suffering from digestive diseases that cause chronic diarrhea are also at risk for zinc deficiency.

The earliest sign of zinc deficiency is poor appetite, followed by weight loss, taste abnormalities, mental lethargy, and slow healing of wounds. With chronic, severe zinc deficiency, these symptoms worsen and are joined by hair loss, diarrhea, skin rashes, depressed immune function and increased susceptibility to infections, delayed fetal development and reduced growth (in children and adolescents), impaired vision, and reproductive dysfunction.

Large doses of zinc (150 milligrams and greater) have been shown to cause nausea, vomiting, and dizziness. Over time, zinc intakes of 150 to 450 milligrams per day result in reduced immune function and reduced levels of HDL ("good" cholesterol) as well. The National Academy of Sciences is currently evaluating the long-term risk of taking zinc supplements.

RECOMMENDED DIETARY ALLOWANCES (RDA) FOR ZINC

AGE/SEX	ZINC (MG)*
Males	
14+ years	11
Females	
14–18 years	9
18+ years	8
Pregnant women	
14–18 years	13
19+ years	11
Lactating women	
14–18 years	14
19+ years	12

Source: The National Academy of Sciences, 2001.
*mg = milligrams.

Caution!

- Do not take more than 15 milligrams of zinc per day unless advised by your doctor for a specific complaint or severe deficiency.
- If you are taking antibiotics, check with your doctor before taking zinc supplements.
- Certain groups of people may not be getting enough zinc. A multivitamin containing zinc should be sufficient for most people and is also safe. Taking zinc for a cold may provide some relief.
- If you have a medical condition or are pregnant or lactating, talk to your doctor before taking any supplement.

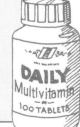

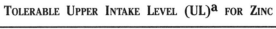

Tolerable Upper Intake Level (UL)[a] for Zinc

Age	Zinc (mg)*
9–13 years	23
14–18 years	34
19+ years	40
Pregnancy	
14–18 years	34
19+ years	40
Lactation	
14–18 years	34
19+ years	40

Source: National Academy of Sciences, 2001.

[a] = The maximum level of daily nutrient intake that is likely to pose no risk of adverse effects.

*mg = milligrams.

CHAPTER 4

Amino Acids: The Body's Building Blocks

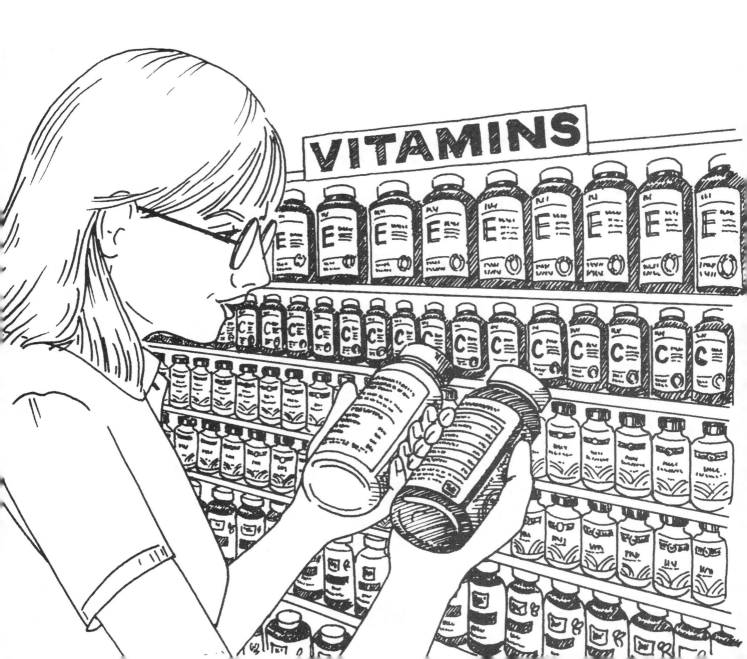

The body requires about 50,000 proteins to make the cells, tissues, organs, enzymes, hormones, and other substances necessary for life. These proteins are made up of amino acids, which can combine in an almost infinite number of ways. Some proteins, such as oligopeptides (*oligo* means "few"), are made up of short amino acid chains, which are composed of just two or three amino acids. Most of the neurotransmitters (chemical substances that send messages to and from the brain) are **peptides**. Other proteins are made up of hundreds of amino acids.

How does the body know which amino acids to link together? Our genetic material (DNA, or deoxyribonucleic acid) has all the "instructions" the body needs. DNA, which is located in each body cell, tells the cells which amino acids to hook together to make whatever protein is needed, when it's needed, and in the amounts necessary. Amazingly, after a protein has done its job within the body, it's broken down by other proteins—recycled so that the amino acids can be used again in other combinations. It's a very complicated, efficient process—and an essential one, not only for humans, but for all species.

Essential and Nonessential Amino Acids

Amino acids are divided into two categories: essential and nonessential. There are nine **essential amino acids** that we must get from food. The remaining **nonessential amino acids** are required for life, but if they aren't supplied by our diets, they can be manufactured by our body's cells. All of the amino acids are vital to good health. In fact, a lack of just one amino acid will, over time, cause serious health problems.

Animal proteins (except for gelatin) contain all nine of the essential amino acids, as well as some nonessential ones. Because of this, meat, poultry, eggs, and milk are commonly referred to as containing **"complete" proteins**. Proteins from plant sources, such as vegetables and grains, are called "incomplete" proteins because they are deficient in one or more of the essential amino acids. The exception to this is the soybean, which is nearly equal to animal protein in amino acid content.

Key Terms Defined

Amino acid: The basic chemical subunit of proteins. Amino acids that are joined together by peptide bonds (strong chemical links) into a "chain" make peptides or proteins. A huge number of proteins can be made by varying the sequence and number of amino acids included in each chain.

Essential amino acids: Essential amino acids are histidine, isoleucine, leucine, lysine, methionine, phenylalanine, threonine, tryptophan, and valine.

Nonessential amino acids: Nonessential amino acids are alanine, arginine,* asparagine, aspartic acid, carnitine,* cysteine, glutamic acid, glycine, proline, serine, taurine,* and tyrosine.

*May be essential in some circumstances.

Peptide: Peptides are chains of amino acids of varying lengths. Polypeptides (*poly* means "many") are chains with 10 to 49 amino acids. Oligopeptides (*oligo* means "few") contain 10 or fewer amino acids. Although not true proteins, peptides have important biological functions, including serving as hormones. For example, oxytocin is a hormone (and a peptide consisting of nine amino acids) that stimulates uterine contractions during labor.

Protein: A peptide chain that contains 50 or more amino acids. The term *protein* is derived from the Greek word *proteious*, which means "of first importance"—fitting because life would be impossible without proteins. Proteins are grouped according to their functions:

Structural proteins: Those that form connective tissues, such as collagen

Transport proteins: Those that move substances around in the body, such as hemoglobin, which transports oxygen

Storage proteins: Those that house important substances or nutrients in the body, such as ferritin, which stores iron in the liver

Defensive proteins: Those that protect the body (antibodies, which fight allergens)

Catalytic proteins: Those that cause or speed up chemical reactions in the body (enzymes)

Contractile proteins: Those that make up muscle tissue fibers

Complementary Proteins

Not all incomplete proteins are deficient in the same amino acids, so by combining different plant foods one can make up for any amino acids that might be deficient. Plant foods that compensate for each other are called **complementary proteins**. Eating complementary protein foods is how strict vegetarians (those who eat no animal products at all) can still get an adequate supply of all the essential amino acids. Interestingly, many traditional cultural food combinations, such as beans and tortillas, peas and rice, tofu and rice—even America's beloved peanut butter sandwiches—are all complementary protein combinations.

It used to be thought that since the body doesn't store amino acids, complementary proteins needed to be eaten at the same time—in other words, at the same meal. That's been found to be unnecessary for adults (but it still may be a good idea for growing children who are vegetarians). Now, we know that one simply needs to eat complementary protein foods within the same day.

Amino Acid Supplements

In general, most Americans get more protein than they need, and therefore get adequate amounts of amino acids. If you're healthy and eating a varied diet, you probably don't need amino acid supplements. However, amino acids may be desirable for therapeutic benefits—those beyond general good health. For example, research suggests that various amino acids (arginine, carnitine, and taurine) are useful in the treatment of heart disease, while glutamine is beneficial for problems of the digestive tract.

There is a danger of the body's amino acids becoming out of balance if single amino acid supplements are routinely taken. For those using amino acids longer than a month, a supplement that provides a variety of amino acids (sometimes called a "complex") is recommended to help keep amino acid intake balanced. In addition, when amino acids are taken for therapeutic benefits, it's wise to do so under a doctor's supervision, especially if you'll be taking them longer than a few months. Never exceed the recommended dose of amino acids, as high doses may be toxic and cause nausea, vomiting, or diarrhea. Finally, pregnant women or anyone with liver or kidney disease should talk to their doctor before taking any amino acid supplements.

L or D?

Amino acid names on supplement labels are frequently preceded by the letters "L" or "D." This refers to the chemical form of the amino acid. Those with the "L" in their name are the most similar to amino acids in the body, and are therefore preferable over the "D" forms.

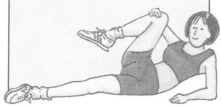

Arginine

Arginine (pronounced AR-ji-neen) is a nonessential amino acid found in a variety of foods. It plays a role in several important body functions, including cell division, wound healing, immune function, and the removal of ammonia from the body. Arginine may also be important during growth periods, since experts believe it may stimulate secretion of human growth hormone.

The Benefits of Arginine

Arginine and Heart Disease

Arginine helps make nitric oxide, which dilates—or relaxes—arteries, making blood flow more freely and thus lowering blood pressure. Nitric oxide also helps prevent clot formation and plaque buildup on artery walls that can lead to a heart attack or stroke. Because of arginine's role in the production of nitric oxide, it has been suggested that the amino acid may be useful as a treatment for a variety of heart conditions. Doses as large as 30 grams of arginine per day have been used to treat congestive heart failure.

Experts have also looked at the role of arginine in intermittent claudication (painful cramping in the calf as a result of poor circulation). Individuals with advanced hardening and narrowing of the arteries often have difficulty walking due to a lack of blood flow to the legs. In one study, individuals who consumed snack food bars containing arginine were able to improve their walking distance. After two weeks of eating two bars per day, the study participants were able to walk 66 percent farther.

Arginine and Other Potential Benefits

Scientists are looking at the possible use of arginine as part of a treatment strategy during angioplasty, coronary bypass, and heart transplantation. Some are also investigating whether arginine may improve sperm function and thereby help treat male infertility. As much as 30 grams of arginine have been given before chemotherapy treatments to help improve immune function in patients with breast and colon cancers. Although these areas of research are

What to Know about Taking Arginine Supplements

- Arginine is found in tablets, capsules, bars, drinks, and protein powders ranging in dosage from 2 to 3 grams per day. Arginine is also found in amino acid combinations.
- Arginine supplements are usually well tolerated, but increased sodium and water losses have been seen in some individuals.
- Since dietary supplements (or claims for them) are not reviewed by the Food and Drug Administration, quality control and potency problems may exist with arginine supplements.

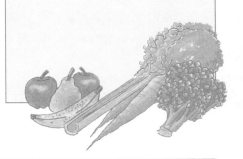

promising, much more research is needed. Despite claims to the contrary, arginine supplementation has not been shown to build muscle, prevent colds, treat impotence, or improve athletic performance.

Arginine in Food

Arginine is found in a variety of foods including dairy products, meat, poultry, fish, nuts, and chocolate.

FOOD SOURCES OF ARGININE

FOOD SOURCES	SERVING SIZE	ARGININE (MG)*
Beef, ground, lean	3¹/₂ ounces	1,499
Garbanzo beans	1 cup	1,369
Beef, prime rib	3¹/₂ ounces	1,362
Atlantic salmon	3 ounces	1,124
Peanuts, roasted	1 ounce	882
Almonds	1 ounce	691
Soy milk	1 cup	524
Rice, brown	1 cup	382
Egg	1 large	375
Milk nonfat	1 cup	301
Bagel	1 (3¹/₂" diameter)	280
Cheese, cheddar	1 ounce	267
Baking, chocolate	1 ounce	165
Figs, dried	10	131

Source: USDA Nutrient Database for Standard Reference, Release 13, 1999.
*mg = milligrams.

When to Supplement with Arginine

Most people get the arginine they need through food or via production in the body, and supplements are not recommended for children. The average U.S. diet provides about 5.5 grams of arginine per day. However, certain conditions can deplete the body's arginine stores, including infections, severe burns, and injuries. Although arginine appears to have some beneficial effects, there have been no long-term studies on the safety of arginine supplementation.

Caution!

- Since arginine deficiency is rare and much more research is needed, supplements are not recommended for the general population. If you are considering supplementing with arginine, consult with your doctor first.
- There is some evidence that consuming large doses of one particular amino acid can negatively affect the amino acid balance in the body.
- If you have a medical condition or are pregnant or lactating, talk to your doctor before taking any supplement.
- Individuals taking lysine to treat herpes should not take these supplements, since arginine may interfere or counteract any potential benefit.

Carnitine

Carnitine (pronounced CAR-na-teen) is not a true amino acid, but rather a water-soluble vitaminlike compound that the body uses to turn fat into energy. Carnitine works as part of an enzyme complex made up of carnitine acyltransferase I, carnitine translocase, and carnitine transferase II. Carnitine is not normally considered essential because the body can make enough of it from the amino acids lysine and methionine.

The Benefits of Carnitine

Carnitine and Heart Disease

Carnitine is primarily used for heart conditions, and research has shown it may be useful in the treatment (along with conventional treatment) for angina, or chest pain. In one study, 200 people with angina were given either 2,000 milligrams of carnitine or a placebo per day—along with their usual medications. Those supplementing with carnitine showed improved heart function, including a greater ability to exercise without chest pain, compared to those receiving the placebo. Moreover, many in the carnitine supplement group were able to reduce the dosage of some of their heart medications—under a doctor's supervision.

Preliminary research indicates that carnitine may also be useful in the treatment of congestive heart failure and intermittent claudication (pain in the legs after walking). Individuals with advanced hardening and narrowing of the arteries, or **arteriosclerosis**, often have difficulty walking due to a lack of blood flow to the legs. The pain can hit after walking less than half a block. Although carnitine does not increase blood flow, it may enable the muscles to function better under difficult circumstances. In a study of 245 people with intermittent claudication, those treated with 2,000 milligrams of carnitine per day showed a 70 percent improvement in walking distance.

Researchers are also looking at the potential role of carnitine in reducing the death rate following a heart attack. Findings from a study of 472 people showed that carnitine may improve survival rate if given within 24 hours after a heart attack.

What to Know about Taking Carnitine Supplements

- Carnitine is available in several different forms: L-carnitine, L-propionyl-carnitine, and acetyl-L-carnitine. Avoid the poorly regulated supplements known as "D-carnitine" or "DL-carnitine," as they may cause angina, muscle pain, and/or loss of muscle function.

- Carnitine is available in tablet and capsule forms, as a single supplement containing 250 to 500 milligrams of carnitine, or in a combination amino acid supplement.

- Although there is no known toxicity seen with dietary sources, carnitine supplementation above 3,000 milligrams per day may cause diarrhea and/or a "fish odor" in those who take it.

- Since dietary supplements are not reviewed by the FDA, quality control and potency problems may exist with carnitine supplements.

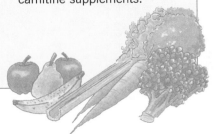

Carnitine and Other Potential Benefits

There are a number of alleged benefits of carnitine supplements, but the scientific research to support such claims is either preliminary, contradictory, or significantly lacking at this time. Examples include the use of carnitine in Alzheimer's, depression in the elderly, and adult-onset diabetes. Researchers are also beginning to look at the role of carnitine in reducing cholesterol and triglyceride levels, but much more research is needed.

Despite claims to the contrary, carnitine has not been shown to be useful for treating Down's syndrome, muscular dystrophy, irregular heartbeat, impaired sperm motility, and the toxicity of the AIDS drug AZT. Nor does carnitine aid in weight loss, endurance performance, or enhanced aerobic or anaerobic exercise performance. Although carnitine does play a role in energy production, amounts in excess of the body's needs do not appear to provide any benefit.

Carnitine in Food

The best source of carnitine is in high-protein foods, such as meat, especially beef, lamb, and mutton. Other foods rich in protein also provide carnitine, including milk, cheese, and poultry. Fruits and vegetables contain negligible amounts of this amino acid.

When to Supplement with Carnitine

Although there is no dietary requirement for carnitine, a small number of individuals have a genetic defect that prevents the body from making this compound. Additionally, liver, brain, and kidney diseases can hinder carnitine production. Certain medications such as antiseizure drugs may also reduce carnitine levels. Infants on formulas that do not contain carnitine (i.e., non-milk-based formulas) should be supplemented with carnitine to the levels found in breastmilk. Carnitine supplements are not recommended for children.

Caution!

- Because the body makes its own carnitine and much more research is needed, carnitine supplements are not recommended for the general population. If you're considering taking this supplement, consult with your doctor first.
- If you have a medical condition or are pregnant or lactating, talk to your doctor before taking any supplement.
- Individuals with liver and kidney diseases should not take carnitine supplements.

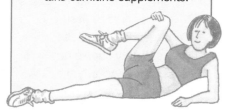

Creatine

Creatine is a nonessential amino acid that's used by the body to meet muscular demands during short bursts of high-intensity exercise, such as a sprint. Since 1992, when the use of creatine by Olympic athletes was publicized, the supplement's popularity has grown enormously—appealing to both men and women. Creatine use is common among professional athletes, and it appeals to recreational athletes, college athletes, and even teens and children. Creatine supplements are marketed as muscle-building supplements that will help the consumer train harder and longer, but they aren't recommended because of their unknown long-term health effects.

The Benefits of Creatine

The benefits of creatine supplementation relate to the amino acid's involvement in energy-providing chemical reactions in the body. During high-intensity exercise, muscles obtain energy from a series of reactions involving adenosine triphosphate (ATP), phosphocreatine (PCr), adenosine diphosphate (ADP), and creatine. ATP provides energy when it changes to ADP. To regenerate ATP requires PCr. Creatine supplements increase the storage of PCr, thus making more ATP available to fuel the working muscles. Stored PCr can fuel only the first 10 seconds or so of a sprint or other similar activity; after that another fuel, such as glucose (blood sugar), must provide the energy to sustain the activity.

Creatine and Exercise Performance

A good number of studies support the use of creatine supplementation for enhancing performance of activities that require short bursts of power and strength, including weightlifting, sprinting, and rowing. Initial studies conducted in the mid-1990s indicated that creatine, taken in the right doses and in conjunction with an exercise program, can result in a 5 to 10 percent increase in strength and power.

Daily creatine supplementation (5 grams per day) increased the intracellular creatine and PCr content of the quadriceps muscle in 17 participants. In addition, exercise increased creatine uptake in

What You Need to Know about Taking Creatine Supplements

- Creatine supplements are available in capsules, chewable tablets, and powder. One teaspoon of creatine monohydrate powder contains 5 grams of creatine.
- Creatine users may want to avoid caffeine, as one study showed that caffeine diminished the strength gains the creatine produced. Caffeine is also dehydrating and may compound the dehydrating effects of creatine.
- Creatine supplements must be taken daily.
- When creatine is combined with simple carbohydrates such as fructose (fruit sugar), it enters the muscles more easily. This is why some supplement manufacturers suggest dissolving creatine powder in juice or a sports drink.
- Since dietary supplements are not reviewed by the FDA, quality control and potency problems may exist.

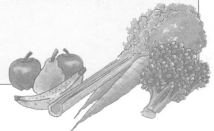

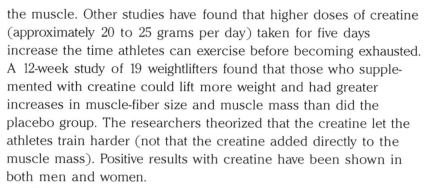

Caution!

- Creatine isn't recommended for athletes or nonathletes. The risk of side effects and its unknown long-term safety record don't justify its use for most people. Although it may work if body stores are low, there's no way to know the status of creatine stores. Don't use creatine therapeutically.

- When taking creatine supplements, it's important to keep well hydrated—drink at least 64 ounces of liquid (preferably water) per day.

- Baseline kidney and liver tests are advised before starting creatine supplementation.

- If you have a medical condition or are pregnant or lactating, talk to your doctor before taking any supplement.

- People with kidney problems should not take creatine supplements.

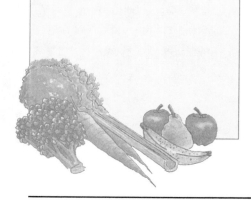

the muscle. Other studies have found that higher doses of creatine (approximately 20 to 25 grams per day) taken for five days increase the time athletes can exercise before becoming exhausted. A 12-week study of 19 weightlifters found that those who supplemented with creatine could lift more weight and had greater increases in muscle-fiber size and muscle mass than did the placebo group. The researchers theorized that the creatine let the athletes train harder (not that the creatine added directly to the muscle mass). Positive results with creatine have been shown in both men and women.

Other studies indicate that creatine is not useful for aerobic activities such as distance running and cycling. It also doesn't appear to help with running speed, and may not be helpful in sprint swimming performance.

Creatine and Other Potential Benefits

Research into therapeutic uses of creatine supplements to help combat muscle losses caused by certain diseases such as muscular dystrophy and amyotrophic lateral sclerosis (ALS, or Lou Gehrig's disease) suggests some gains in strength can be made. One study of 81 people with various neurological diseases (including muscular dystrophy) showed that taking 10 grams of creatine per day for five days, followed by 5 grams for another week, increased strength at various body sites, including the ankle, knee, and hand. Knee strength, for example, increased 11 percent, compared with just over 2 percent for the placebo. This increase may be enough to make a real difference in daily activities and quality of life. However, results are preliminary, and the studies were conducted with very small populations.

When to Supplement with Creatine

Body stores of creatine can be replenished from either food or supplements. The normal dietary intake of creatine is 1 to 2 grams per day, although vegetarians may consume less, since creatine is found only in meat and seafood (see "Foods That

Contain Creatine"). If dietary creatine is limited and no supplements are taken, the body can make it from other amino acids (glycine, arginine, and methionine) at the rate of about 2 grams per day, provided enough protein is consumed.

Body stores of creatine are located in muscle cells, kidneys, sperm cells, and brain tissue. About 60 percent of muscle creatine is in the form of PCr. Saturating the muscle with PCr requires huge amounts of food, so supplements may be the best way to increase body stores of creatine. Most creatine supplement regimens begin with 20 to 30 grams (divided in four equal doses) for one week, followed by a 2-gram-per-day maintenance dose. However, these doses vary a little from supplement to supplement. Excess creatine is eliminated through the urine. It's important to realize that unless body stores of creatine are low, supplementation will not be helpful.

Creatine supplementation is not without side effects, the most common of which relate to water retention. One survey of 28 male baseball players and 24 male football players, aged 18 to 23, found that 31 percent of them experienced diarrhea, 25 percent had muscle cramps, 13 percent had unwanted weight gain, and 13 percent reported dehydration when taking creatine supplements. Proper hydration is important when taking this amino acid in order to prevent the body from holding water within cells. Creatine-associated water retention may also be connected to reports of heat intolerance and dizziness when taking creatine supplements. There have been two published reports of creatine supplementation causing decreased kidney function in people who already had some degree of kidney disease. However, it appears that creatine is safe for those whose kidneys are healthy to begin with.

There are many unknowns with creatine in terms of safety and efficacy. It's not recommended for children at all. It's not known if there is a point of diminishing returns with creatine—that is, there may be a point where enhanced performance levels off from long-term supplement usage. What's more, despite many clinical trials, high-quality research on creatine efficacy is lacking. In fact, there are about equal numbers of studies on both sides—half show it works, half show it doesn't.

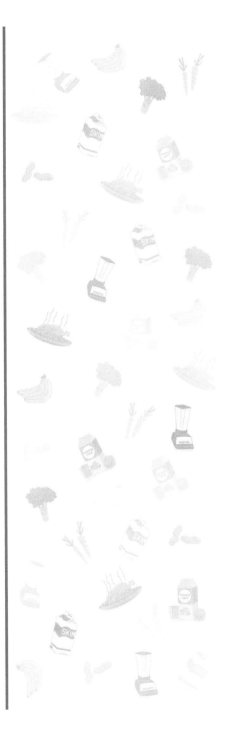

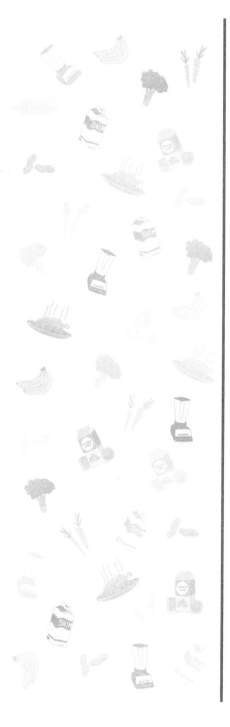

Foods That Contain Creatine

Some foods that naturally contain creatine are:

- Beef
- Chicken
- Pork
- Tuna

- Cod
- Salmon
- Herring

Glutamine

Glutamine (pronounced GLUE-tah-mean) is the most abundant amino acid in the body. Glutamine is a nonessential amino acid, but since the 1980s glutamine has been considered to be "conditionally essential" by some experts. This means that under normal circumstances the body can make adequate quantities of the amino acid. However, the research done on glutamine in the past few decades indicates that in times of stress (such as fever or illness), the body cannot produce as much as it requires. There has been a great deal of research on glutamine in the past few years, and supplementation has been shown to be useful in a number of areas, including gastrointestinal diseases and conditions, HIV/AIDS, burns, chronic wounds and surgical wounds, and combating the side effects of cancer treatments.

The Benefits of Glutamine

Glutamine and Gastrointestinal Conditions

Early research on glutamine examined its effects on the gastrointestinal (GI) system, where it is considered essential for health. Among the GI benefits of glutamine are faster healing after bowel surgery, improved nutritional status in people with Crohn's disease, and improved reabsorption of sodium and water during diarrhea (thereby lessening the detrimental effects of diarrhea). People with inflammatory bowel disease and short bowel syndrome may benefit from glutamine supplementation, since it has been shown to help control diarrhea and help maintain the integrity of the intestines. Additionally, there is some research showing that glutamine enhances the healing of stomach ulcers, but this is still quite preliminary.

Glutamine and Cancer

This area of research is very promising, with many completed and ongoing human studies focused on glutamine supplementation and cancer treatment. Taken prior to and during cancer therapy (chemotherapy or radiation), glutamine has been shown to help restore levels of glutathione (a potent antioxidant), repair damage to the intestines, decrease infection, and reduce some of the side effects from therapy. Research at the University of Arkansas also indicates that glutamine enhances the ability of chemotherapy to kill tumors. Most recently, researchers have shown that glutamine helps decrease the pain associated with radiation and chemotherapy by reducing the duration and severity of irritation to the tissues of the mouth, esophagus, and bowel.

Glutamine and Wound Healing

In people with large burns or chronic wounds, where much healing of tissue needs to be accomplished, glutamine is released from the muscles to support tissue repair, provide energy, and maintain immune response. Supplementation with glutamine for these conditions has been extremely successful. Specifically, glutamine has been shown to increase protein production, promote wound healing, decrease infection, and help restore body protein stores.

Glutamine and HIV/AIDS

Research suggests that glutamine supplementation may help limit muscle loss, decrease diarrhea and malabsorption, enhance immunity, and reduce infection in people with HIV/AIDS. One researcher was able to help patients increase body weight with a glutamine supplement (combined with other nutrients). This is a promising area of study, but much more research needs to be done.

Caution!

- There's no evidence that glutamine supplements provide any benefits for healthy people. In addition, glutamine supplementation is rather complicated, and supplements may not provide enough to be useful.
- In general, taking single amino acid supplements isn't wise because they can cause imbalances in the body that may interfere with absorption of dietary amino acids.
- Glutamine may cause constipation in individuals who are prone to the condition. Eating a diet high in **soluble fiber** and drinking lots of water can help.
- If you have a medical condition or are pregnant or lactating, talk to your doctor before taking any supplement.

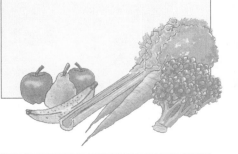

Glutamine in Food

Although meat, poultry, fish, and eggs contain the most glutamine, food in general is not a good source of this nutrient, and cooking quickly inactivates it.

When to Supplement with Glutamine

For GI conditions, cancer, and wound healing, glutamine supplements have proven to be helpful, but taking the supplements is not a simple matter. They are not recommended for children.

First, there is no recommended dose for each specific condition, and medical supervision for people who are ill is very important. Hospitals often give 30 grams of glutamine per day, divided into three to six servings. This is a lot more than most people would consume via supplements at home. Second, it's not yet known how much glutamine is too much. Some safety studies have been conducted, but more need to be done. Third, glutamine should not randomly be added to the diet; it needs to be balanced with protein intake. And finally, glutamine supplements available at health food stores or through mail order usually contain very little of the amino acid, and they aren't the same quality grade as the glutamine used in research.

Glutamine vs. Glutamic Acid

Although glutamine and glutamic acid are very similar, they are not the same. Glutamic acid is a component of glutamine (glutamine is broken down in the body to glutamic acid and ammonia). There is a continuous conversion between glutamate and glutamine in the body. Both amino acids are plentiful in the body.

Lysine

Lysine (pronounced LIE-seen) is an essential amino acid found in both plant and animal foods. Lysine is necessary for proper growth, so it's especially important to get enough of this amino acid during infancy and adolescence.

The Benefits of Lysine

Both cold sores and genital herpes are caused by a virus called herpes simplex. After one is infected with herpes simplex, the virus "hides" and reappears at times of stress. Some preliminary studies suggest that lysine supplements (1 to 3 grams, divided among meals) can reduce the number of herpes flare-ups, and others propose that lysine helps one recover from herpes attacks faster. A study of 52 people with a history of herpes flare-ups showed that those receiving 3 grams of lysine every day had an average of 2.4 fewer flare-ups over six months than those in the placebo group. The lysine-takers' flare-ups were also considered less severe and healed faster.

Test-tube research suggests that lysine fights herpes by blocking arginine, an amino acid that the virus needs in order to replicate. Because of its arginine-blocking effect, lysine may be more effective for herpes treatment when a low-arginine diet is followed. This involves avoiding foods including chocolate, peanuts, tree nuts, and seeds.

Not all studies on lysine and herpes suggest that the supplement is helpful—a number of them showed no benefit from taking the supplements. Most of the research on lysine and herpes is small scale— larger studies need to be done.

Lysine in Food

Good sources of lysine include red meat, poultry, sardines, cheese, nuts, eggs, and legumes. Cereal grains tend to be low in lysine, which is why in these foods lysine is called the "limiting amino acid"—it's the amino acid that's present in the least amount relative to what's needed for the body to make new protein.

When to Supplement with Lysine

This is one of those amino acids for which a deficiency is very rare, if the diet contains sufficient protein. Signs of a lysine deficiency include fatigue, nausea, dizziness, appetite loss, anxiety, decreased immunity, and slow growth. People who have inadequate protein intake, and strict vegetarians (vegans) whose diets lack legumes and don't include a wide variety of foods, may need more lysine—and amino acids in general. In that case, a supplement that provides a combination of amino

What to Know about Taking Lysine Supplements

- Lysine is generally available in 500-milligram capsules and in combination amino acid products in varying amounts.
- For better absorption, don't take lysine supplements with a high-protein meal. Try taking them first thing in the morning or at bedtime.
- Since dietary supplements are not reviewed by the FDA, quality control and potency problems may exist with lysine supplements.
- Calculate your estimated requirement for lysine using the following equation:

Your weight $\div$ 2.2 $\times$ lysine requirement for your age = milligrams lysine needed per day.

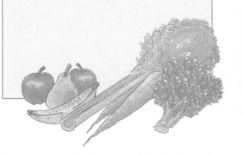

acids would be a better choice than single amino acid supplements. The chances of creating an amino acid imbalance in the body are greater when taking single amino acids, and imbalances can interfere with the absorption of dietary amino acids.

The estimated adult requirement for lysine is 12 milligrams per kilogram of body weight. Again, as with some of the other amino acids, some experts feel that the requirement is set too low. The National Academy of Sciences acknowledges that the state of knowledge concerning amino acid requirements is "unsatisfactory" and expresses the hope that continuing research in the field will yield additional information for consideration. There is no information on the specific amino acid requirements for pregnant or lactating women, and the requirements for older people are considered to be the same as for younger adults.

Lysine supplements appear to be nontoxic, but they're not without side effects—the biggest one being that they can increase cholesterol and triglyceride levels in the blood. People at risk for cardiovascular disease, or who already have elevated cholesterol and triglyceride levels, should definitely talk with their doctors before taking lysine. Children should not take lysine supplements.

FOOD SOURCES OF LYSINE

FOOD SOURCES	SERVING SIZE	LYSINE (MG)*
Soybean nuts, roasted	1/2 cup	2,466
Beef, top sirloin	3 1/2 ounces	2,330
Lamb, ground	3 1/2 ounces	2,186
Halibut	3 ounces	2,085
Bluefish	3 ounces	2,007
Ham steak	3 1/2 ounces	1,658
Milk, 2% fat	1 cup	644
Quinoa	1/2 cup	624
Cheese, cheddar	1 ounce	587
Wheat germ, toasted	1/4 cup	536
Egg, hard boiled	1 large	452
Pistachios	1 ounce	362

Source: *Pennington, Bowes & Church's Food Values of Portions Commonly Used,* 17th Ed., Revised by Jean Pennington, Ph.D., R.D., 1998.
*mg = milligrams.

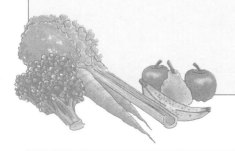

ESTIMATED REQUIREMENTS[a] FOR LYSINE[†]

AGE	LYSINE (MG/KG)*
Infants	
3–4 months	103[b]
Children	
up to 2 years	64[c]
10 to 12 years	44[d]
Adults	12[e]

Reprinted with permission of The National Academy of Sciences, 1989. Courtesy of the National Academy Press, Washington D.C.

*mg = milligrams; kg = kilograms.

[a] = From WHO, 1985.

[b] = Based on amino acid amounts in human milk or cow's milk formulas fed at levels that supported good growth.

[c] = Based on achievement of nitrogen balance sufficient to support adequate lean tissue gain (16 mg N/kg per day).

[d] = Based on upper range of requirement for positive nitrogen balance.

[e] = Based on highest estimate of requirement to achieve nitrogen balance.

[†] = The missing data in this chart demonstrates the unsatisfactory state of knowledge concerning amino acid requirements.

Phenylalanine

Phenylalanine (pronounced fee-nul-AL-uh-neen) is an essential amino acid that occurs in two forms: L-phenylalanine and D-phenylalanine. The "L" form is the one found naturally in proteins and the "D" form is the man-made, laboratory-produced version. Research on the benefits of phenylalanine has used both versions, and sometimes a combination of the two, known as DL-phenylalanine.

Caution

- Phenylalanine supplements are not recommended for the general population. What little research exists on the benefits of phenylalanine supplements is still preliminary, and the long-term safety of the supplements isn't known.
- In general, taking single amino acid supplements isn't wise, because they can cause imbalances in the body that may interfere with absorption of dietary amino acids.

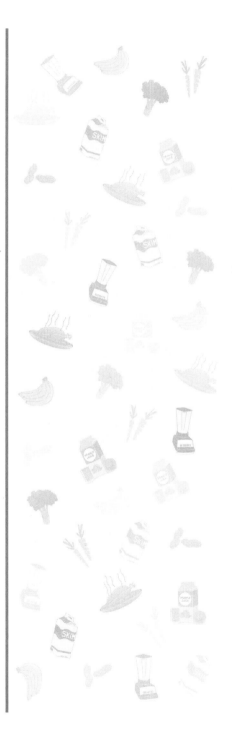

- If you're taking antipsychotic drugs, consult your doctor before taking phenylalanine supplements.
- If you have a medical condition or are pregnant or lactating, talk to your doctor before taking any supplement.
- People with the genetic disorder phenylketonuria, migraine headaches, and high blood pressure, as well as children, should not take phenylalanine.

Taurine

Taurine (pronounced TOR-een) is a sulfur-containing amino acid (as are methionine and cysteine). Body stores of taurine are concentrated in the muscles and central nervous system. The body can make taurine from methionine and cysteine—which is why it's considered nonessential—but it can also be obtained from animal protein foods such as meat, milk, eggs, and fish. Taurine is getting increased attention from researchers who believe it to be a much more important amino acid than previously thought.

The Benefits of Taurine

Taurine and Heart Disease

Not only is taurine a potent antioxidant, but it (along with the amino acids arginine and homocysteine) has been shown to affect some of the risk factors for heart disease. Specifically, taurine seems to lower blood pressure and cholesterol levels. Studies with animals have indicated that LDL ("bad" cholesterol) and triglyceride levels in particular are decreased with taurine supplementation. In addition, in studies where animals were fed a high-cholesterol diet, taurine supplements reduced both blood and liver cholesterol levels.

Another way that taurine may contribute toward cardiovascular health is by reducing the tendency of special blood cells, called platelets, to stick together or **aggregate**. Sticky platelets can form blood clots, which can lead to a heart attack or stroke if they block arteries to the heart or brain. In a study conducted at Brandeis University, platelets from taurine-depleted animals were

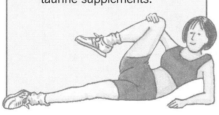

What to Know about Taking Taurine Supplements

- Taurine is generally available in 500-milligram capsules, and sometimes in combination with vitamins or other amino acids.
- Since dietary supplements (or claims for them) are not reviewed by the Food and Drug Administration, quality control and potency problems may exist with taurine supplements.

twice as sensitive to aggregation as platelets from animals receiving taurine. In humans receiving supplemental taurine (even though their taurine status was normal to begin with), resistance to platelet aggregation increased by 30 to 70 percent. In other words, decreased platelet "stickiness" was seen with increased taurine.

Taurine and Cystic Fibrosis

Cystic fibrosis is a genetic disease that affects the pancreas, respiratory system, and sweat glands. People with cystic fibrosis don't absorb fat well because of pancreatic malfunctioning, and the result is chronic fatty diarrhea called steatorrhea. Taurine supplementation has been found in a few studies to decrease steatorrhea. In one study, 22 children with cystic fibrosis and documented steatorrhea received taurine capsules (30 milligrams per kilogram body weight per day). Steatorrhea improved in the 19 participants who completed the study, and in the 10 children with the more severe steatorrhea, the decrease in fat loss approached 20 percent. These studies suggest that taurine supplementation can be a useful therapy in cystic fibrosis patients with fat malabsorption.

When to Supplement with Taurine

Blood levels of taurine have been found to be low in people in some instances. For example, strict vegetarians (vegans) may have low levels of taurine, and studies show that cancer patients also have low levels after they receive chemotherapy or radiation treatments. In addition, people who receive intravenous nutrition (feedings by vein) for long periods of time have been shown to be taurine-depleted.

However, there is no classical taurine deficiency in normal, healthy people because the body can make the amino acid if necessary. Taurine supplements are sometimes marketed as being necessary for the digestion of fats, but there is no research to show that healthy people need additional taurine for fat digestion or utilization by the body.

Caution!

- Taurine supplements are not recommended for the general population. Much of the research has been conducted only with animals, and the research on taurine's cardiovascular benefits is still preliminary.
- In general, taking single amino acid supplements isn't wise because they can cause imbalances in the body that may interfere with absorption of dietary amino acids.
- If you have a medical condition or are pregnant or lactating, talk to your doctor before taking any supplement.
- Taurine supplements are not recommended for anyone, with the possible exception of cystic fibrosis patients, and then only under the direct supervision of a physician.

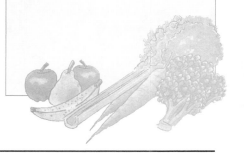

Tyrosine

Tyrosine (pronounced TIE-ro-seen) is an amino acid used to make both skin and hair pigments. The body also uses tyrosine to make a number of neurotransmitters (chemicals that help the brain and nervous system function): L-dopa, norepinephrine, and epinephrine. Tyrosine is not considered essential because the body can make what it needs from the amino acid phenylalanine.

The Benefits of Tyrosine

Little research has been done on the health benefits of tyrosine, and what has been done is either preliminary or contradictory at this time. Examples include the use of tyrosine for attention deficit disorder and depression.

Another area of research has looked at the effects of tyrosine on sleep deprivation. In a preliminary study, 20 marines were deprived of sleep for a night and then tested for alertness throughout the following day. Compared to those receiving a placebo, the group that received 10 to 15 grams of tyrosine twice a day appeared to get a "pickup" for about two to three hours. The findings also showed that tyrosine supplements at this level are relatively harmless.

Tyrosine in Food

Tyrosine is found in dairy products, meats, fish, and beans (see "Food Sources of Tyrosine").

When to Supplement with Tyrosine

Although there is no dietary requirement for tyrosine, individuals with certain forms of kidney disease and those with the rare metabolic disorder phenylketonuria (PKU) may need to supplement. Individuals with PKU must completely avoid foods containing phenylalanine, which in turn can reduce production of tyrosine. Tyrosine supplements are not recommended for children.

What to Know about Taking Tyrosine Supplements

- Tyrosine is available in tablet form, as a single supplement containing about 500 milligrams tyrosine, or in an amino acid formula.
- Although there is no toxicity seen with dietary sources, high doses of tyrosine may cause diarrhea, nausea, or nervousness.
- Since dietary supplements are not reviewed by the FDA, quality control and potency problems may exist.
- Calculate your estimated requirement for tyrosine using this equation:

Your weight ÷ 2.2 × tyrosine = estimated milligrams tyrosine needed per day.

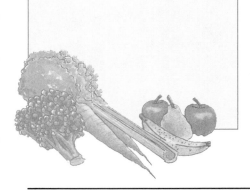

FOOD SOURCES OF TYROSINE

FOOD SOURCES	SERVING SIZE	TYROSINE (MG)*
Cheese, cottage, 2% fat	1 cup	1,654
Soybean nuts, dry roasted	1/2 cup	1,287
Tuna salad	1/2 cup	1,105
Chicken, breast, roasted	3 ounces	900
Beef, ground, lean	3 1/2 ounces	831
Snapper, cooked, dry heat	3 ounces	755
Milk, 2% fat	1 cup	393
Cheese, cheddar	1 ounce	341
Bagel, plain	1 (3 1/2" diameter)	214
Walnuts, black	1 ounce	212

Source: *Pennington, Bowes & Church's Food Values of Portions Commonly Used,* 17th Ed., revised by Jean Pennington, Ph.D., R.D., 1998.
*mg = milligrams.

ESTIMATED REQUIREMENTS FOR PHENYLALANINE PLUS TYROSINE[a],*,[†]

AGE	PHENYLALANINE/TYROSINE (MG/KG)**
Infants	
3–4 months	125[b]
Children	
up to 2 years	69[c]
10–12 years	22[d]
Adults	14[e]

Reprinted with permission of National Academy of Sciences, 1989. Courtesy of the National Academy Press, Washington D.C.
*Since tyrosine can replace about 50 percent of the requirement for phenylalanine, they must be considered together.
**mg = milligrams; kg = kilograms.
[a] = From WHO, 1985.
[b] = Based on amino acid amounts in human milk or cow's milk formulas fed at levels that supported good growth.
[c] = Based on achievement of nitrogen balance sufficient to support adequate lean tissue gain (16 mg N/kg per day).
[d] = Based on upper range of requirement for positive nitrogen balance.
[e] = Based on highest estimate of requirement to achieve nitrogen balance.
[†] = The missing data in this chart demonstrates the unsatisfactory state of knowledge concerning amino acid requirements.

Caution!

- Because the body makes its own tyrosine and much more research is needed, tyrosine supplements are not recommended for the general population. However, it is important to make sure you get enough phenylalanine, so that it can make tyrosine.
- Supplementing with single amino acids may upset the amino acid balance in the body.
- If you have a medical condition or are pregnant or lactating, talk to your doctor before taking any supplement.
- Individuals taking MAO inhibitors should not take tyrosine supplements.

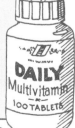

Tryptophan (5-HTP)

Tryptophan is an essential amino acid that is found in a variety of high-protein foods. Tryptophan supplements were banned in the United States in 1990 after contaminated supplements were linked to an outbreak of eosinophilia–myalgia syndrome (EMS), a rare and sometimes fatal muscle disorder. Later it was discovered that the tainted supplements were produced by a single Japanese company. However, tryptophan was known to be associated with significant health risks years before this incident occurred. Now, in response to the banning of tryptophan, a chemical cousin called 5-HTP (short for 5-hydroxytryptophan) is available in supplement form and is touted for much the same reasons that the original tryptophan was.

5-HTP is a derivative of tryptophan—the body makes 5-HTP in the brain from the tryptophan we get from food. The 5-HTP used in supplements comes from the seeds of an African plant *(Griffonia simplicifolia)*. In our bodies, 5-HTP quickly becomes **serotonin**, a neurotransmitter (a chemical that carries messages to and from the brain) that affects sleep cycles, appetite, and mood. Extra tryptophan in our diets leads to extra serotonin in our brains, which is why the supplements are touted as a sleep aid and mood-lifter, among other things.

The Benefits of Tryptophan

5-HTP and Insomnia

The primary use of 5-HTP supplements (and the original tryptophan supplements) is to promote sleep. In Europe 5-HTP has been prescribed by doctors for insomnia for years. There's really no controversy over the effectiveness of tryptophan and 5-HTP at inducing sleep. The mechanism for the effect is well understood and actually quite simple. Dietary tryptophan has to compete with other amino acids for entry into the brain after a high-protein meal is consumed. However, after a high-carbohydrate meal is eaten, insulin causes the competing amino acids to enter the muscles, allowing a greater proportion of the tryptophan to enter the brain and be converted to serotonin. This is why meals that are heavy on carbohydrates (and tryptophan-containing foods) cause us to feel drowsy and high-protein meals don't. 5-HTP has also been shown to improve the quality of sleep

---

What to Know about Taking 5-HTP Supplements

- 5-HTP supplements are typically sold in 50-milligram and 100-milligram capsules or tablets.
- For insomnia, a dose of 100 milligrams of 5-HTP taken about a half hour before bedtime is recommended. However, starting with a smaller dose (50 milligrams), and working up to 100 milligrams if necessary, can minimize side effects.
- Sometimes 5-HTP is combined with herbs or other ingredients that you may not want. Always check supplement labels carefully so you know what you're getting.
- 5-HTP is most rapidly absorbed when taken on an empty stomach.
- Since dietary supplements are not reviewed by the FDA, quality control and potency problems may exist.

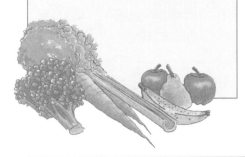

by increasing the amount of time spent in deep sleep and REM sleep (dream sleep). Getting extra tryptophan through 5-HTP supplements can be an effective way to produce more serotonin—and get some shuteye.

5-HTP and Depression

In the 1980s several European studies found that 5-HTP decreased depression in some people, although apparently no more so than traditional antidepressant medications. However, the supplement may work more quickly than antidepressants and produce fewer side effects. The typical dose of 5-HTP for depression treatment is 150 to 300 milligrams per day.

5-HTP and Other Potential Benefits

Preliminary research suggests that 5-HTP may be able to ease migraine headaches, decrease the pain of fibromyalgia (tenderness and pain in the muscles and joints), inhibit anxiety, and curb overeating. However, it's much too early to recommend the supplement for these uses.

5-HTP in Food

5-HTP is obtained through supplements, but tryptophan is found in many protein foods including beef, chicken, fish, and dairy products.

FOOD SOURCES OF TRYPTOPHAN

FOOD SOURCES	SERVING SIZE	TRYPTOPHAN (MG)*
Turkey, light meat, roasted	3¹/₂ ounces	340
Beef, ground	3¹/₂ ounces	320
Cottage cheese, 1% fat	1 cup	312
Chicken thigh, fried	2 ounces	187
Eggnog, nonalcoholic	1 cup	137
Milk, 2% fat	1 cup	115
Almonds, dried	1 ounce	100
Bagel, plain	3¹/₂" diameter	88
Macaroni, cooked	1 cup	85
Hot dog	1 frank	62

Source: *Pennington, Bowes & Church's Food Values of Portions Commonly Used*, 17th Ed., Revised by Jean Pennington, Ph.D., R.D., 1998.
*mg = milligrams.

Caution!

- There's no need to supplement dietary tryptophan with 5-HTP; the only reasons to take it would be therapeutic. Given the potential risks, as well as the fact that there are numerous other supplements and/or medications that have the same effects, taking this supplement just doesn't make sense.
- If you have a psychiatric condition, consult your doctor before taking 5-HTP.
- Do not use 5-HTP for more than two to three months unless you're being monitored by a doctor.
- Before driving or doing dangerous work, find out how 5-HTP affects you. It may make you too sleepy to perform these tasks safely.
- If you have a medical condition or are pregnant or lactating, talk to your doctor before taking any supplement.
- People who supplement with Saint John's wort and people who take antidepressant medications should not take 5-HTP.

When to Supplement with 5-HTP

Although the efficacy of 5-HTP (and tryptophan in general) to promote sleep is well established, use of the supplement remains controversial. Why? Adverse reactions to 5-HTP have been documented. In fact, in 1991 one case of EMS—the same illness that affected so many who used the contaminated tryptophan in 1989—was linked with 5-HTP. And, in 1998 the FDA confirmed that the same impurity that was present in the banned tryptophan supplements was also found in 5-HTP supplements. This impurity, known as "Peak X," was identified in the 1991 EMS case, and similar impurities were implicated in the 1989 outbreak. Although the exact cause of the EMS in all of these cases isn't clear (FDA did not blame it directly on "Peak X"), the fact that this impurity has now also turned up in 5-HTP supplements is definitely cause for concern. FDA is continuing to monitor the supplement and encourages consumers and medical professionals to report any adverse reactions to 5-HTP to the MedWatch program (call 800-FDA-1088).

Aside from the risk of consuming impure 5-HTP, the supplement can cause side effects, though most are generally mild. These include nausea, constipation, intestinal gas, and reduced sex drive. The nausea may diminish within a few days of starting the supplement. 5-HTP is not recommended for children.

Tryptophan and Niacin

About half the tryptophan you consume is converted into the B vitamin niacin—that's why practically no one is ever deficient in niacin. It takes approximately 60 milligrams of tryptophan to make 1 milligram of niacin.

ESTIMATED REQUIREMENTS FOR TRYPTOPHAN[a,†]

AGE	TRYPTOPHAN (MG/KG)*
Infants	
3–4 months	17[b]
Children	
up to 2 years	12.5[c]
10 to 12 years	3.3[d]
Adults	3.5[e]

Reprinted with permission of The National Academy of Sciences, 1989. Courtesy of the National Academy Press, Washington D.C.

*mg = milligrams; kg = kilograms.

[a] = From WHO, 1985.

[b] = Based on amino acid amounts in human milk or cow's milk formulas fed at levels that supported good growth.

[c] = Based on achievement of nitrogen balance sufficient to support adequate lean tissue gain (16 mg N/kg per day).

[d] = Based on upper range of requirement for positive nitrogen balance.

[e] = Based on highest estimate of requirement to achieve nitrogen balance.

[†] = The missing data in this chart demonstrates the unsatisfactory state of knowledge concerning amino acid requirements.

CHAPTER 5

Enzymes and Coenzymes

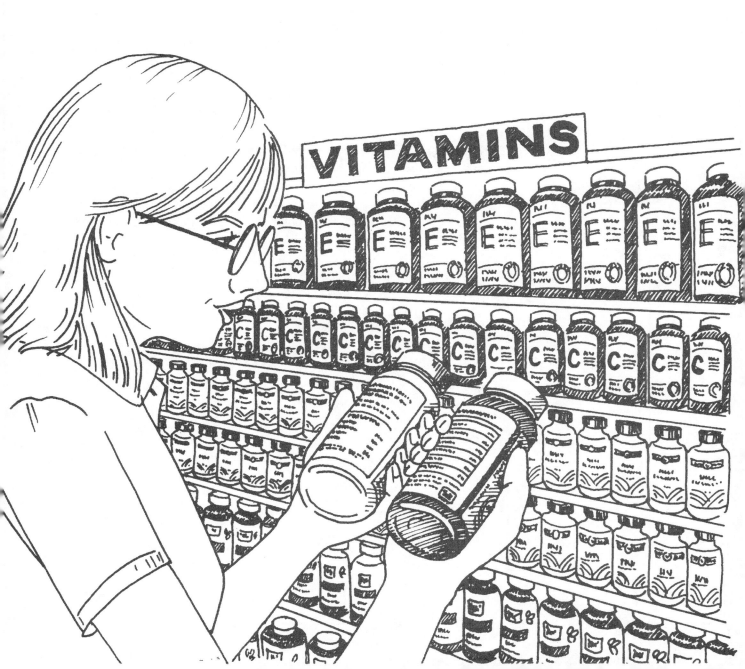

uman enzymes are protein molecules that serve as catalysts. Catalysts speed up many of the chemical reactions
that take place in the body. Thousands of different enzymes
exist in the body's cells, each associated with a specific chemical
reaction. Most of these reactions would proceed very slowly, or not
at all, without enzymes. Some of these reactions include breaking
down proteins, carbohydrates, and fat during digestion, releasing
energy from these nutrients, and disarming dangerous substances,
such as free radicals, in the body.

Literally thousands of different human enzymes have been isolated and studied, but only a few are available in supplement form.
Typical enzyme supplements include the digestive enzymes amylase
(breaks down carbohydrates), protease (breaks down proteins), and
lipase (breaks down fat), as well as lactase (breaks down the milk
sugar, **lactose**). Some plant-derived enzymes, including bromelain
(breaks down protein) and papain, can also be obtained through
supplements. Enzyme supplements are available at the same places
where vitamin and mineral supplements are sold, and are frequently
sold in multiple enzyme formulas.

Enzymes Depend on Vitamins and Minerals

Many vitamins and minerals have important roles in forming or
assisting enzymes. Enzyme cofactors are essential components of
enzymes, while coenzymes are substances that help the enzymes
do their jobs in the body. Examples of minerals that act as cofactors are copper, iron, magnesium, and zinc. Coenzyme nutrients
include niacin, biotin, thiamin, and vitamins B_6 and B_{12}. The following chart lists some enzymes and the nutrients they require to
do their jobs:

ENZYME	FUNCTION	NUTRIENT NEEDED
Alcohol dehydrogenase	Breaks down alcohol	Zinc
Biotinidase	Helps release bound biotin for "recycling" in the body	Biotin
Flavokinase	Helps form flavin mononucleotide (FMN), which is a more complex coenzyme necessary for hundreds of bodily reactions	Riboflavin
Superoxide dismutase	Antioxidant	Copper
Xanthine oxidase	Necessary for growth, development, and proper iron utilization	Molybdenum
Proline hydroxylase	Necessary for the formation of collagen	Vitamin C

In the past, enzymes were named by simply adding the suffix "-ase," to the name of the substance or the name of the reaction. For example, the enzyme that breaks down fat, technically known as "lipid," was called lipase. Later a system of naming was adopted to more accurately describe enzymes. Enzymes were divided into six groups based on the type of reactions they cause. For example, there's one group for enzymes that form chemical bonds (ligases) and another group for enzymes that separate chemicals (lyases).

Coenzyme Q10

Coenzyme Q_{10}, also called ubiquinone or CoQ_{10}, is a naturally occurring compound found in plants and animals. CoQ_{10} is necessary for **mitochondria**—the energy-generating components of all cells—to work properly. Research indicates that certain illnesses and the aging process can decrease CoQ_{10} levels in the body.

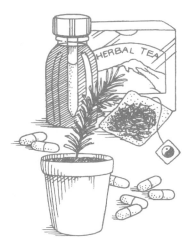

The Benefits of Coenzyme Q10

Coenzyme Q10 and Heart Disease

Because mitochondria are found in great abundance in the cells of heart tissue, much research has been focused on CoQ_{10} and heart disease. For instance, CoQ_{10} has been shown to be useful in abnormalities involving the heart's ability to contract and pump blood effectively, such as congestive heart failure and a number of cardiomyopathies (heart muscle diseases).

In one study, people with cardiomyopathy who took 100 milligrams of CoQ_{10} per day, along with traditional therapy, showed greater improvement than those who took the traditional treatment and a placebo. In fact, the results from the CoQ_{10} group were so positive, the investigators stopped the study because they couldn't ethically give the placebo.

Coenzyme Q_{10} is also a potent antioxidant, and as such, appears to protect vitamin E, which helps prevent the oxidation of low-density lipoprotein (LDL, or "bad" cholesterol). It's believed that oxidized LDL can lead to plaque buildup, clogged arteries, and an increased risk of heart attack or stroke.

In another study, researchers found that CoQ_{10} may reduce the ability of blood to clot, thereby decreasing the chance of a blood clot getting stuck in a clogged artery and causing a heart attack or stroke. Interestingly, some of the drugs commonly taken by heart patients can actually decrease CoQ_{10} levels in the body by interfering with its production. If you're currently on such medications, you might want to talk to your doctor about supplementing with CoQ_{10}.

Other heart-related conditions for which CoQ_{10} supplementation shows promise include hypertension and heart valve replacement. In people who suffer from angina (chest pain), supplementing with CoQ_{10} appears to increase their ability to exercise longer, decrease pain frequency, and reduce the need for nitroglycerin.

Coenzyme Q10 and Cancer

The data on CoQ_{10} and cancer is preliminary at best. There are studies underway looking at the effect of CoQ_{10} on breast and prostate cancers; however, it will be a while before the results are in.

What to Know about Taking Coenzyme Q10 Supplements

- CoQ_{10} supplements come in capsule and tablet forms in dosages ranging from 10 to 130 milligrams.
- Since dietary supplements (or claims for them) are not reviewed by the Food and Drug Administration, quality control and potency problems may exist with CoQ_{10} supplements.

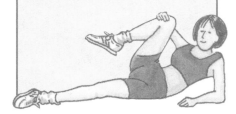

Studies have shown, however, that a chemotherapy agent called adriamycin can be toxic to the heart and interferes with CoQ_{10} in the body. Some researchers believe that supplementing with CoQ_{10} before chemotherapy may reduce the damage from this drug and possibly allow higher doses of adriamycin to be given to patients without causing dangerous side effects to the heart. Other researchers disagree, stating that supplementation with CoQ_{10} might reduce the effectiveness of adriamycin on cancer cells.

Coenzyme Q_{10} and Parkinson's Disease

Scientists are also looking at the effect of CoQ_{10} on Parkinson's disease. Some believe that this coenzyme may actually slow the progression of the disease. The U.S. government recently launched a study to compare three different doses of CoQ_{10} with a placebo in slowing the progression of Parkinson's disease.

Coenzyme Q_{10} and Other Potential Benefits

There are a number of alleged benefits of CoQ_{10} supplements, but the scientific research to support such claims is preliminary, contradictory, or significantly lacking at this time. Examples include the use of CoQ_{10} in periodontal disease, Alzheimer's disease, and improved immunity in HIV/AIDS. Some of the least convincing claims include the use of CoQ_{10} for weight loss, performance enhancement, and to delay the aging process.

Coenzyme Q_{10} in Food

Because CoQ_{10} is not an essential nutrient, there is no RDA. In addition to being produced in the body, CoQ_{10} is found in sardines, mackerel, nuts, organ meats, and vegetable oils. Frying appears to destroy some CoQ_{10}, but boiling does not. CoQ_{10} is fat-soluble, so it should be eaten with foods containing some fat. Other foods that contain CoQ_{10} are beef, broccoli, chicken, oranges, pork chops, salmon, and trout.

Caution!

- Supplementing with 30 to 200 milligrams per day of CoQ_{10} may be warranted for people with heart disease, especially those diagnosed with congestive heart failure or cardiomyopathy. Be sure, however, to talk to your doctor first.
- If you have cancer, consult with your doctor before taking CoQ_{10}.
- If you have a medical condition or are pregnant or lactating, talk to your doctor before taking any supplement.

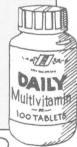

What to Know about Taking Lactase Supplements

- Several drops of liquid lactase added to milk can break down most or all of the lactose present.
- Oral lactase tablets can be taken before eating lactose-containing foods—read the directions on the package for specific dosing information.
- Since supplements are not reviewed by the FDA, quality control and potency problems may exist.

Who Is Most Susceptible to Lactose Maldigestion?

90 percent of Asian Americans
80 percent of African-Americans
62–100 percent of Native Americans
53 percent of Mexican Americans
15 percent of Caucasians

From the National Dairy Council's brochure on lactose intolerance and minorities.

When to Supplement with Coenzyme Q10

The Japanese were the first to take CoQ10 in supplement form and continue to do so today to treat heart failure patients. The supplement first began to garner attention in the United States in the mid-1980s, but there have been no long-term studies conducted for safety and efficacy. In most of the studies to date, supplementing with CoQ10 for up to one year has resulted in no major side effects, although some people have experienced mild gastrointestinal distress. It is not recommended for children.

Lactase

Lactase, an enzyme that is usually produced in the small intestine, is important for its role in breaking down the milk sugar, lactose.

The Benefits of Lactase

The primary benefit of lactase is its ability to break lactose down into simpler forms of sugar that can be absorbed into the bloodstream. When there is not enough lactase present, lactose maldigestion occurs.

The world's most prevalent disorder, lactose maldigestion affects 25 percent of the U.S. population (see "Who Is Most Susceptible to Lactose Maldigestion?"). Interestingly, levels of lactase seem to be highest in the people and regions where there was a long history of herding and domesticating animals and a reliance on these animals for food/milk. For instance, there is very little lactose maldigestion among people from northern Europe, such as Scandinavians, British, Dutch, Irish, French, Poles, Czechs, and northern Italians. The same is true for certain groups of people in the Middle East, including Bedouins, Saudis, and Yemenis. On the other hand, those who did not traditionally domesticate herd animals for food have higher rates of maldigestion, including Chinese, Koreans, Japanese, Jews, most Africans, and Native Americans.

Having lactose maldigestion does not necessarily mean you are lactose intolerant. What's the difference? In many population groups lactase activity begins to drop off between the ages of three and five years. This genetically controlled decline in lactase activity is called lactose maldigestion. Lactose intolerance, on the other hand, occurs when lactose is not digested and reaches the large intestine, where naturally present bacteria ferments it, leading to a variety of symptoms. These symptoms (cramps, gas, bloating, diarrhea, and abdominal pain) usually appear within 30 minutes to two hours after eating or drinking lactose-containing foods. Symptoms vary from person to person and depend on the type and amount of foods eaten.

Studies show that lactose intolerance is actually much less common than many believe. If you think you suffer from lactose maldigestion and/or intolerance, talk to your doctor. A simple blood test or breath hydrogen test can give you the answers you need. People who cannot digest lactose have more hydrogen in their exhaled breath than most people.

Certain medical conditions such as a stomach virus, a parasitic infection, or the use of antibiotics can temporarily wipe out the lactose-digesting bacteria in the intestines. However, over time, the bacteria usually return, and tolerance to milk and other dairy foods returns as well.

Lactase and Lactose in Food

Lactase is an enzyme that is present in the body or available in supplements. Lactose, on the other hand, is found in the food supply primarily in dairy products. Lactose is also added to processed foods such as baked goods, breakfast cereals, instant soup, instant potatoes, breakfast drinks, margarine, nonkosher luncheon meats, salad dressings, candies, and mixes for biscuits, pancakes, and cookies. Other foods that contain lactose are: ice cream/ice milk, milk (whole, low-fat, skim, buttermilk), processed cheese, sour cream, and yogurt.

When to Supplement with Lactase and Lactose

Many people who have problems digesting lactose tend to avoid dairy products, thereby decreasing the calcium content of their diets. Ironically, increasing consumption of lactose-containing foods, such as milk, actually helps lactose maldigestors build up tolerance to lactose. According to experts, drinking a little milk helps the digestive system learn to digest lactose without unpleasant side effects. Consuming dairy foods only once in a while may, in fact, increase symptoms because the digestive system isn't used to these foods. A number of factors,

Caution!

- If adjusting the amount and types of dairy foods does not alleviate lactose intolerance symptoms, you may want to try lactose-free or lactose-reduced dairy products. Another option is to use commercial lactase products such as chewable tablets, capsules, and solutions.
- If you have a medical condition or are pregnant or lactating, talk to your doctor before taking any supplement.

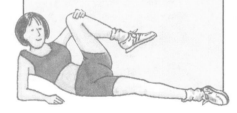

including the amount of lactose consumed at one time and whether or not lactose-containing foods are consumed alone or in a meal, can make a difference in symptoms.

One study showed that lactose maldigesters (many of whom described themselves as lactose intolerant) were able to consume the amount of lactose in two cups of milk, one at breakfast and the other at dinner, without any symptoms. If you suffer from lactose intolerance, try some of the following tips:

- Start with just $1/4$ or $1/2$ cup of milk, two to three times per day, and gradually increase the amount until symptoms begin to appear.
- Drink milk with a meal or a snack. The additional food slows the delivery of lactose to the large intestine, allowing more time for any lactase enzyme to digest it.
- Whole milk and chocolate milk are often better tolerated than lower fat and unflavored milk.
- Most people can tolerate yogurts made with live, active cultures.
- A number of different cheeses such as cheddar, Colby, Swiss, and parmesan, are low in lactose.

NADH

NADH or NAD (sometimes referred to as "coenzyme 1") is known scientifically as nicotinamide adenine dinucleotide. Available since 1995, the supplement is an enzyme form of the B vitamin niacin. NADH triggers energy production in the body, and without it the body would not be able to utilize fats and carbohydrates properly to obtain energy.

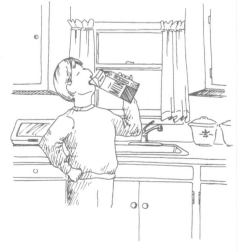

Caution!

- Most people have no need for additional amounts of NADH. What's more, all of the research with this enzyme is preliminary. Save your money until the benefits are proven and safety studies are more conclusive.
- If you have a medical condition or are pregnant or lactating, talk to your doctor before taking any supplement.

The Benefits of NADH

NADH and Chronic Fatigue Syndrome

Chronic fatigue syndrome (CFS) is a disorder characterized by prolonged, debilitating tiredness. A variety of other symptoms include mental dysfunction, weakness, low-grade fever, sore throat, headache, and sleep disturbances. A study conducted at DePaul University estimates that CFS is more common than previously thought, affecting 422 per 100,000 people. The cause of CFS is unknown, and to date there's no established, effective treatment.

A study published in 1999, however, indicates that NADH supplements may have a role in treating CFS. Twenty-six patients with CFS received either 10 milligrams of NADH or a placebo for one month. Eight of them (31 percent) responded favorably to NADH—achieving a 10 percent improvement in symptoms—compared with only two of those (8 percent) receiving the placebo. Minor side effects, including loss of appetite and flatulence (passing gas), were reported with NADH, but none of them caused the participants to drop out of the study. Since this was a small study, the researchers conducted a follow-up study and observed that after one and one-half years of NADH treatment, more than 80 percent of participants experienced improvement in their condition. Another, larger study is now planned.

The use of NADH for CFS is based on the fact that the enzyme is required for the generation of an energy-producing substance in the body. However, whether this substance is lacking in people with chronic fatigue syndrome hasn't been firmly established.

NADH and Other Potential Benefits

Very little published research is currently available on NADH; however, a number of studies are underway. Parkinson's disease is one condition where NADH supplements appear to reduce symptoms—especially in younger, more recently diagnosed patients. The supplement's possible effects on athletic endurance are also being investigated. Marketers of one NADH supplement claim that the enzyme may be beneficial in the treatment of Alzheimer's disease

What to Know about Taking NADH Supplements

- NADH, or nicotinamide adenine dinucleotide, is made in all tissues of the body, and is also one of the main dietary forms of the B vitamin niacin.
- NADH supplements are available in tablet form, in 2.5- to 5-milligram tablets.
- Talk with your doctor before taking NADH for these conditions to determine whether NADH supplements are appropriate for you, and in what dosage.
- Since dietary supplements are not reviewed by the FDA, quality control and potency problems may exist.

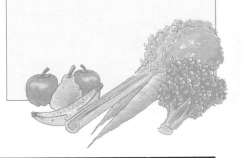

and depression, too. All of these areas of research are ongoing, and results of completed studies are still considered preliminary.

When to Supplement with NADH

People with CFS may wish to discuss NADH supplementation with their doctors, since no other treatments for the syndrome are available at this time. Suggested **therapeutic doses** of NADH for CFS (and Parkinson's disease) range from 5 to 10 milligrams per day.

NADH supplements appear to have few side effects and are believed to be safe. However, no long-term safety studies have been conducted. Children should not take NADH supplements.

Proteolytic (Digestive) Enzymes

There are a number of digestive enzymes available in supplement form. The simplest ones are from tropical fruits: bromelain (pronounced BRO-mah-lain) from pineapple and papain (pronounced PA-pain) from papayas. Enzymes are proteins, and the primary function of these two enzymes is to digest or break down other proteins, which is why they're sometimes called proteolytic enzymes. *Proteolytic* means "to break down proteins"—the suffix *lysis* means "dissolution" or "decomposition." The body makes its own digestive enzymes, too. The main ones are called trypsin (TRIP-sin) and chymotrypsin (KIE-mo-trip-sin). For supplements, trypsin and chymotrypsin are extracted from the pancreas of various animals.

The Benefits of Proteolytic Enzymes

Proteolytic Enzymes and Digestion

Ironically, the primary use for proteolytic enzymes—as digestive aids—is also the area where good research on their effects is lacking. Studies on bromelain suggest that the enzyme may be particularly helpful for digestion because, unlike most digestive enzymes, it's active in both the acidic environment of the stomach and the alkaline environment of the small intestine. Therefore, it can work longer than the other enzymes. A dose of 500 milligrams of bromelain, taken about an hour and a half before each meal, is suggested by some. Although the effect of proteolytic enzymes on digestion is less dramatic than those of comparable pharmaceutical products, they may help one feel less bloated after eating.

Proteolytic Enzymes and Inflammation

There is a growing body of research suggesting that proteolytic enzymes may help decrease bruising, swelling, and inflammation. The most convincing of these studies shows that bromelain brought about mild improvement in swelling of the nose and sinuses. Other related ailments for which proteolytic enzymes are suggested as a treatment—but for which research is scarce—include hemorrhoids and swelling of sutured areas after childbirth.

Proteolytic Enzymes and Arthritis

Arthritis is an area where the research on proteolytic enzymes shows great promise, but there just isn't enough of it yet to draw firm conclusions. A recent Austrian study of 73 people with osteoarthritis of the knee found that those who received a bromelain-containing enzyme mixture experienced a reduction of pain and improvement in knee motion equal to those who received a typical **nonsteroidal anti-inflammatory drug (NSAID)**. The researchers point out that those who received the bromelain did not suffer from the side effects that the NSAID group did, making bromelain a viable alternative to traditional osteoarthritis treatment. Although this study lasted only three weeks, unpublished data from trials lasting up to four years suggest that bromelain is also well tolerated when taken for long periods of time.

Rheumatoid arthritis, which is an autoimmune disorder and not an inflammatory one like osteoarthritis, is another condition under investigation with regard to proteolytic enzymes. Currently, however, there is no real evidence that the enzymes are at all effective in easing the symptoms of rheumatoid arthritis.

Proteolytic Enzymes and Blood Thinning

Bromelain inhibits blood platelets from sticking or clumping together (coagulating). This effect is well documented and is consid-

Caution!

- Healthy people don't need proteolytic enzyme supplements. However, they may be helpful for osteoarthritis (in place of, or in addition to, traditional medicine) or instead of daily aspirin therapy for blood thinning. Don't begin changing your current medical treatments until you've consulted your doctor.
- Because of their anticoagulant property, if you're taking blood-thinning medications (including aspirin therapy), you should consult your doctor before using proteolytic enzyme supplements.
- Consult your doctor about the need for extra folate if you take pancreatin, since the enzyme can interfere with folate absorption.
- If you have gastrointestinal ulcers, proteolytic enzymes may cause further tissue damage.
- If you have a medical condition or are pregnant or lactating, talk to your doctor before taking any supplement.

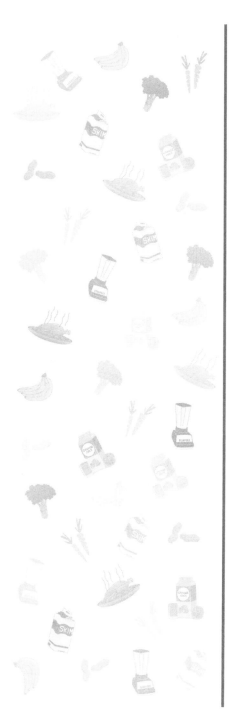

ered to be one of the main medical benefits of the enzyme. In fact, both animal and human studies indicate that bromelain therapy even helps prevent **thrombosis**—the formation of a blood clot—which can lead to a heart attack or stroke if the blood clot blocks arteries to the heart or brain.

Proteolytic Enzymes and Other Potential Benefits

Some alternative medicine practitioners credit proteolytic enzymes with the ability to positively affect a wide variety of health conditions, including food allergies, autoimmune disorders, and breast cancer. In addition, two small studies of athletes suggest that the enzymes can speed the healing of mild sports injuries and bruises. At this time, however, there is not enough evidence to recommend proteolytic enzymes for any of these problems. Finally, steer clear of weight loss and "fat absorber" pills containing bromelain or other proteolytic enzymes—they're completely ineffective and a waste of money. They are not recommended for children.

When to Supplement with Proteolytic Enzymes

There is no physiological need for supplemental proteolytic enzymes, except in rare cases when the pancreas is unable to manufacture them. These supplements have yet to become popular in the United States, although they are widely used in Europe. Perhaps the way they are frequently marketed in this country—as "digestive aids"—isn't especially appealing to consumers. What's more, this function may not even be the enzymes' best benefit. It appears that the most promising properties of proteolytic enzymes are their anticoagulant and anti-inflammatory abilities, although much additional research needs to be done before they're widely accepted for these purposes.

In general, proteolytic enzymes are believed to be quite safe, except perhaps in the case of gastrointestinal ulcers, where there are concerns that the enzymes' digestive capabilities may further irritate exposed tissue. And, although there are numerous pharmaceutical products available that can do the same jobs as proteolytic enzymes, the enzymes generally seem to be free of side effects, while some pharmaceutical products have well known side effects. This is a factor that may be important for some people. Proteolytic enzymes are not recommended for children.

CHAPTER 6

Essential Fatty Acids

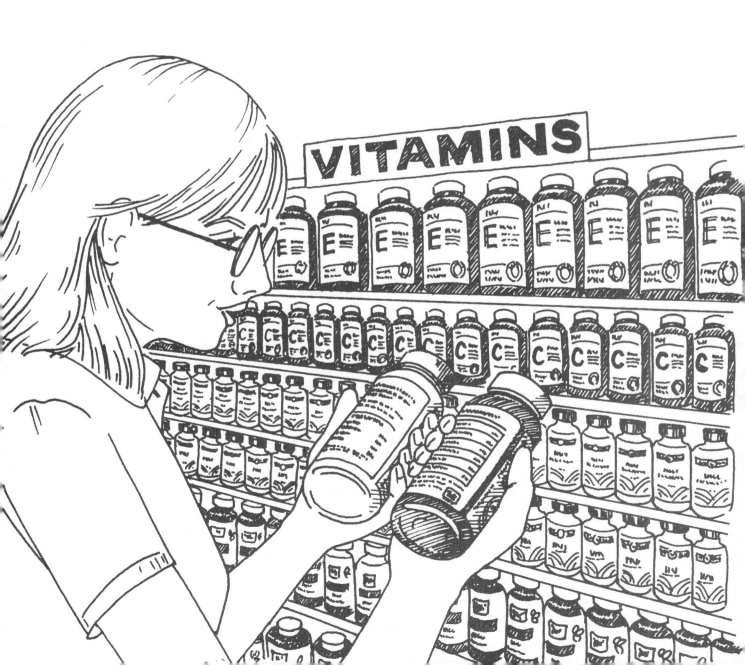

Essential fatty acids are **polyunsaturated fatty acids** (a chain of carbon atoms with hydrogens attached—the type of fats that can help lower LDL, or the "bad" cholesterol). Essential fatty acids cannot be produced by the human body, and, therefore, must be obtained from the diet. These include alpha-linolenic acid (ALA), an omega-3 fatty acid, and linoleic acid (LA), an omega-6 fatty acid. ALA is found in foods such as cold-water fatty fish, walnuts, flaxseed, and leafy green vegetables. LA is found in vegetable oils such as safflower and corn oils.

In the body, alpha-linolenic turns into the long-chain omega-3 fatty acids eicosapentaenoic acid (EPA) and docosahexaenoic acid (DHA). Likewise, linoleic acid can form the long-chain omega-6 fatty acids, gamma-linoleic acid (GLA), dihomogamma-linolenic acid (DGLA), and arachidonic acid (AA). Researchers are studying these fatty acids for potential health benefits. DHA, for instance, may help reduce the risk of heart disease and stroke.

As structural components of membranes, essential fatty acids help form a barrier that keeps foreign molecules, viruses, yeasts, fungi, and bacteria outside of the body's cells, and the cell's proteins, enzymes, genetic material, and organelles (small organs) inside. They also help regulate the traffic of substances in and out of cells via protein channels, pumps, and other mechanisms. Essential fatty acids are required for normal growth and development and should be included in the diet, especially the diets of pregnant women, children, and premature and full-term infants.

Over the years, intakes of omega-6 fatty acids in the United States have risen, while intakes of omega-3 fatty acids have fallen (see "The Rise and Fall of the Omegas" on page 200). This is partly due to the fact that Americans eat more processed foods, which are typically higher in omega-6 fatty acids than in omega-3 fatty acids. This change in the balance of intakes of fatty acids poses a potential problem with regard to health. Although omega-6 fatty acids lower blood levels of total cholesterol and LDL ("bad" cholesterol), one particular omega-6 long-chain fatty acid, called arachidonic acid, may actually increase the risk of heart disease by promoting vasoconstriction (constriction of the arteries) and platelet aggregation or "stickiness." Moreover, omega-6 fatty acids

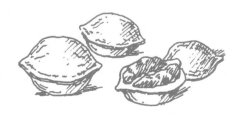

can also interfere with the conversion of ALA into EPA and DHA—by as much as 40 percent. Therefore, experts recommend replacing some of the omega-6 fatty acids in the diet with omega-3 fatty acids.

Most of the research on essential fatty acids has focused on the omega-3 family of fats. Therefore, the remainder of this chapter will primarily highlight the potential health benefits of alpha-linolenic acid and its derivatives, DHA and EPA.

The Benefits of Essential Fatty Acids

Essential Fatty Acids and Cardiovascular Disease

Since the 1970s, experts have known that people living in fishing populations in Alaska, Greenland, and Japan have lower rates of coronary heart disease, despite the high fat content of their diets. It turns out that, although the fat content of their diets is similar to the U.S. diet, their intakes of EPA and DHA (from marine fish and mammals) are significantly higher. These particular long-chain omega-3 fatty acids have been shown to reduce triglyceride levels, increase HDL (the "good" cholesterol) levels, lower blood pressure, and reduce platelet reactivity—all of which can reduce the risk of heart disease and stroke.

In a study of individuals who had previously had a heart attack, those who followed a Mediterranean diet—lots of plant foods, nuts, and fish—rich in alpha-linolenic acid (ALA) experienced nearly a 70 percent reduction in repeat heart attacks and cardiac deaths. These results were achieved without a decrease in blood cholesterol and triglyceride levels, compared to a control group who ate a typical Western diet that was not high in ALA.

Similar findings were seen in the Health Professionals Follow-up Study, in which men who consumed a greater percentage of calories from ALA had a lower risk of heart attack and cardiac deaths. Comparable findings have also been seen in women.

In another study, researchers gave more than 11,000 Italians, who had recently had heart attacks and were taking medication, daily supplements of 1 gram of fish oil, 300 milligrams of vitamin E, both, or neither. After three-and-a-half years, those who supplemented with

ALA, DHA, and EPA

ALA, or alpha-linolenic acid, is the omega-3 fatty acid found in plant foods such as walnuts, flax, and algae. ALA converts to DHA and EPA in the body. However, you can get DHA and EPA directly from fish such as salmon, mackerel, and sardines. There is a lot of interest from the scientific community in the potential health benefits of DHA and EPA. As a result, many supplement manufacturers are now selling DHA supplements. Until more data is collected, though, you're better off increasing the amount of omega-3 fatty acids in your diet by simply eating more fish and plant foods. It may likely turn out, for instance, that we need *both* EPA and DHA in order to reap the health benefits.

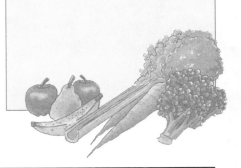

Caution!

- Americans get more than enough omega-6 fatty acids in their diets, but could use more omega-3 fatty acids. If you can't reach recommended levels, you might want to consider a supplement.
- Fish oils act as a blood thinner. Therefore, if you are on any kind of anticoagulation medication (including aspirin) or have a clotting disorder, talk to your doctor before supplementing with omega-3 fatty acids. Additionally, if you are supplementing with vitamin E, garlic, or gingko biloba, talk to your physician as well, since these supplements also act as blood thinners.
- Individuals prone to falls or undergoing surgery should not take omega-3 fatty acid supplements.
- If you have a medical condition or are pregnant or lactating, talk to your doctor before taking any supplement.

fish oil experienced 15 percent fewer heart attacks, strokes, and deaths than the controls. Interestingly, the group who took vitamin E did not have a significant reduction in risk. The researchers suggest that this may have been because the vitamin E dose was too low, because the study was too short, or because the Italians were already eating a vitamin E–rich Mediterranean diet.

Data from looking at the relationship between fatty acids and disease indicates that omega-3 fatty acids typically provide a slight increase in HDL and a marked decrease in triglycerides, and have no consistent effect on LDL. The big story, however, may be the effect of omega-3 fatty acids on inflammation and thrombosis (clot formation) in the development of coronary heart disease—an area that has only recently been studied. And, it is in this arena that omega-3 fatty acids have the most potential to affect coronary heart disease (CHD) risk.

Atherosclerosis, which is essentially the buildup of cholesterol on the arterial walls, is a type of CHD involving a number of different processes. One process that has been examined is the "response to injury." Initially, there is an injury to the arterial wall; then, platelet aggregation or clumping occurs, followed by cholesterol deposition and plaque formation. This can then lead to a heart attack or stroke. Preliminary research indicates that omega-3 fatty acids may interfere at several points in this process, resulting in a decreased risk of stroke and heart attack.

Omega-3 fatty acids may also protect against arrhythmias (abnormal heart rhythms), the leading cause of death after heart attacks. Every year in the United States, nearly a quarter million people die within one hour of having a heart attack, mostly due to arrhythmias. Omega-3 fatty acids may provide protection by enhancing the stability of the heart cells and increasing their resistance to becoming overexcited. In the Physicians' Health Study, those who ate fish just one to two times per week had a 40 percent reduction in sudden deaths from cardiac arrhythmias.

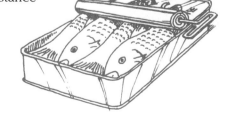

Essential Fatty Acids and Blood Pressure

Several studies have looked at the role of omega-3 fatty acids in blood pressure. The findings indicate that high doses of fish oil can reduce both systolic (the top number in a blood pressure reading) and diastolic (the bottom number) blood pressure in individuals with mildly elevated blood pressure. Some experts believe it may be the DHA component of fish oil that is exerting the protective effects.

Essential Fatty Acids and Cancer

Omega-3 fatty acids may also play an important role in the prevention and treatment of cancer. Animal studies show that omega-3 fatty acids may delay tumor formation and decrease the rate of growth, size, and number of tumors. In studies with mice, omega-3 fatty aids in fish oil appear to increase the sensitivity of cancer cells to oxidative damage by certain chemotherapy drugs, which in turn causes the cells to die. However, normal cells are able to protect themselves from this damage.

In humans, researchers have found that the omega-3 fatty acid ALA in breast fat tissue may help reduce tumor metastasis, or spreading. Low levels of alpha-linolenic acid in breast tissue near the site of the cancer was associated with increased risk of lymph node involvement and the spread of cancer.

In an Italian study, researchers compared the diets of 10,000 people with various cancers to those of 8,000 people without cancer over a 13-year period. At the end of the study, researchers found that those who ate fish once a week had a 20 to 30 percent lower risk of cancers of the mouth, stomach, esophagus, pancreas, colon, and rectum than those who ate less than one serving of fish per week. The risk of cancer was reduced even further, to 30 to 50 percent, in people who ate two or more servings of fish per week. The researchers suggest that the protective effect of the fish may be due to its omega-3 fatty acid content. Although these findings are intriguing, much more research is needed.

Essential Fatty Acids and Infant Growth and Development

The role of omega-3 and omega-6 fatty acids in pregnancy has only recently been studied in humans. Because the greatest amount

Vegetarians and Omega-3s

Just because you don't eat fish doesn't mean you have to supplement with omega-3 fatty acids. Foods such as walnuts, walnut oil, flaxseed, flaxseed oil, canola oil, and dark green, leafy vegetables all provide alpha-linolenic acid, which can convert into DHA and EPA in the body.

of DHA accumulation occurs during the last trimester of pregnancy, the amount of DHA available to premature infants is critical. Prior to the 1990s, infant formula in the United States did not contain alpha-linolenic acid (ALA), much less AA, EPA, or DHA, whereas breastmilk contains all of the essential fatty acids. Studies show that infants fed DHA-rich formula develop visual acuity faster than those fed standard formula.

Experts now agree that omega-3 fatty acids, and DHA in particular, are essential for optimal development of the nervous system and eyesight in both premature and full-term infants. Unfortunately, simply adding ALA to formula may not be enough. Very low birth weight infants are unable to convert ALA into sufficient quantities of EPA or DHA. As a result, several manufacturers are now working on formulas that will contain DHA.

Essential Fatty Acids and Depression

Preliminary but exciting new research suggests that omega-3 fatty acids may help decrease symptoms of bipolar disorder (or manic depression). Researchers at Harvard University observed 30 men and women with the disorder for four months. Half the group was given seven fish oil capsules twice a day (totaling nearly 10 grams of fish oil per day), while the other half of the group received a placebo. At the end of the study, nine of the 14 people who took the fish oil pills reported relief of symptoms, compared to only three of the 16 who received the placebo.

The researchers suggest that omega-3 fats may interfere with the brain signals that trigger the characteristic mood swings seen with bipolar disorder. Interestingly, the investigators reported unusually high patient interest and acceptance of omega-3 fatty acids as mood stabilizers. The supplements were viewed as "natural" compounds with few side effects. If these findings hold true in future studies, omega-3 fatty acids may have implications for treating other psychiatric disorders such as depression and schizophrenia.

Essential Fatty Acids and Other Potential Benefits

Preliminary research indicates that omega-3 fatty acids may inhibit the inflammatory process, thereby aiding in the treatment of

---

What to Know About Omega-6 Fatty Acids

Omega-6 fatty acids are found primarily in vegetable oils such as soybean, sunflower, corn, cottonseed, and safflower oils. These types of oils are commonly used in processed foods such as crackers, cookies, mayonnaise, and salad dressings. Try to limit intake to 6 grams per day, or no more than four times the omega-3 intake.

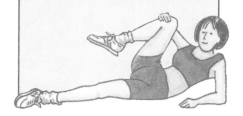

inflammatory diseases such as rheumatoid arthritis, psoriasis, ulcerative colitis, and autoimmune disorders. And, researchers have begun to look at possible benefits of omega-3 fatty acids on premenstrual syndrome. Scientists in Denmark studied the effects of 2 grams of fish oil capsules per day, compared to 2 grams of another fat, in 42 female adolescents. Those who received the fish oil reported greater relief from symptoms. Although both of these areas of research show promise, much more is needed.

Omega-3 Fatty Acids in Food

Omega-3 fatty acids are found in cold-water fatty fish, walnuts, walnut oil, flaxseed, canola, soybeans, leafy green vegetables, and the seeds of most plants. Just two to three servings of fatty fish per week provide approximately 3 grams of fish oil. If you choose to use fish oil supplements, be sure to buy capsules that state "distilled" or "molecularly distilled" on the label. This will assure you that the oil inside does not contain contaminants such as mercury, PCBs, and lead, which have a tendency to accumulate in some fish.

See the table below for more food sources of omega-3.

FOOD SOURCES OF OMEGA-3 FATTY ACIDS

FOOD SOURCES (100 GRAM SERVINGS)	ALA (GRAMS/SERVING)	EPA (GRAMS/SERVING)	DHA (GRAMS/SERVING)
Butternuts, dried	8.7	0	0
Walnuts, English	6.8	0	0
Walnuts, black	3.3	0	0
Soybeans, green, raw	3.2	0	0
Soybean sprouts, cooked	2.1	0	0
Soybean kernels, roasted	1.5	0	0
Sardines, canned, drained	0.5	0.4	0.6
Purslane	0.4	0	0
Lake trout	0.4	0.5	1.1
Beans, navy, pinto, cooked	0.3	0	0
Salmon, chinook	0.1	0.8	0.6
Pacific herring	0.1	1.0	0.7
Atlantic sturgeon	Trace	1.0	0.5
Bluefin tuna	0	0.4	1.2

What to Know about Taking Omega-3 Fatty Acid Supplements

- The fish oil used in supplements comes from sardines, tuna, salmon, or anchovies, and is sold in softgel capsules or as a liquid oil. Manufacturers are now also selling concentrated sources of DHA and EPA.

- Store the supplements in the refrigerator.

- Supplements provide 180 to 300 milligrams of EPA and 120 to 200 milligrams of DHA per capsule, with an RDA ranging from 1 to 10 grams.

- Although there is no set upper limit for omega-3 fatty acids, the FDA concluded that intakes of up to 3 grams of DHA and EPA per day from fish oil are safe. Some people experience a fishy smell and gastrointestinal upset when taking fish oil supplements.

- High intakes of fish oil can cause nosebleeds, easy bruising, and an increased risk of bleeding in the brain, or stroke.

The Rise and Fall of the Omegas

Both omega-6 and omega-3 fatty acids are essential for good health, and it's important to get them in balanced amounts. In the past century, consumption of omega-6 has grown significantly.

New technologies expanded the vegetable oil industry and increased consumption of linoleic-rich oils. At the same time, alpha-linolenic acid content was reduced in soybean and canola oils because of flavor problems, which also prevented the large-scale use of flaxseed (or linseed) oil. The use of vegetable oils, which supply omega-6 and lower serum cholesterol, led to an increase in fat in the diet and an increase in omega-6 at the expense of omega-3.

Today's fish are raised via aquaculture and contain less omega-3 fatty acid because they don't have access to omega-3-rich microalgae—the source of DHA in the food chain. Also, animals are now raised on feeds that are high in omega-6 and short on omega-3. It's no wonder consumption of omega-3 has declined!

When to Supplement with Omega-3 Fatty Acids

Although there are no formal recommended intakes for essential fatty acids in the United States, many experts believe that an optimal intake for omega-3 fatty acids is 800 to 1,100 milligrams per day for alpha-linolenic, and 300 to 400 milligrams per day for both EPA and DHA (the equivalent to about two fatty fish servings per week). The current American diet generally provides only 50 milligrams EPA and 80 milligrams DHA per person per day. As you might expect, the best way to improve your intake of omega-3 fatty acids is to make healthy changes in your diet (see "Food Sources of Omega-3 Fatty Acids").

The concept of essential fatty acid deficiency is well known, yet its incidence has been considered to be rare and limited to premature infants and patients with severe malabsorption, short bowel syndrome, or those only receiving food intravenously. Symptoms of essential fatty acid deficiency include impaired growth, abnormal skin and hair, impaired immune function, liver and kidney disease, and premature death. Until recently, essential fatty acid deficiencies were rarely identified because of low methodological sensitivity—in other words, the deficiency was below all methods of detection. With the advent of new technology, EFA deficiency or insufficiency may be redefined.

However, as a result of a lack of deficiency identification, the role of essential fatty acids in the cause of coronary heart disease, for example, was dismissed and emphasis shifted to decreasing dietary saturated fat and cholesterol. Many argue that current clinical emphasis on restricting dietary saturated fat and cholesterol is misplaced, and that it's the sufficient level of essential fatty acids that regulates the balance of saturated fat in the cells and blood cholesterol.

The USDA Dietary Guidelines for Americans advocate a low-fat diet, with the bulk of the calories coming from pastas, breads, and grains. These foods contain few, if any, essential fatty acids. And, essential fatty acids are difficult to obtain in processed foods, as food manufacturers generally remove them from plant products because they shorten shelf life. Ideally, people should eat foods that are low in fat and saturated fat, high in essential fatty acids, and that provide protein, fiber, vitamins, and minerals.

CHAPTER 7

Fiber

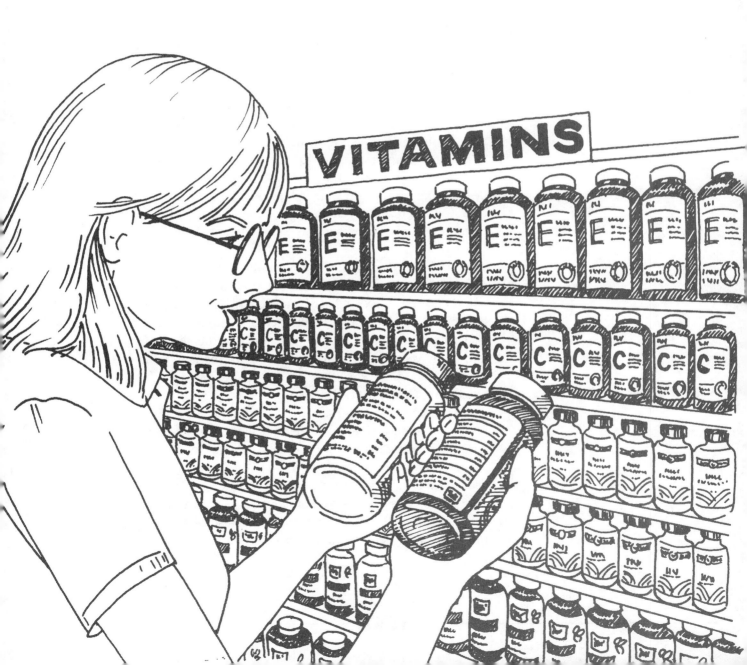

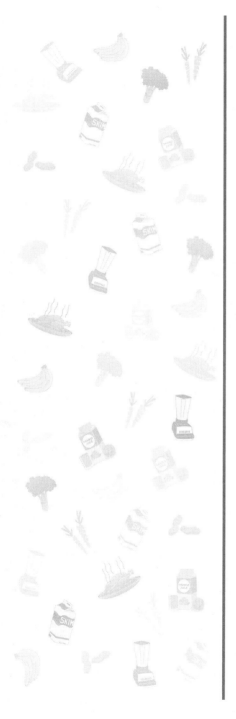

Fiber Facts

Nutrition experts recommend getting 20 to 35 grams of **dietary fiber** every day. However, most Americans eat only 14 to 15 grams a day. Fiber is found only in plant foods, such as fruits, vegetables, and grains, and it's the part of the plant that is not digested in the human body. There are two types of dietary fiber—soluble and insoluble. Both forms are necessary for good health. Most foods rich in dietary fiber contain both soluble and insoluble forms.

Soluble fiber is the "sticky" form of fiber that thickens the contents of the intestines, thereby slowing the digestion/absorption process and making you feel full for a longer period of time. Soluble fiber also appears to play a protective role against diabetes and heart disease. Examples of soluble fiber sources include pectin, gums, and mucilages, found in peas, dried beans, some fruits and vegetables (oranges, apples and carrots), oats and oat bran, psyllium, flaxseed, and barley, as well as canned peas or beans such as kidney beans, white beans, and black beans.

Insoluble fiber aids in the prevention of constipation, **diverticulosis**, hemorrhoids, and some forms of cancer such as colon and rectal. Examples of insoluble fiber include cellulose, hemicellulose, and lignin, found in whole grains and cereals—especially wheat bran, barley, and oats, and the skins of fruits and many vegetables (cauliflower, green beans, and potatoes).

Fiber and Heart Disease

High blood cholesterol is a risk factor for heart disease. Studies have shown that soluble fiber can lower total blood cholesterol (TC) levels by 2 to 6 percent, and low-density lipoprotein (LDL or "bad" cholesterol) levels by 2 to 29 percent in people with normal or high cholesterol levels. High intakes of some soluble fibers, such as dried beans and oat bran, can lower TC and LDL levels significantly, even in people whose diets contain as much as 37 percent of calories from fat.

Fiber and Diabetes

Researchers at the University of Texas Southwestern Medical Center in Dallas studied the effect of fiber on 13 **obese** individuals with Type 2 diabetes (non-insulin-dependent diabetes). After consuming a high fiber diet (50 grams of fiber—half soluble and half insoluble), the study participants experienced lowered glucose (blood sugar) levels, by as much as 10 percent, and lower insulin and blood lipid levels. The results from this study support previous findings.

Fiber and Cancer

Can fiber reduce the risk of colon cancer, too? According to recent headlines—no. In two different studies, researchers looked at the effects of fiber on adenomatous polyps, or growths from which colon cancer often develops. Many expected the studies to show that a high fiber diet would result in fewer polyps—it didn't. So does this mean we should forgo our fiber?

No. Because colon cancer develops over many years, a longer time frame for the studies may have been needed. In addition, not all adenomatous polyps eventually turn into cancer. It's possible that fiber plays a role later in the cancer process, by slowing or preventing benign adenoma growths from becoming cancerous. The type of fiber may also make a difference. In an Italian study, colorectal cancer was reduced by 32 percent in people who ate more vegetable fiber rather than fruit or cereal fiber.

What's more, although fiber may not be the magic pill for cancer, it has been shown in numerous studies to reduce the risk of heart disease, diabetes, and high blood pressure. And the benefits of fiber go beyond life-threatening diseases—it is essential for normal function of the gastrointestinal tract.

Chitosan

Chitin (KITE-in) is a substance that comes from the shells of crustaceans such as shrimp, lobster, and crab. When chemically treated, chitin becomes chitosan, which has the ability to bind fat and prevent its absorption. Some marketers claim that chitosan-containing

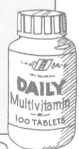

How to Increase Your Fiber Intake

- Eat more fruits, vegetables, grains, and cereals. The National Cancer Institute recommends getting at least *five* servings of fruits and vegetables a day—they're high in fiber and fat-free.
- Eat *whole* vegetables and fruits, since much of the fiber is in the skin.
- Look for whole-grain breads and cereals such as psyllium, oat bran, oatmeal, whole wheat pasta, etc.
- If you're still having trouble meeting your fiber needs, you might want to consider a supplement.

products not only aid in weight loss, but can decrease cholesterol levels as well.

The Benefits of Chitosan

Chitosan and Weight Loss

In theory, taking chitosan supplements should aid weight loss because it absorbs fat. Unfortunately, two recent studies have found that this is not the case. In a study conducted in Europe, 30 overweight volunteers who received four capsules of either chitosan or a placebo for 28 consecutive days were told to eat their normal diet. At the end of the four weeks, neither group had lost weight. In another study that lasted eight weeks, the chitosan-supplemented group had no greater weight loss than those taking the placebo.

If chitosan does absorb some fat, then why don't these supplements help people lose weight? First of all, the capsules absorb only tiny amounts of fat. For example, a 400 milligram capsule of chitosan, taken three times per day (as many products specify), would only absorb about 4.8 grams of fat—roughly equal to 43 calories of fat. That's not much, considering that an average jelly doughnut contains nearly 16 grams of fat.

Chitosan and Cholesterol

Some of the same studies that examined chitosan and weight loss also looked at the ability of the supplements to lower cholesterol levels. Again, the amount of chitosan present in the supplements was too small to have an effect on cholesterol levels.

When to Supplement with Chitosan

Although chitosan-containing supplements are safe, there's no scientific evidence that shows they'll aid in weight loss or cholesterol reduction. In fact, manufacturers and marketers of these products have recently come under fire for advertising unsubstantiated claims for chitosan supplements.

In 1997, the maker of a chitosan product sold in the United Kingdom was cited for advertising the product's ability to prevent

Caution!

- Don't bother with chitosan supplements—they don't work and there are too many potential drawbacks associated with their use.
- Avoid taking chitosan supplements if you have a shellfish allergy.
- If you have a medical condition or are pregnant or lactating, talk to your doctor before taking any supplement.
- Chitosan supplements are not "magic bullets," as many weight loss ads may say, and they may not help you lose weight at all. But, they are safe. What works? The tried and true methods—eating less and exercising more.

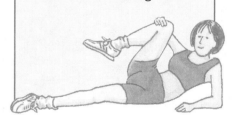

weight gain. The British Advertising Standards Authority concluded that there wasn't enough evidence that the product absorbed enough dietary fat to affect energy balance in humans, and the company had to change their advertising pitch.

In the United States, various marketers of chitosan capsules have been forced by the Federal Trade Commission to refund money to purchasers of their products. In addition, these companies are no longer permitted to make unsubstantiated advertising claims for their supplements. Some of these claims included weight control without dieting or exercise, prevention of fat absorption (they don't completely eliminate all fat absorption), increased metabolism, and the "burning" of fat.

Another point to consider when evaluating whether or not to take chitosan supplements is the supplement's impact on fat-soluble nutrients and fat-containing medications. Because the supplement binds with all types of fat, it has the ability to impair the absorption of fat-soluble vitamins (A, D, E, and K) as well as certain beneficial phytochemicals and valuable fatty acids, such as omega-3 fatty acids found in fish. Chitosan may also affect the absorption of fat-based medications, including birth-control pills, steroids, hormone replacements, and some cholesterol-lowering drugs, if it's present in the digestive system at the same time. Chitosan supplements are not recommended for children. Finally, keep in mind that anything that prevents absorption of fat can result in gas, bloating, and diarrhea.

Oat Bran

The bran of the oat grain is the outermost layer of the oat kernel. This layer is where much of the fiber and many nutrients are located. Whole oats and products made with whole oats contain the bran, but some processed oat products require the removal of this layer.

The late 1980s saw oat bran rise from relative obscurity to "super food" status when research revealed that it was an effective cholesterol reducer. Media attention and skyrocketing sales of oatmeal and oat bran products, as well as a rapid increase in scien-

What to Know about Taking Chitosan-Containing Supplements

- Chitosan is available in capsules or tablets and may also be an ingredient in other weight loss products.
- Do not exceed the manufacturer's recommended dosage.
- In order to bind fat, chitosan supplements must be present in the digestive system at the same time as fat-containing foods, so supplements should be taken with meals.
- Consider taking a multivitamin in order to offset some of the nutrient losses that may occur when taking chitosan supplements. Do not take the multivitamin at the same time as the chitosan.
- Since dietary supplements are not reviewed by the FDA, quality control and potency problems may exist.

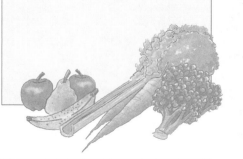

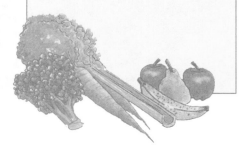

tific attention to the once lowly oat, carried oat bran to nationwide fame. Then, just as quickly, oat bran fell from popularity. Why? A Harvard University study was released that indicated that oat bran eaters were no better off than those who ate white flour products—as far as cholesterol was concerned. The public response was swift and definite. Sales of oat bran–containing products plummeted.

This dramatic public response to oat bran, dubbed by some as the "oat bran craze," was unfortunate but typical. Foods—and supplements—are not "magic bullets" or quick cures. However, in the case of oat bran and oat products in general, there's still much to recommend.

The Benefits of Oat Bran

Oat Bran and Cholesterol Reduction

Despite the contradictory Harvard study and the considerable loss of public interest in oat bran, it still is an excellent source of soluble fiber, which has been repeatedly shown to help decrease blood cholesterol levels when consumed in adequate amounts. Keeping blood cholesterol levels in control (preferably less than 200 milligrams/deciliter) is important for a healthy heart and circulatory system. Excess cholesterol in the blood can clog arteries and lead to heart attack and stroke.

In 1992, an analysis of 10 research studies on oat bran and oatmeal showed that eating 3 grams of soluble fiber per day (the amount contained in two bowls of oatmeal or one cup of cooked oat bran) reduced cholesterol moderately—by six points in three months. The authors note that the higher the blood cholesterol levels, the more dramatic the results observed from oat products. Other researchers have found that the benefits of oat bran drop considerably in people whose cholesterol level is less than 180 milligrams/deciliter. Numerous additional studies on oat products have found that the cholesterol-lowering effect of soluble fiber not only reduces total blood cholesterol concentrations, but targets LDL (the so-called bad cholesterol) specifically, while leaving HDL (good cholesterol) alone. Incidentally, these results are also seen with other soluble fiber sources, such as pectin and psyllium.

Based on the amount of research that shows overwhelmingly that oat products produce a moderate decline in cholesterol levels when eaten regularly, the FDA announced in 1997 that food manufacturers who used oats in their products could make the health claim, "May reduce the risk of heart disease," on their products.

How does soluble fiber lower cholesterol? It's quite complicated, and there is some scientific disagreement over the mechanism of this effect. However, a simple explanation is this: the effective soluble fiber in oats (and also in barley), called beta-glucan, forms a gel that traps bile acids, which contain a lot of cholesterol, and carries them out of the body. In response, your liver makes more bile acids, which requires it to take more cholesterol out of your blood. Research into how fiber consumption (both soluble and insoluble) helps decrease cardiovascular disease risk is ongoing.

Oat Bran in Food

Whole oats have their bran layer still intact and therefore are a good source of oat bran. Whether you choose steel-cut oats (the most roughly cut and least processed), rolled or "old-fashioned" oats, quick oats, or instant oats is your choice. All types of oats are effective at reducing cholesterol. Keep in mind that you need to eat more oats and oatmeal than oat bran, which is concentrated. Oat bran that is removed from the whole oat is sold in the cereal aisle of the supermarket, alongside the oatmeal, and in health food stores.

In order for an oat-containing food product label to make the claim that it helps lower cholesterol and prevent heart disease, the food must contain at least three-quarters of a gram of soluble fiber in one serving.

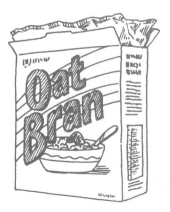

To get the daily 3 grams of soluble fiber recommended for cholesterol lowering, you'll need to eat:

2 ounces of oat bran ($2/3$ cup dry or about $1^1/2$ cups cooked)
or
3 ounces of oatmeal (1 cup dry or 2 cups cooked)

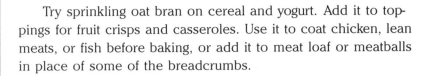

Try sprinkling oat bran on cereal and yogurt. Add it to toppings for fruit crisps and casseroles. Use it to coat chicken, lean meats, or fish before baking, or add it to meat loaf or meatballs in place of some of the breadcrumbs.

When to Supplement with Oat Bran

This is one of the few supplements that could be helpful for nearly everyone. Most Americans don't get nearly enough fiber in their diets, and many of us can use all the help we can get to lower our cholesterol levels. Also, although eating oatmeal and other oat bran–containing products is desirable because foods contain other things we need, such as nutrients and phytochemicals, taking an oat bran supplement is an inexpensive, quick, and easy way to get some additional soluble fiber. However, it is not recommended for children.

Psyllium

Psyllium (pronounced SIL-lee-um) is a plant used as a grain, similar to corn, wheat, and oats. A natural fiber, psyllium comes from the seed husks of *Plantago ovata,* a weedlike plant grown in the Mediterranean and India. Psyllium is made up of 86 percent dietary fiber (71 percent is soluble fiber and 15 percent is insoluble), 5 percent protein, 3 percent fat, and insignificant amounts of vitamins and minerals. In fact, psyllium has 14 times more soluble fiber than the once highly touted oat bran. It is this high amount of soluble fiber that has led researchers to investigate its effect on cholesterol levels.

Psyllium Health Claim

The benefits of soluble fiber, and psyllium in particular, are so great that the FDA announced in 1998 that it would allow foods containing psyllium to make a health claim. Foods such as certain breakfast cereals that contain soluble fiber from psyllium seed husk (PSH) may claim that, as part of a diet low in saturated fat and

---

What to Know about Taking Oat Bran Supplements

- Oat bran is available both in grain form and in supplement form as a tablet.
- Adding oat bran specifically to your diet, or taking oat bran supplements, will probably be more effective than eating baked goods (breads, muffins, etc.) containing oat bran. Most baked goods contain very little oat bran, and may also contain high amounts of fat and calories.
- Getting at least 3 grams of soluble fiber per day is recommended for the best cholesterol-lowering effects.
- Because dietary supplements are not reviewed by the FDA, quality control and potency problems may exist with oat bran supplements.

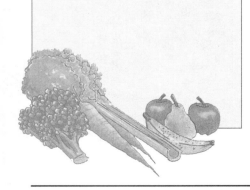

cholesterol, they may reduce the risk of coronary heart disease. This health claim is an amendment to the earlier health claim allowing products containing whole oats to advertise that the soluble fiber in whole oats can reduce the risk of heart disease.

Foods carrying the psyllium health claim must provide at least 1.7 grams of soluble fiber from PSH per serving.

Some foods containing psyllium can potentially cause dangerous blockages in the throat or intestines. Therefore, foods carrying the health claim must also have a label statement advising the need to consume foods with adequate amounts of liquid and to avoid eating the food if one has difficulty swallowing.

The Benefits of Psyllium
Psyllium and Heart Disease

Approximately 52 million Americans have elevated cholesterol levels. A number of studies have reported a significant decline in death due to coronary heart disease (CHD) as a result of lowering blood cholesterol levels in the population. Reductions in total cholesterol of as little as 3 percent could reduce CHD deaths in the United States by as much as 6 to 12 percent, potentially affecting as many as 840,000 lives per year.

Over the past 30 years, more than 55 studies have linked psyllium intake to blood cholesterol. Only three of these studies did not show a reduction in cholesterol levels. The studies ranged in duration from as little as nine days to as long as 29 months and showed a cholesterol-lowering effect on people with diets at varying fat levels.

A recent analysis of 12 studies, involving 404 adults, looked at the effects of about 10 grams of psyllium per day (providing approximately 7 grams of soluble fiber). People who ate psyllium-enriched cereal experienced a 5 percent reduction in total cholesterol and a 9 percent reduction in LDL cholesterol (low-density lipoprotein or "bad" cholesterol) compared to those who ate a control cereal. High-density lipoprotein (HDL or "good" cholesterol) levels were not affected. The evidence was so strong that

Caution!

- Individuals with trouble swallowing or with a known allergy to psyllium dust, such as health-care workers, should not take psyllium supplements.
- If you have a medical condition or are pregnant or lactating, talk to your doctor before taking any supplement.
- Research is underway to look at the benefits of psyllium for individuals with diabetes and genetic fat disorders.

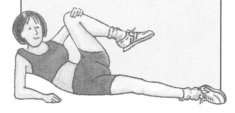

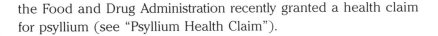

What to Know about Taking Psyllium Supplements

- Psyllium is sold in powder, wafer, and capsule forms, usually as a laxative. Most supplements provide 500 to 650 milligrams per serving and must be taken three to four times per day.
- Since dietary supplements (or claims for them) are not reviewed by the Food and Drug Administration, quality control and potency problems may exist with psyllium supplements.
- Research is underway to look at the benefits of psyllium for individuals with diabetes and genetic fat disorders.

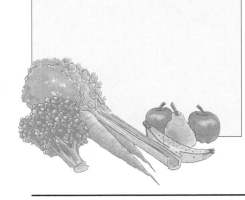

the Food and Drug Administration recently granted a health claim for psyllium (see "Psyllium Health Claim").

Psyllium and Ulcerative Colitis

Psyllium seeds may be a preferable alternative to drugs in the treatment of ulcerative colitis (inflammation of the lining of the colon). In a study of 105 people in remission from the disease, one-third received 20 grams of psyllium seeds (different from psyllium husks) per day, a third received the standard drug therapy, and one-third got both. After one year, the relapse rate in all three groups was the same—30 to 40 percent.

Psyllium seeds contain a fermentable fiber that encourages the growth of beneficial bacteria in the colon. This is believed to increase production of the fatty acid butyrate, which has anti-inflammatory actions that may relieve symptoms of ulcerative colitis.

Psyllium and the Digestive System

Psyllium is the active ingredient in several bulk laxative products, and it's commonly recommended for the treatment and prevention of constipation and/or diarrhea. The use of psyllium may also be useful for people suffering from a number of bowel disorders, including diverticulosis (small pockets in the lining of the intestines that can trap digested foods and become inflamed), **irritable bowel syndrome**, and hemorrhoids. Although bulk-forming laxatives containing psyllium are usually well tolerated, some people may experience gastrointestinal discomfort and nausea when first using these products.

Psyllium in Food

Psyllium is available in the American diet in breads, pastas, grains, snacks, and ready-to-eat cereals. It's also available in bulk-forming laxatives such as Metamucil. Now that there's a health claim for psyllium, it will probably be added to more foods and should be listed on the label.

When to Supplement with Psyllium

Since most Americans do not get the recommended 25 to 30 grams of fiber per day, adding psyllium-containing foods or supplements can help boost fiber intake. About 10 grams of psyllium per day will provide enough soluble fiber to help reduce total and LDL cholesterol levels in a healthy diet. Be sure not to exceed 30 grams of supplemental fiber, unless you're under a doctor's supervision. Too much psyllium may reduce the absorption of certain minerals. Children should not take psyllium supplements.

There are some reports of allergic reactions to psyllium, but most are occupationally related. A number of psyllium allergy complaints were heard in the early 1980s following the initial launch of psyllium food products. Following these complaints, researchers at Johns Hopkins University found that all of the reported reactions were in health professionals, primarily nurses who had dispensed psyllium-based laxatives, or workers in plants manufacturing psyllium products. The researchers were then able to identify the allergenic protein in psyllium and dramatically reduce or eliminate the protein from psyllium. Since then allergies have been largely eliminated.

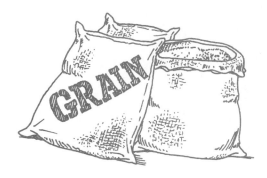

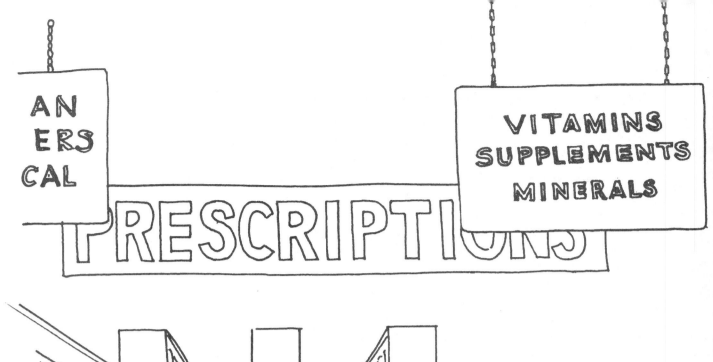

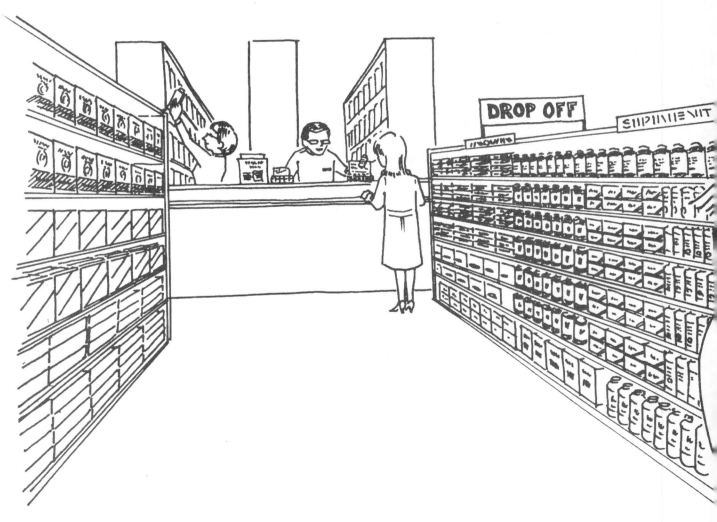

CHAPTER 8

Hormones in a Pill: Too Good to Be True?

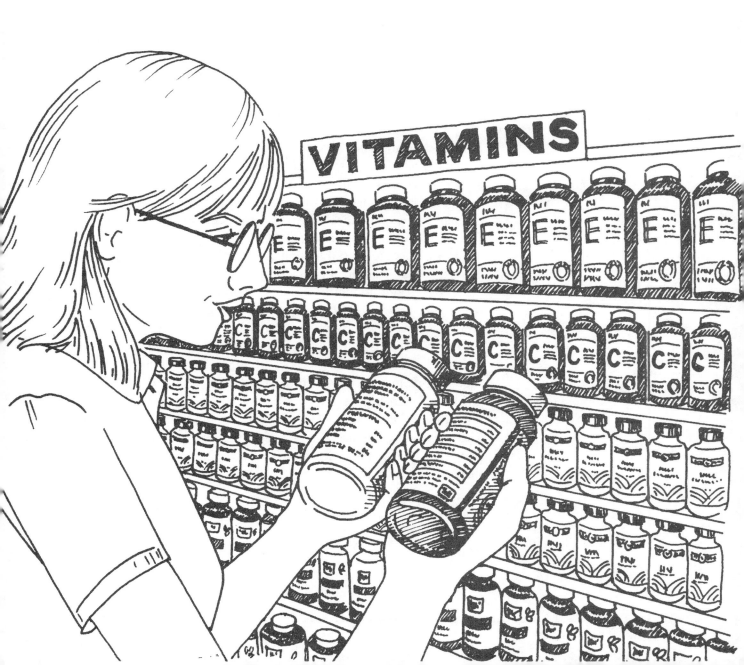

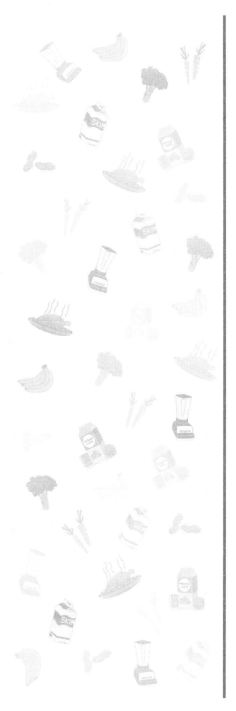

More and more baby boomers are entering "middle age" every day, and not surprisingly, interest in "anti-aging" products is also on the rise. The hormone supplement industry is thriving with products such as melatonin and DHEA (dehydroepiandrosterone). But can these products really turn back the clock?

Many consumers seem to think so, but unfortunately, "anti-aging" pills may not be what they seem. In April 1997, the National Institute on Aging (NIA) launched a media campaign to warn consumers about "anti-aging" hormone supplements.

Contrary to popular belief, none of these hormones, including estrogen and testosterone, have been shown to prevent or reverse the effects of aging, such as wrinkles, decreased energy and immune function, hair loss, and vision problems. While research is currently underway to study the effects of these supplements, consumer demand is pushing the market ahead of the science. Aside from estrogen and testosterone, these hormones have not been examined in controlled, long-term studies. And, the research that has been done is often shaky at best.

Hormones are powerful chemicals produced in the body by glands, (cells or groups of cells that have the ability to make a secretion, or hormone, that is discharged and used in some other part of the body). They are released into the bloodstream and are carried to different parts of the body where they influence the way organs and tissues work. As we age, the levels of some hormones decrease. However, these levels can be increased by taking hormone supplements in the form of a pill, shot, or medicated skin patch. Unfortunately, researchers do not know if hormones produced by the body work the same way as supplemented hormones. The specific arguments for and against the use of two hormones in particular—DHEA and melatonin—are discussed in greater detail in their respective sections.

DHEA

DHEA (dehydroepiandrosterone) is the latest anti-aging hormone to hit drugstore shelves and the media. Considered the "mother hormone," DHEA is the precursor to all other hormones in the body, including estrogen and testosterone. It is made by the adrenal glands, tiny sacs that sit on top of each kidney. DHEA production peaks at puberty and remains high until age 30 or so, when it begins to drop off with age.

The Benefits of DHEA

DHEA and Lupus

DHEA may provide relief from lupus, a chronic inflammatory disease of connective tissue that affects the skin, joints, kidneys, nervous system, and mucous membranes. In a 12-month study of 50 female patients with lupus, who took 50 to 200 milligrams of DHEA per day, DHEA was well tolerated and appeared clinically beneficial. Although the data is promising, further studies are needed.

DHEA and Other Potential Benefits

Researchers at the University of California, San Diego, have found in preliminary studies that DHEA, in appropriate replacement doses, appears to have an effect in increasing muscle strength and lean body mass, improving immune function, and enhancing quality of life in aging men and women. These findings have fueled many of the claims that DHEA can prevent heart disease and cancer, improve both mood and the immune system, and melt away body fat. Although the data looks promising, subsequent studies have shown that DHEA is very complex in the way it works. Many of the claims regarding DHEA are unproven. In fact, the experts who have studied DHEA believe that much more research is needed.

When to Supplement with DHEA

There have been some early signs indicating that DHEA supplementation may lead to liver damage, even when taken briefly.

Caution!

- Consumers need to use caution when considering the use of hormones. After all, supplementing can be harmful. When estrogen was first prescribed for postmenopausal women, there were quite a few side effects until doctors realized it was often better to prescribe a combination of estrogen and progesterone. Talk to your doctor.
- Hormone supplementation should not be taken lightly. Before taking any hormone, check with your physician.
- If you have a medical condition or are taking prescription medications, talk to your doctor before taking any supplement.
- Individuals with prostate, breast, or ovarian cancer, or those with a strong family history of these diseases should not take DHEA.
- Women who are pregnant or lactating and individuals under 40 years of age should not take DHEA.

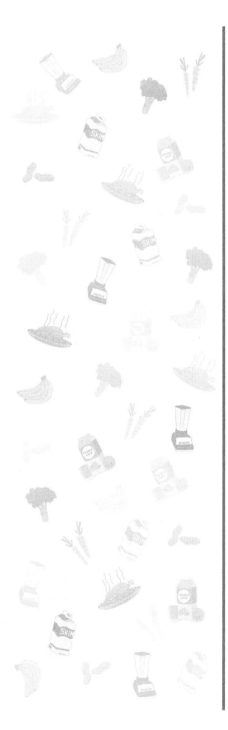

Researchers are also concerned that DHEA supplements may cause high levels of testosterone and estrogen in some people. High testosterone levels have been associated with a greater risk of prostate cancer, and elevated estrogen levels have been suspected of increasing breast cancer risk.

Preliminary research indicates that DHEA may also lower levels of heart-healthy HDL (high-density lipoproteins—the "good" cholesterol). In one study, women who took 25 milligrams of DHEA per day over six months had a 13 percent drop in HDL. Moreover, the dosage used in this study is equal to that found in most supplements.

DHEA is not recommended for children.

What to Know about Taking DHEA Supplements

- Women who choose to supplement with DHEA should take the smallest dose possible and have frequent checkups to measure their liver function, testosterone levels, and cholesterol levels. Excess DHEA can cause hair growth in women, deepening of the voice, and mood changes.
- DHEA supplements generally come in 10- or 25-milligram capsules or tablets. It is also sold in cream form.
- Since dietary supplements (or claims for them) are not reviewed by the Food and Drug Administration, quality control and potency problems may exist with DHEA supplements.

Melatonin

The hormone melatonin is made by the pineal gland (an organ the size of a pea located in the middle of the brain) to help our bodies keep time. At night the eye perceives darkness and sends a signal to the brain to release melatonin. In the morning, sunlight shuts down the hormone trigger. As we age, melatonin production slows down, which may explain why older people often have a harder time falling asleep at night. According to some estimates, about 33 percent of people over age 65 suffer from chronic insomnia.

The Benefits of Melatonin

Melatonin as a Sleep Aid

In recent years melatonin has been touted as the safe and "natural" sleep aid, especially for travelers. Some studies have shown that melatonin supplementation may help decrease the effects of jet lag and may induce sleep. However, a study at Columbia University found otherwise. Researchers assigned 257 Norwegian physicians, who were visiting New York for five days, to one of four regimens: (1) 0.5 milligrams of melatonin at bedtime, (2) 0.5 milligrams of melatonin on a shifting schedule, (3) 5 milligrams of melatonin at bedtime, or (4) a placebo. Interestingly, none of the melatonin treatments eased symptoms any better than the placebo. Another study showed that melatonin also failed to help regulate the sleep schedules of Space Shuttle astronauts.

Melatonin and Other Potential Benefits

Much of the research to date on melatonin and cancer has been conducted in animals, and its long-term safety in humans is not yet known. Preliminary data indicates that the hormone may be beneficial in an advanced reproductive-organ cancer—under a physician's care. Melatonin is not recommended for patients with autoimmune disorders, lymphoma, or leukemia.

Although melatonin may act as an antioxidant, and thereby reduce the harmful aging effects of free radical damage, claims that it acts as an anti-aging remedy are far from proven. Studies of melatonin have been much too limited to support these claims and have focused on animals, not people.

When to Supplement with Melatonin

Although no major medical problems have been associated with the short-term use of melatonin for jet lag, experts recommend against chronic use of the hormone until data regarding long-term supplementation is available (it is not recommended at all for children). Occasional use of $1/2$–1 milligram of melatonin appears to be safe. The dose of melatonin often found in supplements—3 milligrams—is too much and can result in accumulations in the blood up to 40 times higher than normal. The effects of these levels are still unknown.

What to Know about Taking Melatonin Supplements

- Melatonin supplements are available in capsule, tablet, softgel, lozenge and liquid forms in 1- to 3-milligram doses.
- When supplementing with melatonin, be sure to use synthetic brands. Be wary of those made from animal glands, because of the risk of contamination or disease.
- Melatonin taken at the wrong time of day can disrupt the sleep/wake cycle.
- Side effects may include confusion, drowsiness, and headache the next morning.
- Since dietary supplements (or claims for them) are not reviewed by the Food and Drug Administration, quality control and potency problems may exist with melatonin supplements.

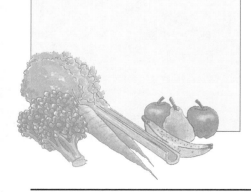

CHAPTER 9

Phytochemicals: A New Tool for Prevention?

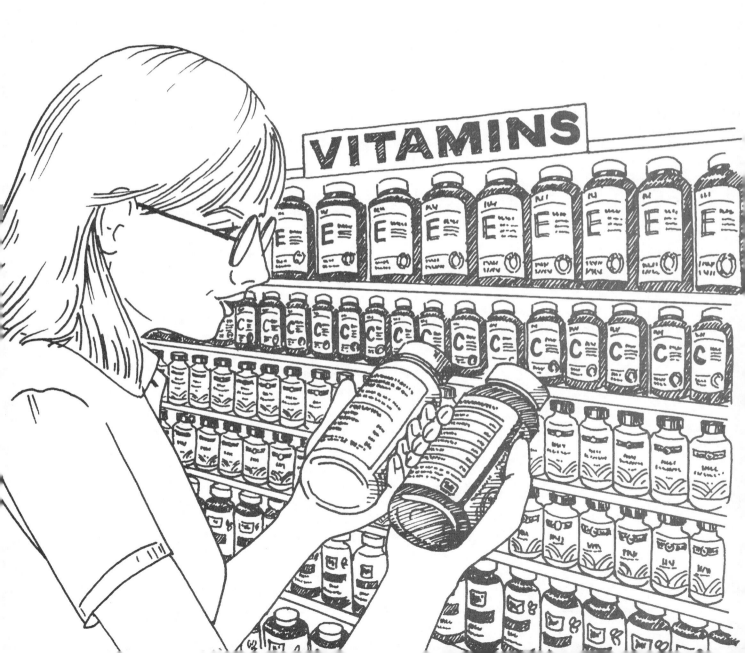

Many experts feel that the majority of the antioxidant capacity in fruits and vegetables may actually come from a variety of phytochemicals—chemical compounds found in plants. These compounds are not vitamins or minerals, and therefore are not considered essential for life. As pigments, oils, flavors, and microstructures, phytochemicals appear to work both alone and together, alongside other nutrients in food. They have been associated with the prevention and/or treatment of at least four of the leading causes of death in the United States: cancer, heart disease, diabetes, and high blood pressure. Because there are so many phytochemicals (approximately 4,000), they are separated into different groups (see "Phytochemicals in Foods"). In this book we review some of the more popular and well researched groups of phytochemicals.

Carotenoids

Of the thousands of different phytochemicals, one particular group of natural pigments, known as carotenoids, has a lot of antioxidant potential. These pigments give fruits and vegetables their yellow, orange, and red colors (in green leafy vegetables such as spinach, the carotenoid pigments are masked by green chlorophyll). A large body of evidence suggests that high blood levels of carotenoids may reduce the risk of cancer, heart disease, cataracts, and macular degeneration, the leading cause of irreversible blindness in old age. Although hundreds of different carotenoids have been identified in plants, only a handful are used in significant ways by the body: alpha- and beta-carotene, lutein, lycopene, zeaxanthin, and beta-cryptoxanthin.

The only proven function of carotenoids in the body is vitamin A activity. Fewer than 10 percent of carotenoids are provitamins, which can turn into vitamin A in the body. These include alpha-carotene, beta-carotene, and beta-cryptoxanthin, and they provide approximately 25 percent of the vitamin A in the diet. Most dietary carotenoids, both with and without provitamin A activity, are absorbed from the intestine. They are found primarily in adipose (fat) tissue and the liver, but are also in the kidney. Alpha-carotene, beta-carotene, beta-cryptoxanthin, lycopene, and lutein are the predominant carotenoids found in the body. Beta-carotene, the most

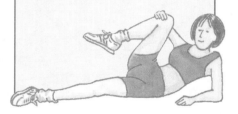

Phytochemicals in Supplement Form

The most common phytochemicals found in supplements are the carotenoids, including beta-carotene, lycopene, and lutein. Isoflavones are also available in combination and as single DHA and EPA supplements. And, you can find flavonoid supplements that contain quercitin. No doubt, as more research is conducted, many more supplements will appear on the market.

studied, comprises 15 to 30 percent of total serum (blood) carotenoids. Interestingly, women tend to have higher serum concentrations of beta-carotene and cryptoxanthin than men, but equal concentrations of lutein and lycopene.

Beta-carotene is unique because it is the most abundant carotenoid that humans can metabolize to vitamin A. Until recently, only beta-carotene was examined in human dietary studies. However, with new food composition data for a number of carotenoids, researchers have been able to go back to studies originally done on beta-carotene alone, and reanalyze the same data for a number of carotenoids. Now they can look at 24-hour recalls (people's recall of their diet for the previous 24 hours), for example, and analyze foods containing lycopene, lutein, etc. Before, they could only analyze foods for their beta-carotene content.

Although the exact mechanism by which carotenoids provide health benefits is not known, they may protect cells from oxidative stress by extinguishing free radicals capable of causing damage to cells. Another theory is that carotenoids may stop cancer at its earliest stage by altering the way cells communicate.

According to scientists, carotenoids enhance communication between premalignant—or precancerous—cells and normal cells. This enables the premalignant cells to receive growth-regulating signals from normal cells, thereby suppressing tumor growth. This positive effect seems to be independent of either the provitamin A or antioxidant properties of carotenoids.

Few studies have been conducted on specific carotenoids, although previous research has shown repeatedly that protection from various diseases is achieved by a diet that includes a variety of fruits and vegetables—rather than a diet made up of foods rich in a single carotenoid. In fact, a growing number of laboratory studies suggest cancer-inhibiting properties for a number of other phytochemicals besides carotenoids.

Phytoestrogens

A group of phytochemicals that are grabbing headlines are the **phytoestrogens**—and **isoflavones** in particular. Found primarily in soy products, phytoestrogens are the plant version of the female

Flavonoids, Flavones, and Isoflavones

Flavonoids are the largest group of phytochemicals. Within the flavonoid group are two subgroups called anthocyanins (blue, red, and purple pigment molecules) and **anthoxanthins** (white, yellow, and colorless molecules). The anthoxanthin subgroup is further divided into classes (or types), and flavones and isoflavones are two of those classes. Flavones and isoflavones are found predominantly in vegetables, legumes, and soy foods.

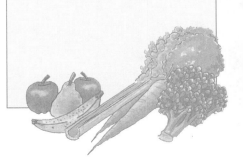

hormone estrogen. Researchers are looking at a potential role of phytoestrogens in the fight against cancer, heart disease, and osteoporosis. They're also investigating the use of isoflavones in the treatment of menopausal symptoms such as hot flashes and night sweats.

Just five years ago less than half of the phytochemicals identified today were known to exist. With more than 600 different carotenoids and many more phytochemicals, it's best not to put all of your money on just one or two of them. As many experts suggest, "Practice moderation in all things except variety."

When to Supplement with Phytochemicals

Most experts recommend getting phytochemicals in the diet. Why? Because there is not enough research on phytochemicals in foods, let alone the supplement versions. In addition, many warn that phytochemicals should not be considered nutrients in isolation. Research indicates that these compounds work better when in combination with other nutrients found in foods.

PHYTOCHEMICALS IN FOODS

PHYTOCHEMICALS	FOOD SOURCES
Allyl sulfides	Onions, garlic, leeks, chives
Carotenoids	Yellow-orange and red vegetables and fruits, green leafy vegetables
Ellagic acid	Strawberries, raspberries, nuts, grapes
Flavonoids	Tea, most fruits and vegetables, nuts
Glucosinolates	Cabbage, kale, turnips, Brussels sprouts, cauliflower, broccoli
Indoles	Broccoli, cabbage, cauliflower
Isoflavones	Soy products
Phenolic acids	Grapes, berries, nuts, citrus fruits, whole grains
Phytoalexins	Wine, grapes, peanuts, spices
Saponins	Legumes, oats, quinoa, asparagus, beans, citrus, herbs
Terpenes	Citrus, licorice, spices, cherries

Beta-Carotene

Beta-carotene is probably the most recognized carotenoid, giving fruits and vegetables their bright red, orange, and yellow coloring. It is believed to potentially decrease the risk of cancer, heart disease, and cataracts, and enhance immune function. Like all carotenoids, beta-carotene is fat-soluble and is therefore found in fatty tissues in humans.

Beta-carotene is one of the few carotenoids that is a vitamin A precursor, meaning it can turn into vitamin A in the body. It is also an antioxidant, although there has been much debate of late on whether or not beta-carotene acts as an antioxidant in the body.

The Benefits of Beta-Carotene

Beta-Carotene and Cancer

Twenty-six out of 28 recent studies have shown that diets rich in beta-carotene, fruits, and vegetables are linked to lower cancer rates, especially for lung cancer. But when researchers in three large studies took this a step further and gave individuals beta-carotene supplements, they found that the supplements did not help. All three studies included individuals who smoked and in all three trials, beta-carotene provided no protection against lung cancer. In fact, in two of the studies the risk of lung cancer increased. Male smokers who took 20 to 30 milligrams of beta-carotene a day saw more new tumor growth and deaths (mostly from lung cancer or heart disease) than those taking a placebo. Interestingly, the increased risk was only seen in smokers, not in nonsmokers.

In research on animals, experts have found that high doses of beta-carotene, as much as 10 times the amount found in a typical U.S. diet, reacted with oxygen in the lungs. This reaction produced substances that destroyed protective vitamin A and stimulated a tumor promoter called AP-1. Cigarette smoke worsened the oxidative effects on animals and, in the end, increased the risk of cancer. Although this theory is intriguing, much more research is needed.

In a recent study of nearly 40,000 women, beta-carotene supplements were found to be neither beneficial nor harmful. The women were divided into two groups and received either 50 milligrams of beta-carotene or a placebo on alternate days during the two years of treatment. After two years of follow-up, there were no differences in the rates of cancers of the breast, lung, colon, and ovaries. And, unlike the two previous studies, beta-carotene supplementation did

Caution!

- Beta-carotene supplementation can neither substitute for a good diet nor compensate for a bad diet. Furthermore, high doses of one carotenoid may decrease absorption of other carotenoids. You should increase beta-carotene-rich *foods* in your diet and avoid supplements above 6 milligrams per day. The exceptions are those individuals with erythropoietic protoporphyria or people at risk of vitamin A deficiency, who may need beta-carotene.
- Individuals who smoke should not take beta-carotene supplements.
- If you have a medical condition or are pregnant or lactating, talk to your doctor before taking any supplement.

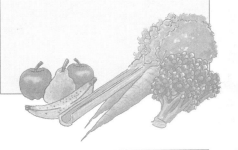

Alpha-Carotene: The Next Media Darling?

Unlike its famous cousins, alpha-carotene has not received much publicity. But in a study of 763 men diagnosed with lung cancer, alpha-carotene showed more promise than beta-carotene. Among the men that were currently, or had been recently, smoking, a beta-carotene-poor diet increased the risk of lung cancer by 60 percent. An alpha-carotene poor diet, on the other hand, nearly doubled the risk of cancer.

Both carotenoids are usually found in the same foods. However, seven of the men in that study had consumed a diet high in beta-carotene-rich foods (spinach and other leafy greens) and low in foods rich in both carotenoids (carrots, sweet potatoes, etc.). All seven men got lung cancer. Investigators warn that much more research is necessary.

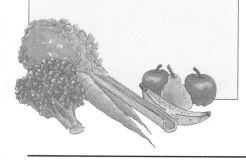

not increase cancer risk in smokers. Some have argued, though, that the duration of the study may not have been long enough to produce similar results.

Beta-Carotene and Heart Disease

Studies on beta-carotene and heart disease have yielded mixed results. The same studies that showed no benefits from beta-carotene in cancer found no protective effect from the carotenoid on heart disease. In fact, beta-carotene had a negative impact on smokers with heart disease.

Beta-Carotene and the Immune System

Carotenoids in general have been studied for potential benefits to the immune system. One study with beta-carotene showed that long-term supplementation enhanced "killer" cell activity in men ages 65 to 85 years, but not in men ages 51 to 64. A later study, however, did show benefits in the latter age group. Obviously, much more research is needed in this area.

Beta-Carotene and Erythropoietic Protoporphyria (EPP)

EPP is an inherited light-sensitive disease characterized by burning, redness, and swelling of the skin when exposed to the sun. Beta-carotene supplements are used therapeutically at extremely high doses (180 milligrams per day) to treat the photosensitivity disorder. In a large, seven-year study of 133 people with EPP, 84 percent of the participants increased their ability to tolerate sunlight exposure without developing symptoms after supplementing with beta-carotene.

Beta-Carotene and Cystic Fibrosis

Cystic fibrosis (CF) is an inherited disease of the exocrine glands that affects the pancreas, respiratory system, and sweat glands. CF usually begins in infancy, and individuals with the disease often suffer from respiratory infections, decreased function of the pancreas, and heat intolerance. The cause of the disease is unknown, and although new antibiotics help to prolong the lifespan of these patients, there is still no cure.

Researchers in Austria recently investigated the use of beta-carotene supplements in a group of 24 CF patients and 14 healthy age-matched participants (the controls), in order to optimize their antioxidant status and respiratory function. Half of the group received 1 milligram of beta-carotene per kilogram of body weight (with a maximum of 50 milligrams of beta-carotene per day) for the first 12 weeks, followed by 12 weeks of a reduced dosage of 10 milligrams of beta-carotene per day. The other half of the group received a placebo. At the beginning of the study the CF patients had much lower plasma beta-carotene concentrations than the controls. In the CF supplemented group, beta-carotene plasma levels were significantly increased after the first 12 weeks of high-dose supplementation. However, the levels dropped during the next 12 weeks when beta-carotene supplementation was decreased. During the high-dose treatment, respiratory problems could be corrected significantly. The researchers concluded that CF patients given 1 milligram of beta-carotene per kilogram of body weight (not to exceed 50 milligrams per day) could achieve plasma beta-carotene levels similar to those of healthy controls and minimize oxidative stress, thereby improving their quality of life.

Beta-Carotene in Food

Beta-carotene is found in a variety of fruits and vegetables, especially those that are bright yellow or orange, and dark, leafy greens. Interestingly, beta-carotene absorption is much better from cooked produce than from raw. Steaming vegetables will increase the availability of beta-carotene, although overcooking can destroy this carotenoid. Because the carotenoids are fat-soluble, eating beta-carotene with a little fat or oil will also increase absorption.

Many people get sweet potatoes and yams mixed up because they do resemble each other. However, their beta-carotene content is as different as night and day. Unlike sweet potatoes, which are an excellent source of this carotenoid, yams contain little, if any, beta-carotene.

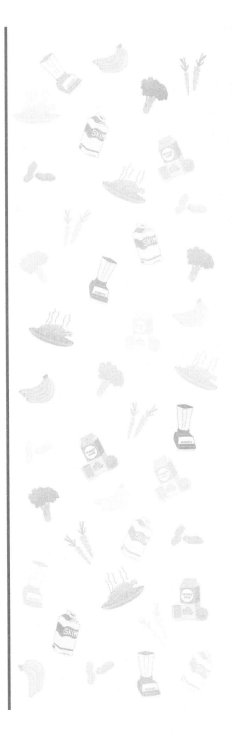

FOOD SOURCES OF BETA-CAROTENE

FOOD SOURCES	BETA-CAROTENE (MG PER 3^{1}/$_{2}$-OUNCE SERVING)*
Sweet potato, cooked	9.4
Carrots, raw	8.8
Pumpkin, canned	6.9
Spinach, raw	5.5
Collard greens, cooked	4.4
Collard greens, raw	3.3
Peppers, sweet, red, raw	2.3
Cantaloupe	1.5
Broccoli, raw	0.7
Grapefruit, pink and red, raw	0.6
Mangos, raw	0.4
Zucchini, raw	0.4
Tomatoes, raw	0.3
Watermelon	0.2

Source: USDA, Carotenoid Database, 1998.
*mg = milligrams.

When to Supplement with Beta-Carotene

No formal recommendation for carotenoids has yet been set, but many experts recommend 5 to 6 milligrams of beta-carotene per day. Although this is double the current USDA intake, it is the amount one would get if following the menus recommended by the Dietary Guidelines or the National Cancer Institute—both of which advocate at least five to six servings of fruits and vegetables per day.

The current U.S. and international guidelines encourage plant-based diets with less emphasis on animal products. Following this type of eating plan would mean getting 90 percent of vitamin A from provitamin A carotenoids such as beta-carotene. This is a far cry from the current U.S. dietary patterns, in which less than 40 percent of vitamin A comes from carotenoids in fruits and vegetables.

Beta-Carotene and Medication/Nutrient Interactions

A diet low in fruits and vegetables will decrease the amount of beta-carotene in the body, but certain medications can also decrease carotenoid absorption. For instance, lipid-lowering drugs can decrease beta-carotene levels in the blood by as much as 65 percent. Plant sterol–enriched margarines, used to help lower cholesterol levels, and dietary pectin supplements can also decrease beta-carotene by interfering with absorption.

Supplementing with two or more carotenoids at the same time can also affect absorption. Individuals who received either 12- or 30-milligram beta-carotene supplements every day for six weeks had significantly lower lutein levels than those who consumed both beta-carotene and lutein from food sources. It seems that supplemental beta-carotene may reduce the amount of lutein that is absorbed from foods.

Although many Americans do not get the carotenoids they need, certain groups are at greater risk, including adolescents and smokers. Most smokers have lower blood levels of beta-carotene and other carotenoids than do nonsmokers. And, the more cigarettes smoked per day, the greater the difference. In light of recent studies, smokers should try to increase their carotenoid and beta-carotene intakes through food rather than supplements. Like tobacco, alcohol is also associated with decreased intakes of beta-carotene. This may be due in part to the fact that most alcoholics have poor dietary intakes.

Beta-carotene is better absorbed in supplement form than in foods, so the risk of getting too much beta-carotene is more of a supplement issue. However, unlike other fat-soluble nutrients, carotenoids, and beta-carotene especially, are nontoxic (except in people who smoke). Too much beta-carotene will cause carotenodermia—yellowing of the skin, particularly the hands and feet. This may be unattractive, but it is not a health threat. The condition has been seen in people supplementing with 30 milligrams of beta-carotene per day or more for an extended period of time. Consuming high levels of carotenoid-rich foods, such as carrots, can also cause carotenodermia. Simply reducing intake of carotenoid-rich foods and/or supplements will make the color disappear within a week or so.

What to Know about Taking Beta-Carotene Supplements

- Beta-carotene supplements are available individually or combined with other carotenoids or antioxidants, such as vitamins C and E. It is available in doses ranging from 90 to 300 milligrams in either the synthetic form (all-trans beta-carotene) or the natural form (all-trans beta-carotene and 9-cis beta-carotene). Most of the research has used the synthetic form.
- To boost absorption, beta-carotene supplements should be taken with food containing some fat.
- Since dietary supplements are not reviewed by the FDA, quality control and potency problems may exist.

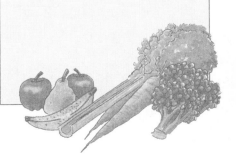

Isoflavones

Isoflavones are part of a group of compounds called phytoestrogens—plant compounds that act like the hormone estrogen in the body. Although isoflavones are found in a number of plants, only soybeans provide a significant amount of phytoestrogens.

The Benefits of Isoflavones

Researchers have long realized that the female sex hormone, estrogen, is associated with improved bone health and cardiovascular disease in women. As a woman ages and goes through menopause, estrogen levels naturally decrease, thereby increasing her risk of heart disease, stroke, and osteoporosis. Although some women opt to use standard **hormone replacement therapy (HRT**—a combination of estrogens and a synthetic progesterone), the majority of women choose not to, or do so only for a short period of time. One reason many women shy away from HRT is that it is associated with an increased risk of estrogen-dependent cancers such as breast, ovarian, and endometrial. Getting phyto-estrogens through the diet—isoflavones specifically—may be an acceptable alternative for many of these women.

Soybeans contain several types of isoflavones, including genistein, daidzein, and to a lesser extent, glycetein. Both genistein and daidzein are structurally similar to estradiol, the main form of estrogen produced by the ovaries. All three of these isoflavones have weak estrogen activity—1/10,000th to 1/1,000th the activity of estrogen. In addition, phytoestrogens can act both as estrogens and antiestrogens in the body. For women with low estrogen levels, adding isoflavones to the diet may increase protection against certain chronic diseases. For women with normal or high levels of estrogen, isoflavones may act as antiestrogens by binding to estrogen receptor sites in the body—giving estrogen less of an opportunity to do so. This may be beneficial for women at risk for estrogen-dependent cancers.

What to Know about Taking Isoflavone Supplements

- Soy supplements are available in capsule, tablet, and powder forms as well as bars, and are sold in health food stores, through catalogs, and through on-line outlets.
- Isoflavone supplements range in dosage from 25 to 50 milligrams.
- Genistein can have toxic effects at high intakes.
- Since dietary supplements are not reviewed by the FDA, quality control and potency problems may exist with isoflavone supplements.

Isoflavones and Cancer

The low breast cancer rate in Japan—where women eat much more soy than do women in the United States—has prompted researchers to look at the potential health benefits of soy isoflavones. A number of studies have shown that soy intake is associated with a decreased risk of breast cancer in premenopausal women (not postmenopausal women). Some experts believe that soy may increase the length of the menstrual cycle, which in turn may reduce the risk of breast cancer. However, not all studies support this theory.

Even though isoflavones are weaker than estrogen, many experts feel that isoflavones may help to reduce estrogen-dependent cancers—but this remains to be proven. Much more research is needed in order to answer definitively whether or not soy foods should be consumed by women with estrogen-sensitive breast tumors, and whether soy food consumption can decrease risk of estrogen-sensitive cancers.

Several animal studies have indicated that isoflavones may also play a protective role in prostate cancer. Preliminary research on humans has found that soy milk and tofu consumption are associated with a decreased risk of this cancer. And in a recent study, researchers found that both genistein and combined isoflavones suppressed tumor growth in patients with urinary tract cancer.

Interestingly, some of the greatest benefits of isoflavones may have nothing to do with their estrogenic effects. First, isoflavones are antioxidants and may protect against the damaging effects of oxidation. Secondly, laboratory research on cancer cells shows that the isoflavone genistein inhibits the growth of hormone and nonhormone-dependent cancers. In fact, most genistein research has focused on the isoflavone's ability to inhibit enzymes that are involved with cell growth and regulation.

Isoflavones and Heart Disease

According to experts, soy protein appears to help prevent heart disease by lowering blood cholesterol levels; decreasing blood clots and platelet "clumping" or aggregation (both of which can increase the risk for a heart attack or stroke); improving the elasticity of

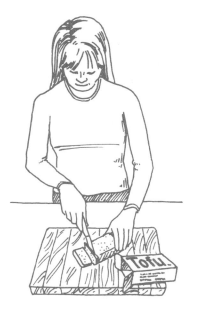

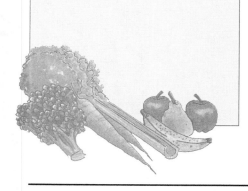

arteries (which makes blood flow better); and reducing oxidation of low-density lipoprotein (LDL or "bad" cholesterol), which can lower the risk of plaque formation. Researchers suspect that the beneficial effects from soy protein are due to the isoflavones, but more research is needed. There is some evidence to suggest, however, that isoflavones may raise high-density lipoprotein (HDL, or the "good" cholesterol) levels.

Whether or not it's the isoflavones in the soy that are helping to prevent heart disease remains to be seen, but the protective ben-efits of soy are tremendous. In fact, the Food and Drug Administration is so convinced of soy's benefits that the agency approved a health claim for soy protein and heart disease in October 1999 (see "Making the Claim for Soy").

Isoflavones and Bone Health

One of the effects of reduced estrogen levels in the body is a decrease in the activity of osteoblasts—the cells that build bone. Two different studies on humans have shown that isoflavone-rich soy protein may increase bone mineral density and reduce bone loss at the spine. And, unlike animal proteins, soy 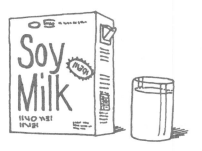 protein does not induce urinary loss of calcium from the body. However, another study showed that isoflavones in postmenopausal women had no effect on bone health. Long-term studies are now underway and may provide a clearer picture of the role of isoflavones in this arena in the future.

Researchers first became interested in the potential benefits of phytoestrogens on osteoporosis after the drug Ipriflavone (a synthetic, or man-made, isoflavone similar in structure to diadzein) was found to be very effective in slowing bone loss in postmenopausal women. In a study of 56 women who had recently gone through menopause, those who supplemented with 200 milligrams of Ipriflavone three times per day maintained their bone density after two years, com-pared to women who received a placebo. Interestingly, both groups also received 1,000 milligrams of calcium per day.

Isoflavones and Menopause

With their weak estrogen effect, isoflavones may help reduce the symptoms of menopause, including hot flashes, night sweats, vaginal dryness, and mood swings. It's known that Japanese women suffer far fewer menopausal symptoms than American women, which has prompted much of this research. Unfortunately, the findings to date are contradictory and inconclusive.

While the jury is still out on whether or not soy is as effective as hormone replacement treatment, many experts feel eating a serving or two of soy foods every day can't hurt and may help in most cases. Of course, women who have estrogen-receptor positive tumors are advised to talk to their doctors before adding soy foods or supplements to their diet.

Isoflavones in Food

Isoflavones are present in a variety of foods such as alfalfa, garbanzo beans (chickpeas), red clover, and soybeans. Miso, regular soymilk, roasted soy nuts, tempeh, tofu, soy flour, and textured vegetable protein are rich in isoflavones, but soy oil and soy sauce are not. Isoflavones are found in the greatest concentration in soy foods.

Food Sources of Isoflavones

Food Sources	Total Isoflavones (mg per 3½-ounce serving)*
Soy flour, defattened	131
Isolated soy protein	97
Miso	43
Tofu, firm	31
Soy cheese	31
Tofu, regular	24
Soy hot dog	15
Soymilk	10
Soy veggie burger	8
Peanuts	<1
Flaxseed	0
Kidney beans, cooked	0

Source: USDA-Iowa State University Database on the Isoflavone Content of Foods, Release 12, 2000.
*mg = milligrams.

Making the Claim for Soy

On October 20, 1999, the FDA announced that it had approved a health claim regarding the association between consumption of soy protein and the reduced risk of coronary heart disease. Food products that contain a minimum of 6.25 grams of soy protein per serving will be allowed to claim on their labels:

"Twenty-five grams of soy protein a day, as part of a diet low in fat and cholesterol, may reduce the risk of heart disease."

This health claim is based on scientific evidence from more than 50 independent studies. Research has shown that soy protein can lower blood cholesterol levels by 5 to 10 percent, which may reduce the risk of heart disease.

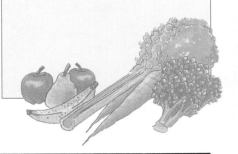

When to Supplement with Isoflavones

Currently, there are no formal RDAs for isoflavones, but studies show that 60 to 90 milligrams per day is needed for bone health, 50 to 80 milligrams per day to reduce symptoms of menopause, and 30 to 90 milligrams per day for potential cancer benefits. Approximately three servings of soy foods per day would provide the upper levels of these recommendations. It is not recommended that children take soy supplements. Although this may not seem like a lot to some people, even consuming just one serving of soy may be a hurdle for most. Fortunately, many experts believe that as little as one serving of a soy food per day may be enough to reap some of the beneficial effects of the isoflavones.

Lutein

Lutein (pronounced LOO-teen) is a phytochemical (naturally occurring chemical components found in fruits, vegetables, legumes, and grains) and one of two major carotenoids found in the human eye in the retina. The other such carotenoid is zeaxanthin.

The Benefits of Lutein

Lutein and Eyesight

Lutein, along with zeaxanthin, is believed to function as an antioxidant, protecting the underlying eye tissues from phototoxic damage by filtering out ultraviolet light in sunshine, and blocking harmful free radicals in the eye. This damage may be a factor in both cataracts and **age-related macular degeneration (ARMD)**, the leading cause of blindness in the United States. Increasing foods rich in lutein and zeaxanthin may decrease the risk of developing advanced or exudative ARMD, the most visually disabling form of macular degeneration among older people. Experts believe antioxidant nutrients, including lutein, not only may help to prevent eye diseases, but may help prevent further deterioration of existing conditions.

What to Know about Taking Lutein Supplements

- The supplements usually contain 6 milligrams of lutein and frequently contain zeaxanthin as well.
- As with other carotenoids, to boost absorption lutein supplements should be taken with food containing some fat.
- Since dietary supplements (or claims for them) are not reviewed by the Food and Drug Administration, quality control and potency problems may exist with lutein supplements.

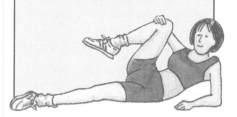

In a recent study, researchers looked at the effect of carotenoid intakes and risk of cataract extraction in more than 77,000 female nurses (part of the Nurses' Health Study). Women with the highest intakes of lutein and zeaxanthin had a 22 percent lower risk of cataract extraction than those with the lowest intakes. The study concluded that lutein and zeaxanthin, and foods rich in these carotenoids, may decrease the risk of cataracts severe enough to require extraction.

Similar findings were also found in men in the Health Professionals Follow-up Study. Men with the highest intakes of lutein and zeaxanthin had a 19 percent lower risk of cataract extraction compared to those with the lowest intakes.

Lutein and Colon Cancer

New findings indicate that lutein may play a protective role in reducing the risk of colon cancer. In one study, researchers looked at two separate groups of people. The first group was made up of individuals known to have colon cancer, and the second group was a control group representative of the population as a whole with no cancer. Researchers gathered information on what foods the participants had eaten two years prior to diagnosis of cancer, or in the case of the controls, in the previous two years before the study.

Interestingly, only one carotenoid—lutein—showed an inverse association with colon cancer. And the protective effect was greater in those who were younger when their cancer was diagnosed, and for those whose tumors were located in the upper part of the colon.

When to Supplement with Lutein

Most Americans consume about 1.2 milligrams of lutein and zeaxanthin every day. However, researchers recommend closer to 4 milligrams per day. Most of the research to date has looked at lutein-rich foods; however, if you don't eat many dark leafy greens, you might want to consider eating more of them or taking a supplement (they are not recommended for children, however).

Lutein in Food

Lutein is found in a variety of fruits and vegetables, especially dark leafy greens (see "Food Sources of Lutein"). When comparing data from 1987 and 1992, researchers found a decrease in the intake of lutein by 18 percent among white women, and 16 percent among adults aged 40 to 69 years. The authors suggest that the decline in lutein intake (from dark green leafy vegetables), particularly in white women, may have public health implications as a result of the recognized association between carotenoid intake and disease risk.

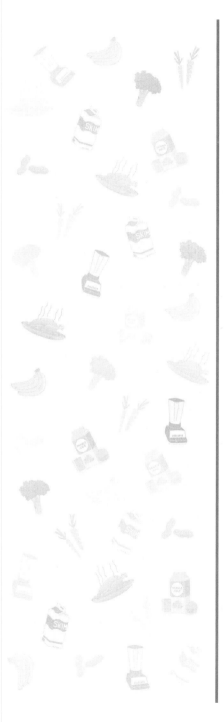

FOOD SOURCES OF LUTEIN AND ZEAXANTHIN

FOOD SOURCES	LUTEIN & ZEAXANTHIN (COMBINED MG PER 3¹/₂-OUNCE SERVING)*
Kale, cooked	15.0
Spinach, raw, chopped	11.0
Turnip greens, cooked	8.0
Collard greens, cooked	8.0
Romaine lettuce, shredded	2.6
Broccoli, cooked	2.2
Zucchini, raw	2.1
Corn (yellow), cooked	1.8

Source: USDA-NCC Carotenoid Database for U.S. Foods, 1998.
*mg = milligrams.

Lycopene

Lycopene (pronounced LIE-co-peen) is a carotenoid, or natural pigment, that gives tomatoes their deep red color. It is the predominant carotenoid in the body—found in human blood and tissue—but it's derived entirely from food sources. Lycopene is also a powerful antioxidant and phytochemical. Studies show that phytochemicals (naturally occurring chemical components found in fruits, vegetables, legumes, and grains) may reduce the incidence and severity of certain diseases. For instance, a growing body of research suggests that lycopene may help reduce the risk of heart disease and some cancers.

The Benefits of Lycopene

Lycopene and Cancer

Lycopene first made headlines in 1995. Researchers at Harvard University studied 47,894 men and found that eating 10 or more servings a week of tomato products, such as tomato sauce, reduced the risk of prostate cancer by as much as 34 percent.

A recent scientific review of 72 research papers indicates that eating five to seven servings a week of lycopene-rich tomato products may protect against certain cancers. Evidence was strongest for cancers of the lung, stomach, and prostate, and was suggestive for cancers of the breast, colon, and cervix, among others.

Lycopene and Heart Disease

Numerous studies have also shown a protective effect of antioxidants on heart disease, and lycopene is no exception. In a recent study, men who had the highest amount of lycopene in their body fat were half as likely to suffer a heart attack as those with the least amount. The level of lycopene in body fat is a good indicator of the amount of lycopene consumed in the diet.

Researchers at the University of Toronto found that daily consumption of at least 40 milligrams of lycopene for only one week (from tomato sauce, tomato juice, or a lycopene supplement) was enough to boost blood levels of the carotenoid. Moreover, oxidized LDLs (the "bad" cholesterol), which can lead to heart disease, were greatly reduced.

Lycopene and the Immune System

Lycopene also helps the immune system by protecting immune cells from oxidation, according to Italian researchers. In a recent study, 10 healthy women ate a diet containing 2 ounces of tomato puree (rich in lycopene) every day for three weeks, either preceded by or followed by a three-week tomato-free diet. The researchers measured blood levels of lycopene and looked for cell damage caused by oxidation before and after each phase. They found that cell damage dropped by 33 to 42 percent after consuming the tomato diet.

When to Supplement with Lycopene

According to data from the 1992 National Health Interview Survey, the average daily lycopene intake for men is 2.3 milligrams, and 2.1 milligrams for women. Most of the research to date has used lycopene-rich foods, so until we have more data, eating tomatoes and tomato products is still your best bet. However, if you don't eat tomatoes, you might want to consider a supplement (they are not recommended for children).

In a recent study, men with prostate cancer who took 30 milligrams of lycopene per day (equal to about $1/2$ cup of spaghetti sauce), for three weeks, had a reduction in tumor size and malignancy.

Lycopene in Food

Since lycopene is not produced in the body, we can only get its beneficial effects by consuming it in the diet. Tomatoes and tomato products, such as tomato sauce, tomato paste, ketchup, and tomato soup, are by far the number one source of lycopene in the diet. In fact, these foods provide more than 85 percent of the lycopene consumed in the American diet. However, it is also found in lesser amounts in watermelon and pink grapefruit (see "Food Sources of Lycopene").

Interestingly, studies show that lycopene is better used by the body when it's consumed in processed tomato products, rather than fresh tomatoes. In one study lycopene was absorbed 2.5 times better from tomato paste than from fresh tomatoes. Remember, lycopene, like all carotenoids, is fat-soluble. When eating a processed tomato product or fresh tomatoes, be sure to include a little fat in the preparation to increase lycopene absorption.

What to Know about Taking Lycopene Supplements

- Lycopene supplements are available as singles or combined with vitamin E or other carotenoids, such as beta-carotene or lutein.
- The supplements usually come in 5- to 10-milligram capsules. Although there is no recommended amount, 10 to 15 milligrams per day is about what you'd get in a typical tomato-based food.
- To boost absorption, lycopene supplements should be taken with food containing some fat.
- Since dietary supplements (or claims for them) are not reviewed by the Food and Drug Administration, quality control and potency problems may exist with lycopene supplements.

The risk of getting too much lycopene is more of an issue with supplements than with foods. However, unlike other fat-soluble nutrients, carotenoids are nontoxic (except in people who smoke). Too much lycopene will cause lycopenodermia—a deep orange discoloration of the skin. This may be unattractive, but it is not a health threat. Because lycopene is a more intensely colored pigment than the other carotenoids, it may take less lycopene to cause this side effect than other carotenes. Consuming high levels of lycopene-rich foods such as tomatoes can also cause lycopenodermia. Simply reducing intake of lycopene-rich foods and/or supplements will make the color disappear within a week or so.

FOOD SOURCES OF LYCOPENE

FOOD SOURCES	LYCOPENE (MG PER 3½-OUNCE SERVING)*
Tomato paste	29
Catsup	17
Spaghetti sauce	16
Tomato sauce	16
Tomato soup (condensed)	11
Tomato juice	9
Watermelon	5
Raw tomato	3
Pink grapefruit	1

Source: USDA-NCC Carotenoid Database for U.S. Foods, 1998.
*mg = milligrams.

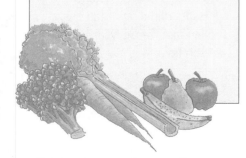

CHAPTER 10

Prebiotics and Probiotics

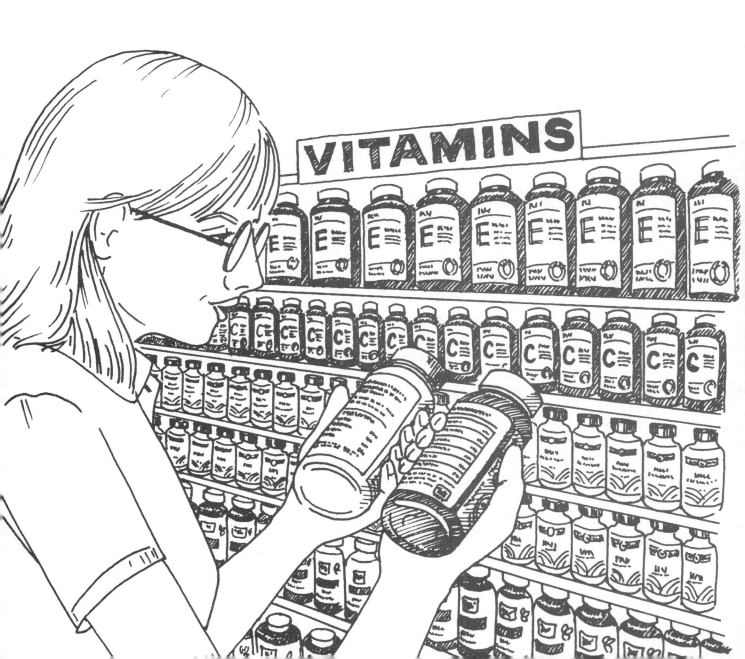

Bacteria That Are Good for You

Humans have used bacterial cultures for thousands of years to ferment various foods and beverages. About a century ago, nutritional scientists began focusing on how bacterial cultures may benefit human health. Since then, a lot has been learned about the specific advantages of various prebiotic and probiotic products.

The term **probiotics** (meaning "pro-life") was coined in the 1930s when the first clinical trials of probiotic foods began. Probiotics are foods that introduce beneficial live organisms into the gut (the gastrointestinal tract—stomach and intestine) in order to favorably alter the balance of bacteria there. Yogurt with live, active cultures is a common probiotic food. The most frequently used bacteria in probiotic products are *Lactobacillus* and *Bifidobacterium* species. Within these species are a number of bacterial strains, not all of which are commonly used in probiotic products (see "Probiotic Bacteria").

Prebiotics are nondigestible food substances that act as food for beneficial microorganisms that are already present in the gastrointestinal tract. As prebiotics, these substances encourage the growth and/or stimulate the activity of "friendly" bacteria species such as *L. acidophilus* and various types of *Bifidobacterium*. Fructooligosaccharides (pronounced FROOK-toe-oh-lee-go-SACK-a-rides and commonly known by the acronym FOS) are an example of a prebiotic substance.

Health Benefits of Prebiotics and Probiotics

There are many alleged health benefits of consuming prebiotic and probiotic products. In general, those benefits for which the most substantial supportive scientific evidence exists include the general maintenance of gastrointestinal (GI) health (including the treatment of diarrhea), the reduction of lactose intolerance symptoms, enhanced mineral absorption, and the treatment of GI disorders including inflammatory bowel syndrome and colitis (pain and inflammation of the intestines).

The mechanisms by which probiotics may enhance GI health include the stimulation of immunity, competition with "unfriendly" bacteria for nutrients, prevention of pathogenic bacteria from

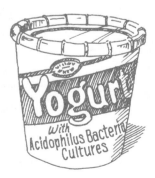

attaching to the intestinal walls, and the production of antimicrobial substances. The specific benefits of *L. acidophilus*, *Bifidobacterium*, and FOS are discussed in greater detail in their respective sections.

Acidophilus

A "friendly" bacteria species, *Lactobacillus acidophilus*, is found naturally in the human gastrointestinal tract, as well as the mouth and vagina. Generally known by its nickname, *acidophilus* (pronounced AS-i-dah-FIL-us) was first mentioned as being potentially beneficial back in the early 1900s. It wasn't until the mid-1980s, however, when *acidophilus* was suggested to have cholesterol-lowering effects, that interest in the bacteria really blossomed. Since then, research has identified additional health benefits associated with this culture. In fact, *acidophilus* is now recognized as one of the most beneficial of the 500 bacteria species that inhabit the body.

The Benefits of *Acidophilus* Bacteria

Gastrointestinal Health

Acidophilus is considered a "good" bacterium, as opposed to various "bad" bacteria such as *E. coli* and *Salmonella*. Probiotic foods, which bring beneficial live organisms into the gut in order to favorably alter the balance of bacteria there, often contain *acidophilus* cultures. In order to have probiotic effects, however, the bacteria must survive the stomach and make it through to the intestines. Research shows that *acidophilus* survives the journey well—better than the bacteria species used to make yogurt, but probably not as well as *bifidobacteria*.

In the gastrointestinal tract, it's more healthful when the good bacteria outnumber the bad. "Bad," or pathogenic (potentially disease-causing), bacteria can produce toxins and other compounds that decrease the body's ability to fight disease, and some are known to be carcinogens (cancer-causing substances). Studies have shown that *acidophilus* is active against a number of pathogenic bacteria including strains of *Shigella* and *Salmonella*, as well as

Probiotic Bacteria

Lactobacillus species
 L. acidophilus
 L. casei
 L. fermentum
 L. gassen
 L. johnsonii
 L. lactis
 L. paracase
 L. plantarum
 L. reuteri
 L. rhamnosus
 L. salivarius

Bifidobacterium species
 B. bifidum
 B. breve
 B. lactis
 B. longum

Streptococcus species
 S. thermophilus

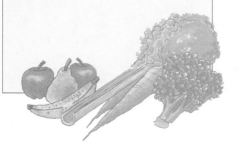

Acidophilus Bacteria in Food

Acidophilus bacteria cultures can be found in supplements, yogurts, and certain milk products. Health food stores often carry a wider variety of *acidophilus*-containing foods than regular supermarkets. Because high heat kills *acidophilus* cultures, they're usually added after pasteurization.

Acidophilus can also be found in some brands of fermented milks, such as kefir, yogurt with live, active cultures, and yogurt drinks.

Improper storage of *acidophilus* supplements (any form) can kill the bacteria. Keep *acidophilus* away from heat or freezing temperatures. Store supplements in a cool, dry place. Liquid supplements should be kept in the refrigerator.

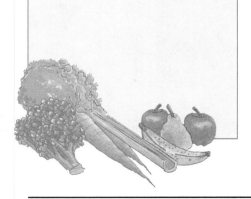

Helicobacter pylori, which has been implicated in the development of ulcers. In some cases, a mixture of *acidophilus* along with *L. casei* cultures showed a greater effect against pathogens than did either of the single strains alone.

The benefits of "good" bacteria such as *acidophilus* go beyond keeping the growth of bad bacteria in check; they also help digest food and promote regularity. The vitamins B_{12}, K, thiamin, and folic acid are also supplied by *acidophilus* cultures.

Acidophilus and Antibiotic Treatment

Antibiotics are effective at killing bacteria and stopping bacterial infections from becoming life-threatening. Unfortunately, antibiotics kill good bacteria as well as bad bacteria. As the intestines recover from the antibiotics, the good and bad bacteria fight for dominance in the gut. *Acidophilus* supplements can help introduce a good supply of beneficial bacteria into the intestines. What's more, the *acidophilus* cultures create an acidic environment that bad bacteria don't like.

Acidophilus and Yeast Infections

There have been a number of studies showing that *acidophilus* taken either orally or topically (as a douche) is an effective treatment for vaginal infections caused by the bacteria *Candida albicans*. This effect may be especially helpful for women who have a tendency to develop yeast infections when taking antibiotics. One researcher reported a threefold decrease in the recurrence of yeast infections in women who ate a cup of *acidophilus*-containing yogurt every day for six months. It's suspected that the additional *acidophilus* grow in the vaginal canal, leaving no room for the yeast to grow. Although in general this area of research is considered quite preliminary, a few other studies have found similar results.

Acidophilus and Diarrhea

A number of studies have tested the effectiveness of *acidophilus* supplements and *acidophilus*-containing diary products in preventing viral diarrhea in children, antibiotic-related diarrhea, and traveler's diarrhea (caused by bacterial contamination). Some studies show that *acidophilus* shortens the duration of symptoms and that, the higher the dose, the better the effects. However, in general, results have been inconsistent, which isn't surprising given the varied causes of diarrhea. This may be an area where a combination of bacterial cultures are necessary for the best effects. *Acidophilus* cultures can, however, help good bacteria establish new "colonies" in the GI tract after a bout of diarrhea cleans out the system, so it may be helpful to take the supplements or consume foods containing *acidophilus* while experiencing diarrhea and for a few days afterward.

Acidophilus and Lactose Intolerance

Lactose intolerance is a condition in which drinking milk or eating most dairy products triggers gas, bloating, cramping, and diarrhea. It's caused by a deficiency of the enzyme (lactase) that is needed to break down the milk sugar called lactose. (For more information on lactose intolerance, see the Lactase section in Chapter 5.)

Some studies have shown that *acidophilus* helps people digest lactose, minimizing the uncomfortable symptoms, while others have shown no effect. The inconclusive results of research in this area led researchers to speculate that perhaps other strains of *Lactobacillus* bacteria would be more effective, or that *acidophilus* needs to be taken for longer than the time periods used in the studies. Research on yogurt, which frequently has *acidophilus* cultures added to it, indicates that the combined-bacteria theory may be correct.

Acidophilus and Cholesterol Levels

High levels of blood cholesterol are one of several risk factors for cardiovascular disease. Ever since it was noted in 1974 that Masai warriors in Africa drank 2 liters of fermented milk per day yet still had low blood cholesterol levels, researchers have been curious about the cholesterol-lowering effect of the milk.

Existing evidence from animal and human studies suggests a moderate cholesterol-lowering action of fermented dairy products. The probable mechanism for this effect relates to the bacteria's consumption of FOS. When the bacteria metabolize the FOS, the production of certain fatty acids is increased, and these acids decrease the blood cholesterol concentrations either by inhibiting

---

Yogurt and Acidophilus Bacteria

Yogurt, the traditional source of *acidophilus*, has been used as a folk medicine for many years. It is known that yogurt is more easily digested by people with lactose intolerance than milk or other dairy products are. By law, yogurt must be produced using two strains of bacteria: *Lactobacillus bulgaricus* and *Streptococcus thermophilus*. These cultures produce lactase, which increases the level of the enzyme in the small intestine. With more enzymes present, the body can more easily digest the lactose in the yogurt. The lactase enzyme in yogurt is better than commercially produced lactase (available in tablets) at alleviating lactose intolerance symptoms. The addition of live *acidophilus* cultures to yogurt may also help, since some experts believe that combinations of cultures are more effective at digesting lactose than either one of them alone.

Caution!

- The strongest case for taking *acidophilus* supplements is the GI benefits and yeast infection fighting abilities of the bacteria. Supplements are generally safe, but eating *acidophilus*-containing dairy products is always an option.
- *Acidophilus* is safe for children, but don't delay in getting medical treatment for diarrhea that lasts longer than one day.
- If you suspect you have your first vaginal infection, consult your doctor before treating yourself with *acidophilus*. The bacterium only works on one type of yeast, *Candida albicans*, and could worsen symptoms of other infections.
- If you have a medical condition or are pregnant or lactating, talk to your doctor before taking any supplement.

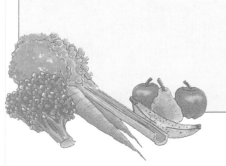

the liver's production of cholesterol, or by redistributing cholesterol from the blood back to the liver. In addition, increased bacterial activity in the large intestine destroys the structure of bile acids, which are made from cholesterol. In order to replace the bile acids, the body pulls more cholesterol from the blood, thereby lowering blood cholesterol levels.

Test-tube studies conducted with *acidophilus* have shown that the bacteria assimilate, or take up, cholesterol into their own cells. This effect has yet to be demonstrated in humans, however. Animal studies have given inconsistent results, with some showing a decrease in blood cholesterol and others showing no effect with *acidophilus*-containing milk. Studies that used supplemental *acidophilus* without the milk did indicate overall reductions in cholesterol levels.

There haven't been a lot of human studies on this topic. One recent study examined the effect of yogurt containing added *acidophilus*, FOS, and vegetable oil in 30 men with elevated cholesterol levels. The men consumed 125 grams (about 4 ounces) of the yogurt three times per day for 21 days. Both total cholesterol and LDL ("bad" cholesterol) levels were reduced (by about 5 percent and 6 percent, respectively) compared to traditional yogurt. However, it's not known exactly which element of the product produced the results—or if it was a combination of all the elements.

When to Supplement with *Acidophilus* Bacteria

Acidophilus supplements should guarantee living cultures at the time of purchase, not just at the time of manufacture. A supplement with no live cultures is worthless. Since it's impossible for a consumer to determine if a supplement contains live cultures, it's best to choose an *acidophilus* supplement from a reputable manufacturer, or choose a food form—the bacteria may be more likely to be alive.

Acidophilus is frequently combined with *bifidobacteria* in supplements, and combination supplements may be more effective for some purposes. Taking FOS in addition to *acidophilus* and *bifi-dobacteria* may also enhance benefits. In general, there are no side effects from *acidophilus*, although very large quantities may cause a temporary increase in digestive gas or diarrhea.

What to Know about Taking *Acidophilus* Supplements

- *Acidophilus* bacteria are available in capsule, tablet, powder, and liquid forms for oral consumption. Douches and suppositories containing *acidophilus* are also available for topical vaginal treatment.

- Dosages of *acidophilus* are expressed in terms of billions of organisms—not in grams or milligrams like many supplements. A typical daily dose should supply about 3 to 5 billion live organisms. Check the product label for the expiration date.

- Taking the supplements (or eating a food that supplies *acidophilus*) regularly—every day or every other day—is important for maintaining the cultures in the digestive tract.

- For gastrointestinal purposes, one to two capsules (containing at least one billion live bacteria) taken one to three times per day is sometimes suggested. For all other forms, check the product label for usage and preparation instructions.

- Take *acidophilus* at least a half hour before eating, and if taking antibiotics, take them at separate times of the day.

- Douching with *acidophilus* (powder mixed with warm water) should be reserved for treating vaginal yeast infections (or when taking antibiotics) and not performed on a regular basis, since excessive douching may irritate the vagina.

- Since dietary supplements (or claims for them) are not reviewed by the Food and Drug Administration, quality control and potency problems may exist with *acidophilus* supplements.

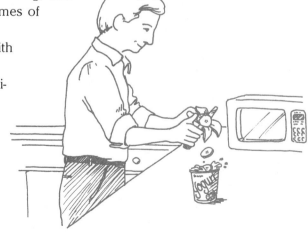

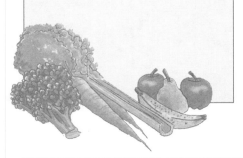

Bifidobacteria

Considered one of the "good" or "friendly" bacteria, *bifidobacteria* are normal inhabitants of the gut. *Bifidobacteria* were first described in 1899. Then, in the early 1900s it was discovered that *bifidobacteria* were the main type of bacteria in the gastrointestinal (GI) tracts of breastfed infants. Given this observation and the fact that breastfed infants generally experience fewer bouts of diarrhea than formula-fed infants, it was speculated that infant diarrhea could be treated by giving doses of *bifidobacteria* orally. Since that time, investigations have indicated that *bifidobacteria* may provide important health benefits for the GI system.

The Benefits of *Bifidobacteria*

Bifidobacteria and Gastrointestinal Health

In order for bacteria to serve a probiotic function, they have to make it to the GI tract alive. Many do not. Research shows that *bifidobacteria* survive the stomach well—about 24 to 38 percent make it through to the intestines.

A number of studies have shown that consuming *bifidobacteria* leads to an increase in GI *bifidobacteria* levels in both infants and adults. Research shows that when consumption of *bifidobacteria*-containing dairy products or supplements is stopped, the level of *bifidobacteria* in the intestinal tract drops back down to normal.

According to one study, mild constipation in women can be partially corrected by the regular consumption of *bifidobacteria*. Sixty participants consumed 125 grams (about 4 ounces) of yogurt containing *bifidobacteria* three times per day. Transit times were decreased, meaning food traveled through the system faster. This effect was not observed with regular yogurt as a control, thus demonstrating that the *bifidobacteria* were responsible for the increased intestinal motility.

Bifidobacteria and Diarrhea

Supplementing the food of infants with *bifidobacteria* may prevent diarrhea. This effect seems to be the most significant against diarrhea caused by **rotavirus** in infants and young children, which suggests that an immunological mechanism is responsible. However, further study is necessary to determine the actual mechanism for this beneficial effect.

Bifidobacteria and Other Potential Benefits

Cancer is an area of current research with regard to *bifidobacteria* and FOS. There's considerable evidence to suggest that the balance of bacteria in the gut is a factor in colon cancer risk. Recent studies demonstrate that cultures of *bifidobacteria* suppress the development of precancerous lesions and tumors in the colons of rats. Some of the most effective studies used both *bifidobacteria* and FOS supplements. Although study results have been promising, much additional research is needed in order to determine whether similar effects occur in humans.

There are a few preliminary studies in humans that relate the consumption of *bifidobacteria* to increased immunity. One study of older people indicated that a mixture of *bifidobacteria* and acidophilus bacteria decreased chronic inflammation of the colon and increased immunity. Others have shown increases in various measures of immune status.

Bifidobacteria in Food

Bifidobacteria cultures can be found in supplements and as added ingredients in certain fermented milk products. (See "Food Sources of *Bifidobacteria*"). Health food stores often carry a wider variety of bacteria-containing foods than regular supermarkets. *Bifidobacteria* can also be found in some brands of fermented milks, such as kefir, yogurt with live, active cultures, and yogurt drinks.

When to Supplement with *Bifidobacteria*

A supplement with no live cultures is worthless. Probiotic supplements should guarantee living cultures at the time of purchase, not just at the time of manufacture. It's impossible for a consumer to determine if a supplement contains live cultures. Choose a supple-

Caution!

- Clearly, *bifidobacteria* provide GI benefits, which are important for everybody's general health. Supplements are generally safe, but eating *bifidobacteria*-containing products is always an option—and one that delivers not only probiotic potential, but nutrition, too.
- *Bifidobacteria* are safe for children, but don't delay in getting medical treatment for diarrhea. If diarrhea in a child lasts longer than one day, consult a pediatrician.
- If you have a medical condition or are pregnant or lactating, talk to your doctor before taking any supplement.

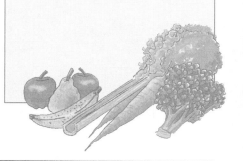

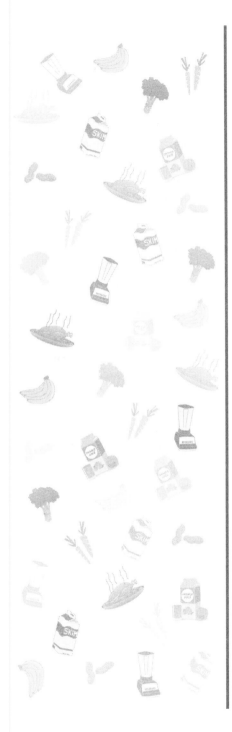

ment from a reputable manufacturer, or choose a food containing *bifidobacteria* to increase the odds that you'll get live cultures.

A combination supplement, or a food product containing *bifidobacteria* as part of a variety of bacterial cultures, may be more effective for some uses and would help "cover all bases" with regard to the health benefits of probiotic cultures.

In general, there are no side effects from *bifidobacteria*, although very large quantities may cause a temporary increase in digestive gas or diarrhea.

FOS (Fructooligosaccharides)

The concept of "prebiotics," in which nondigestible food ingredients are consumed in order to stimulate the growth or activity of beneficial bacteria already present in the gastrointestinal system, was developed in Japan more than a century ago. Researchers there discovered a substance that they called neosugar. After much research using animals and human participants, the product is now accepted as beneficial by the Japanese Ministry of Health and is added to many food products including infant formulas. Neosugar is a regular food component in other countries, such as Belgium, Denmark, Luxembourg, and Portugal, as well. Here in the United States, neosugar is a branded fructooligosaccharide that's beginning to be recognized as a beneficial food ingredient and dietary supplement.

FOS are indigestible carbohydrates (fiber). The chemical structure of FOS is such that it travels through the small intestine without being digested, reaching the large intestine intact. There, FOS acts as food for various "good" bacteria and stimulates their growth.

Although FOS has always been a part of the human diet, recent research suggests that increased FOS consumption (i.e., through supplements or fortified foods) may provide significant health benefits. FOS consumption has been associated with lowered blood cholesterol, reduced free radical formation, better bowel function, and an improved balance of bacteria in the digestive tract.

The Benefits of FOS

FOS and Gastrointestinal Health

Because FOS is not digested in the small intestine, it reaches the large intestine intact, where it has a big impact on the bacteria living there. The large intestine contains both beneficial bacteria and pathogenic (potentially disease-causing) bacteria. *Bifidobacteria*, which are considered beneficial and are the major "good" bacterium inhabiting the gut, begin growing in an infant's gastrointestinal tract within the first few days after birth. *Bifidobacteria* prefer FOS as food and respond to it by multiplying. For example, one study found that 1 gram per day of FOS led to a nearly seven-fold increase in *bifidobacteria*. A number of other studies have found that 4 to 15 grams per day of FOS, taken for as little as two weeks, can significantly increase *bifidobacteria* levels. Larger amounts of FOS, such as 30 grams per day, are also effective, but can cause GI side effects in some people. FOS also encourage the growth of *lactobacillius* bacteria, another beneficial type found in the GI tract.

At the same time that FOS increases the "good" bacteria in the gut, it helps decrease the "bad" bacteria. This is due, in part, to the acidic environment created in the gut when the good bacteria break down the FOS. The growth of pathogenic bacteria (see "Bacteria Found in the Large Intestine"), including *E. coli* and *Clostridium*, is hindered by the acidic environment.

Another beneficial aspect of keeping the bacteria cultures of the gut in balance is that flatulence (passing gas) can likely be decreased. If excessive gas is a problem, it's suggested that FOS supplements be taken along with *acidophilus* and *bifidobacteria* supplements. These friendly bacteria keep the growth of gas-producing bacteria in control, while the FOS promotes the growth of the friendly bacteria.

Caution!

- FOS supplements and foods enriched with FOS are considered safe, and appear to help maintain the health of the GI tract, and aid in calcium absorption. However, don't count on FOS to help with the other potential benefits yet—more research is needed.

- Although FOS supplements have not been shown to be dangerous for children, the GI side effects are likely to occur at much lower doses in children. Reduce dosages accordingly, and discuss the use of FOS with the child's pediatrician prior to giving it to your child.

- If you have a medical condition or are pregnant or lactating, talk to your doctor before taking any supplement.

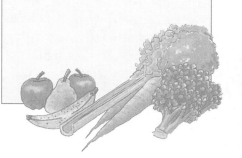

FOS and Mineral Absorption

Human studies conducted with healthy male adults and adolescents showed that consumption of FOS in amounts of 15 grams per day (for nine days) and 40 grams per day (for four weeks) increased calcium absorption by 26 percent and 58 percent, respectively. Given the importance of calcium in the maintenance of bone health and prevention of osteoporosis (and the inadequate calcium consumption many Americans have), increasing the ability of the body to absorb the mineral is clearly beneficial.

FOS and Diarrhea

Growth of the bacteria *Clostridium difficile*, which is responsible for antibiotic-associated diarrhea, is inhibited by FOS.

FOS and Cholesterol Reduction

Initial research suggests that supplemental FOS can lower total and LDL cholesterol (the "bad" type) and possibly triglyceride levels to some degree. Although the exact mechanism of action for this effect is unknown, it may be that FOS increases the amount of cholesterol eliminated from the body. This is an ongoing area of research and should not yet be considered a primary benefit of FOS supplementation.

FOS and Colon Cancer

There's considerable evidence to suggest that the balance of bacteria in the gut is a factor in colon cancer risk. Recent studies demonstrate that cultures of *bifidobacteria* suppress the development of precancerous lesions and tumors in animals. The studies that yielded the best results used both FOS supplements and *bifidobacteria* supplements. Although this is a promising area of research, much additional study is needed in order to determine if similar effects occur in humans.

BACTERIA FOUND IN THE LARGE INTESTINE

BENEFICIAL BACTERIA	PATHOGENIC BACTERIA
Bifidobacterium	Campylobacter
Lactobacillus	Clostridium
	Escherichia
	Listeria
	Salmonella
	Shigella

FOS in Food

Fructooligosaccharides are already being added to various medical nutritional products in the United States, and the market for the FOS-containing food products and supplements appears to be growing rapidly.

So far, nutritional meal replacement drinks are the main products to which FOS is added, but new products are under development. FOS is found naturally in small quantities in a number of fruits, vegetables, and grains, including Jerusalem artichokes, onions, garlic, leeks, peaches, bananas, and tomatoes, but not in quantities sufficient to provide real health benefits. For example, it would take 22 bananas or 383 cloves of garlic to get the same amount of FOS found in 1 teaspoon of an FOS supplement.

When to Supplement with FOS

Although much of the research on FOS seems preliminary, in general there is a substantial body of research that documents its beneficial effects with regard to gastrointestinal health. A dose of 2 to 15 grams of FOS should be sufficient for GI health purposes, although much more can be taken (up to 25 grams per day) without side effects. At doses higher than about 25 grams per day, side effects including excessive gas, bloating, and diarrhea have been reported.

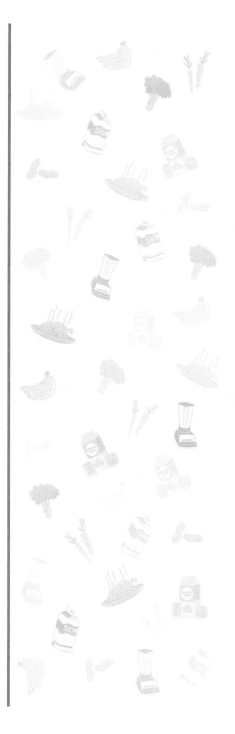

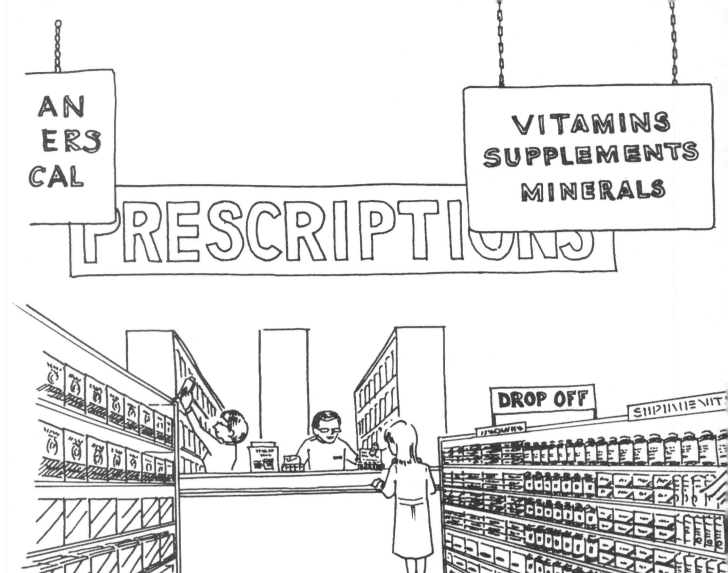
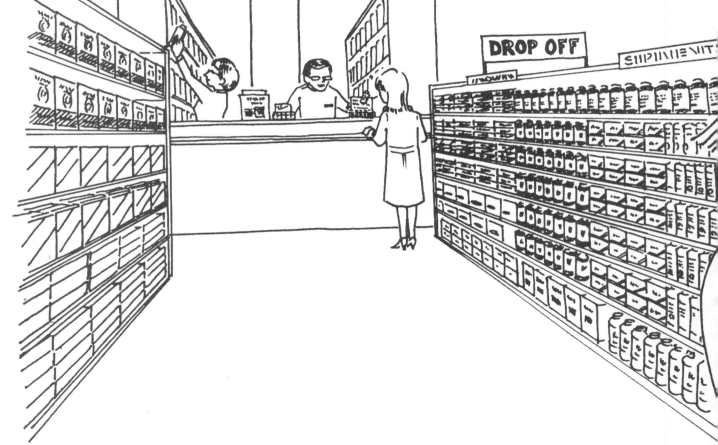

CHAPTER 11

Popular Commercial Supplements

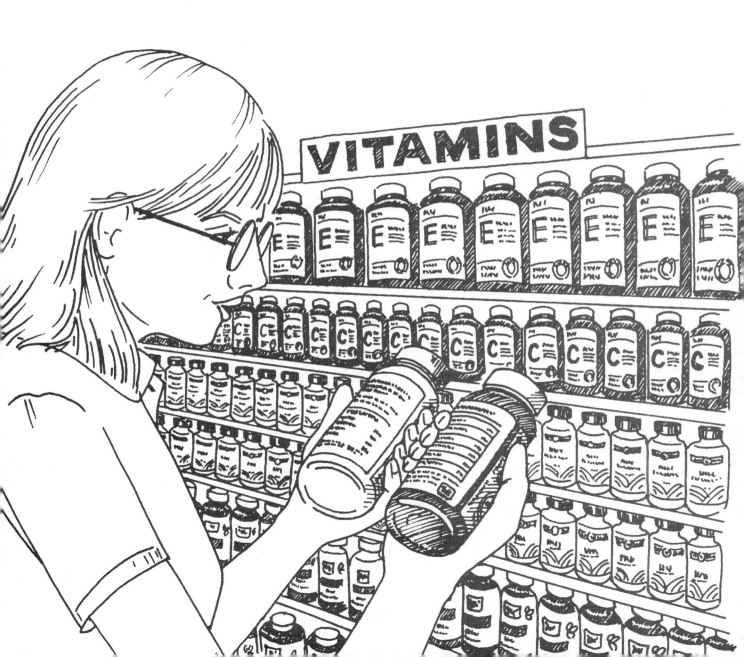

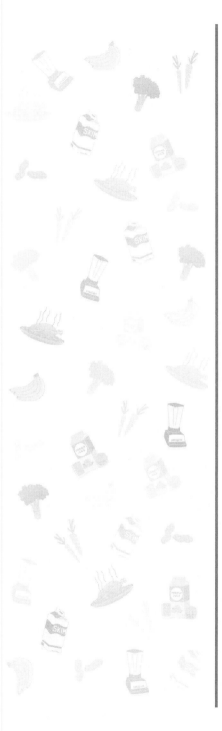

Alpha-Lipoic Acid

Alpha-lipoic acid, also called **thioctic acid** or simply lipoic acid, is a nonessential, vitaminlike compound that was first discovered in the 1950s. The body makes the tiny amounts of lipoic acid that it needs to turn food into energy. In the late 1980s researchers discovered that lipoic acid is also a very powerful antioxidant, and that it may help conserve other antioxidants such as vitamins C and E. Antioxidants are special compounds that fight free radicals—unstable oxygen molecules that can damage body cells and may lead to heart disease, cancer, stroke, and other health problems. Lipoic acid plays an important role in the complicated process that recycles glutathione—another major antioxidant in the body. Many of the claims made for lipoic acid—that it may be helpful for diabetes, cataracts, HIV, and other conditions—hinge on its glutathione connection.

The Benefits of Alpha-Lipoic Acid

Lipoic Acid and Diabetes

There are a number of ways in which lipoic acid may be beneficial for people with Type 2 (non-insulin-dependent, or adult-onset) diabetes. The most promising research is in the area of diabetic neuropathy. Neuropathy is a fairly common nerve condition among diabetics that's characterized by tingling, numbness, and pain in the extremities.

In a 1999 study conducted in Germany, 328 people with Type 2 diabetes received daily intravenous (given by vein) doses of varying amounts (1,200 milligrams, 600 milligrams, or 100 milligrams) of lipoic acid for three weeks. A rating scale was used to measure the changes in the intensity of the pain they experienced. All groups experienced improvement with lipoic acid; however, more participants from the group who received 600 milligrams of lipoic acid per day reported relief than from any other group. Unfortunately, the researchers used injected lipoic acid—a form that most people don't have access to, and shouldn't be using on

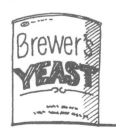

their own anyway. Another study, which used oral lipoic acid supplements, followed 65 participants for two years and showed that a number of measures of nerve function were improved. The few other small studies that utilized oral lipoic acid have shown mixed results.

In Europe, lipoic acid is often prescribed by doctors for treating diabetic neuropathy, with the usual doses being quite high—600 milligrams or more. Because lipoic acid appears to be quite effective in this regard, additional studies are underway. It may be that lipoic acid is effective with nerve damage in general—not just when it's associated with diabetes.

There's some indication that lipoic acid also helps the body utilize glucose better. One medium-sized study showed blood glucose improvements in participants who received 600 milligrams or more of lipoic acid daily. Preliminary animal studies suggest that lipoic acid may help prevent cataracts from forming (sometimes a problem in people with diabetes), although additional research is necessary.

Lipoic Acid and HIV/AIDS

A number of test-tube studies have shown a beneficial role for lipoic acid in helping to fight human immunodeficiency virus (HIV). Some indicate that lipoic acid inhibits a substance that's believed to help activate the virus, thereby reducing its ability to reproduce. Another study showed that immune and liver function in AIDS patients was improved with lipoic acid supplementation. Very few human studies have been conducted in this area to date, so no firm conclusions about the efficacy of lipoic acid supplementation as a therapy for HIV/AIDS can be drawn at this time.

Lipoic Acid and Other Potential Benefits

Several studies have suggested that lipoic acid can be used as a therapeutic agent in a number of conditions relating to liver disease because it helps the liver remove harmful substances from the body. Alcohol-induced liver damage, mushroom poisoning, and metal toxicity are a few of these conditions. So far, however, this benefit remains speculative, because some of the research was flawed and results haven't been conclusive.

Caution!

- Lipoic acid shows great promise, especially for diabetes-related conditions. However, more research on the efficacy and safety of oral lipoic acid supplements is needed.
- Because lipoic acid can improve glucose utilization, people with diabetes may need to adjust their insulin or medications. If you have diabetes, consult with your doctor before taking lipoic acid supplements.
- If you have hypoglycemia (low blood sugar levels), lipoic acid supplements may worsen your condition.
- If you have a medical condition or are pregnant or lactating, consult your doctor before taking any supplement.
- Although some manufacturers and marketers of lipoic acid say it decreases fat storage or slows aging, there isn't a shred of scientific evidence to support these claims.

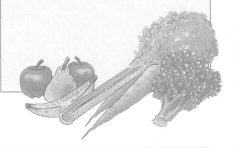

Other uses of lipoic acid supplementation include treatment of radiation injury, neurodegenerative diseases, and brain damage caused by an insufficient blood supply (such as with a stroke). Much of this research has been conducted in test tubes only, or is considered preliminary.

Alpha-Lipoic Acid in Food

Red meat, especially organ meat (liver, kidney, heart), is a source of lipoic acid, as are broccoli, spinach, and brewer's yeast. Supplements are necessary in order to obtain therapeutic dosages.

Should You Supplement with Lipoic Acid?

No one has yet determined how much lipoic acid we need, and since our bodies make it, there is no recommended amount to consume from food or supplements. However, some experts believe that the body only makes enough lipoic acid for the metabolic, or energy-producing, function and that not enough is left over for antioxidant functions. Therefore, these experts suggest that dietary sources and/or supplements may be necessary in order for lipoic acid to achieve its full antioxidant capabilities.

Lipoic acid doses of up to 2,000 milligrams per day appear to be well tolerated. Mild stomach upset and allergic-type skin rashes, although rare, have been reported as side effects. Lipoic acid is not recommended for children.

Bee Pollen, Royal Jelly, and Propolis

We're not talking about honey here, but about bee pollen, royal jelly, and propolis—products that are collected from bees and are widely marketed in health food stores and through supplement catalogs. The most familiar bee product is bee pollen. After the bees collect pollen from plants, they compress it into pellets, which beekeepers then collect from the beehives. Royal jelly is a white, gelatinous substance produced by the salivary glands of worker bees as a food

---

What to Know about Taking Lipoic Acid Supplements

- Lipoic acid is available in both pill and capsule forms. Although most studies have used dosages of 100 to 800 milligrams per day, supplements generally contain much less—usually 50 milligrams or 100 milligrams per pill. Lipoic acid is also available as part of an antioxidant combination supplement.
- Lipoic acid supplements can be taken with or without food.
- Since dietary supplements are not reviewed by the FDA, quality control and potency problems may exist with lipoic acid supplements.

source for the queen bee. Royal jelly is a concentrated protein and mineral source, but only for bees—not humans. Propolis, also called "bee glue," is a sticky resin that bees collect from the buds of pine trees and use to repair cracks in their hives.

The Benefits of Bee Products

Propolis and Cold Sores

Propolis has very limited benefits, and even these aren't well documented or effective across the board. Sometimes topical application of a salve containing propolis is suggested as a remedy for cold sores. But, although it's true that propolis contains some antibacterial compounds, these compounds aren't as effective as standard antibiotics or over-the-counter antibiotic ointments.

Bee Pollen and Pollen Allergies

Although there's no nutritional need for bee pollen in the human diet, some scientists believe that ingesting small amounts of bee pollen prior to allergy season can desensitize people to pollen, thus curing seasonal allergies such as hay fever. To be truly effective, some recommend that the bee pollen come from local bees so that one becomes desensitized to the pollens in one's local area. For allergy relief, it's recommended that one start taking just a few granules of bee pollen, or part of a tablet each day, then gradually increase the amount. Research has yet to prove whether this use of bee pollen is effective at all. Also, the potential for a severe allergic reaction to bee pollen is real if one is allergic to bee stings.

Medicinal Uses of Honey

Honey has been used topically to help heal skin problems since ancient times. In fact, Hippocrates, the Greek physician, made many honey-based treatments for skin disorders such as cuts, sores, and burns. Because of its high sugar content, its low protein content, and its relatively high acidity, honey is an effective antimicrobial agent against certain bacteria, yeast, and molds. In addition, when used topically, honey's ability to draw moisture from the air

Caution!

- There is very little good scientific literature to back up the claims associated with these products—and absolutely no nutritional reason to consume these supplements. Save your money.
- People with asthma or allergies to bee stings should exercise extreme caution when using any bee products.
- If you have a medical condition or are pregnant or lactating, talk to your doctor before taking any supplement.

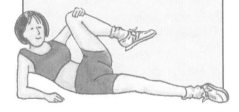

helps promote skin healing, decreases scarring, and keeps the injured area from sticking to a bandage.

Should You Supplement with Bee Products?

Although bee pollen contains protein, B vitamins, and carbohydrates, it isn't a good source of any of these nutrients, and there's always the risk of allergic reaction. What's more, there are no known dosages for any bee products, and the supplement formulations are arbitrary. As for royal jelly, the claimed benefits of consuming royal jelly (growth enhancement, fertility, and longevity) don't transfer to humans. The topical application of propolis appears safe, but may not be effective for all.

What to Know about Taking Bee Product Supplements

- Bee products are available in a myriad of forms: tablets, capsules, softgels, liquids, powders, creams, lozenges, and both dried and fresh pollen. The amounts of each substance provided varies widely.
- Since dietary supplements (or claims for them) are not reviewed by the Food and Drug Administration, quality control and potency problems may exist with bee products.

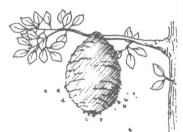

Blue-Green Algae

Blue-green algae is not one specific type of algae, but rather a group of algae. Other algae groups are brown algae and green algae. Algae are single-celled plants that grow in water. The blue-green algae used in supplements is generally harvested from algae "farms" and not from the wild. Two of the most commonly marketed types of blue-green algae are spirulina (rhymes with "ballerina") and aphanizomenon (pronounced ah-FAN-ih-ZO-ma-non). In

Bee Products and Potential Allergic Reactions

Bee products pose a real threat to people who are allergic to bee stings. Cases of asthma, hives, and anaphylactic shock after ingesting the bee pollen or royal jelly have been documented, and in some cases using these products has proven fatal. Those with bee sting allergies should definitely avoid bee products. It's also been discovered that some people who aren't allergic to bee stings may have allergic reactions to bee pollen. This is because bee pollen contains pollen from ragweed (to which many people are allergic) and other plants that may cross-react with ragweed, such as dandelions, sunflowers, or chrysanthemums. In other words, even if the bee hasn't collected pollen from ragweed, other plants that are biochemically similar may cause a ragweedlike allergic reaction. The best bet is to avoid these products completely.

addition to promoting their nutritional content, proponents of blue-green algae tout a wide variety of benefits for the supplements.

The Benefits of Blue-Green Algae

Spirulina and Bad Breath

Spirulina is one of nature's most effective breath fresheners—as long as the bad breath is not due to gum disease or chronic sinusitis. The chlorophyll (green plant pigment) content of spirulina is the key ingredient. In fact, a number of commercial chlorophyll breath fresheners contain spirulina.

Blue-Green Algae as a Concentrated Source of Nutrients

Blue-green algae is a concentrated source of protein—by weight. Sometimes algae is included in vegetarian and macrobiotic diets because of its protein content, since people following restrictive diets may consume too little protein. Most Americans, however, get plenty of protein, and the amount of protein contained in the supplements is not enough to make a real dietary difference. For example, a typical serving size of spirulina would not meet the legal requirements to be considered a source of protein at all. Six spirulina tablets generally contain fewer than 2 grams of protein, while a moderate portion of meat, poultry, or seafood contains about 21 grams of protein.

Blue-green algae also contains several vitamins, such as folic acid, and is a fairly good source of vitamin B_{12} and carotenoids—especially beta-carotene. But again, when considered per serving, these amounts are negligible.

Blue-Green Algae and Other Potential Benefits

The claimed benefits of blue-green algae supplements are numerous and wide ranging—usually a tip-off that the supplement is too good to be true. Some of these "benefits" include increased energy, "detoxification" of the body, correction of hypoglycemia (low blood sugar levels), improved sleep, relief from fatigue, weight loss, enhanced immunity, cancer-fighting and infection-fighting ability—even suppression of AIDS and HIV. To hear the marketers of blue-green

What to Know about Taking Blue-Green Algae Supplements

- Blue-green algae is available in many forms: capsules, tablets, powders, and liquids.
- Blue-green algae supplements may cause nausea or diarrhea in some people. To minimize this side effect, take them with food, decrease the dose, or stop taking them completely.
- To treat bad breath, mix 1 teaspoon of spirulina powder into 4 ounces of water, swish the liquid in the mouth, and then swallow it. Or, chew one spirulina tablet completely, then swallow it. Repeat up to a few times per day as needed.
- Since dietary supplements are not reviewed by the FDA, quality control and potency problems may exist with blue-green algae supplements.

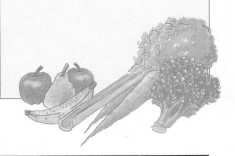

algae, you'd think these supplements can cure practically any health problem! Unfortunately, there are very few studies on blue-green algae at all, and human research in any of these areas is severely lacking. Many of the claims are linked to anecdotal reports and testimonials—not science. Needless to say, there's no evidence that blue-green algae will help with any of these health conditions.

Should You Supplement with Blue-Green Algae?

Most of the research on blue-green algae to date has been conducted with test tubes or animals only. There is no nutritional reason to take algae supplements—there are less expensive and better-tasting ways to get the same nutrients into the diet. And, aside from a treatment for bad breath, there's nothing else to recommend these supplements. Children should not take them regardless.

There's some concern about the safety of blue-green algae products. Some types of blue-green algae grow in the same water as algae that are known to produce highly toxic substances called microcystins. Microcystins are similar to the red tides that sometimes occur in the ocean, killing large numbers of fish. In large doses, microcystins produce acute liver failure, brain damage, and even death. No one knows at what level the microcystins in algae become unsafe. The World Health Organization (WHO) has set upper limits for microcystins in drinking water, and one Canadian study found samples of blue-green algae that contained microcystin levels 50 times higher than the WHO limit. In another study, the Oregon Health Department found microcystins in 35 of 36 blue-green algae products. The Food and Drug Administration has received reports of several adverse reactions from blue-green algae supplements, but it hasn't been established that these effects are due to microcystins.

Choline and Lecithin

Choline (pronounced KOH-leen) and lecithin (pronounced LESS-a-thin) are closely related substances. In fact, lecithin is a source of choline (in the form of phosphatidylcholine). Lecithin is a phospho-

Caution!

- Blue-green algae supplements offer nothing nutritionally that isn't available from regular foods, its numerous claims have not been substantiated scientifically, and its safety is questionable. Skip them unless you want an expensive, "natural" breath freshener.
- If you have a medical condition or are pregnant or lactating, talk to your doctor before taking blue-green algae supplements.
- Never harvest your own algae from the wild. It may be contaminated with wastes and contain dangerous toxins.

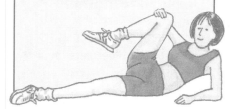

lipid—a fatty-like substance—and as such, reacts with both water and fats. This characteristic makes phospholipids an important part of cell membranes. Choline is important for nerve function and the transport and breakdown of fats and cholesterol in the body. It also speeds up the production and release of **acetylcholine**, an important neurotransmitter (a chemical that carries messages to and from the brain) involved in memory storage, muscle control, and many other functions.

Lecithin is not an essential nutrient because the body can make all that it needs. Choline, on the other hand, is essential, although the Adequate Intake for it was only recently established. Although it's sometimes referred to as a B vitamin, choline isn't really a vitamin. However, it does work in conjunction with the B vitamin folic acid. Choline is needed to make the neurotransmitter acetylcholine, and to help break down fats in the body.

The Benefits of Choline and Lecithin

Lecithin/Choline and Gallbladder Disease

Lecithin helps to stabilize the cholesterol in bile, a fat-digesting substance produced in the liver and stored in the gallbladder. Low levels of lecithin are known to encourage the formation of gallstones, while lecithin or choline supplements may help prevent gallstone formation by improving the flow of fats and cholesterol through the liver and gallbladder.

Lecithin/Choline and the Liver

Choline is often included in various "liver complex" supplements because it's needed to metabolize fats properly, and without it fats can accumulate in the liver. These supplements (which also include other liver-specific nutrients such as the amino acid methionine and the B vitamin inositol) may be helpful for viral **hepatitis** and combating the effects of chemotherapy on the liver. In Europe, choline is already used to treat liver diseases.

Chronic consumption of alcohol can cause cirrhosis of the liver, a condition in which the structure of the liver is damaged and liver function is diminished. A good deal of research on choline supple-

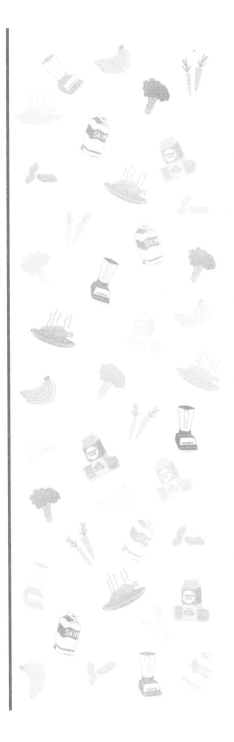

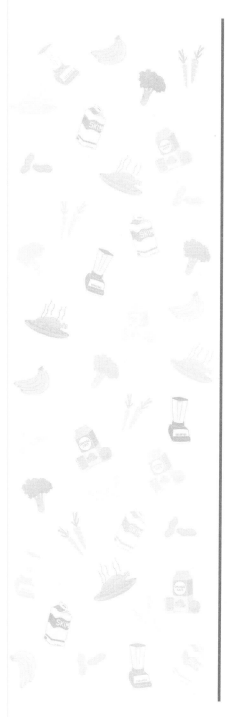

ments and liver disease in baboons shows that the development of alcoholic liver cirrhosis is prevented by choline. More recent research has found that other early changes brought on by alcohol consumption, such as "fatty" liver, are also slowed by choline supplementation. Researchers are hopeful that the beneficial effects of choline, taken at the initial stages of alcoholic liver injury, may prevent or delay the progression to more advanced forms of liver disease. Although these studies have been conducted in animals only, it's believed that the results may also apply to humans.

Lecithin/Choline and Cholesterol

One researcher found that oral lecithin supplements increased HDL ("good" cholesterol) in people, but the results were not reproduced in other studies. Because lecithin contains polyunsaturated fatty acids, many experts feel that any cholesterol-lowering effect these supplements might have can be attributed to the fatty acids, rather than unique properties of lecithin itself. A recent study of 23 men with high blood cholesterol levels found that lecithin had no significant effects on any measure of blood cholesterol, including total cholesterol, HDL, LDL, and triglycerides.

A study examining oral choline supplements revealed moderate reductions in blood cholesterol, and choline has also been used to lower high homocysteine concentrations in both humans and animals. (High levels of homocysteine, an amino acid–like substance, are linked with heart disease.) Although it appears that dietary choline intake might be associated with cardiovascular disease risk, more studies are needed.

Lecithin/Choline and Neurological Diseases

Choline is an essential part of the neurotransmitter acetylcholine, which relays messages between nerve cells in the areas of the brain responsible for memory and learning. Research suggests that choline and lecithin supplementation increases the levels of acetylcholine in specific parts of the brain and may enhance communication between nerve cells. Extensive studies have shown that choline and lecithin supplementation can reduce the symptoms of tardive dyskenesia—tics or twitches sometimes brought on by the use of certain psychological drugs.

The first long-term, well controlled trial of lecithin supplements for Alzheimer's disease was conducted in 1985. Fifty-one participants were given 20 to 25 grams of supplemental lecithin for six months and were then followed for another six months or more. Although there were no differences between the placebo group and the lecithin group, a subgroup of lecithin takers did show improvement. These subjects were older, suggesting that the effects of lecithin may be more evident in older patients, or that there is a "therapeutic window" for lecithin—a specific time period in which taking the supplements is effective. The most recent studies have investigated the possibility that choline supplements may be a useful treatment for Huntington's disease, Parkinson's disease, schizophrenia, and other neurological conditions, but so far no firm conclusions can be made.

Animal studies suggest that dietary choline intake early in life can affect memory and the severity of dementia (loss of mental faculties as a result of Alzheimer's disease or other brain impairments) in older animals. Human studies on choline and dementia were designed to investigate treating, rather than preventing, the symptoms of dementia. More studies are needed to determine whether dietary choline intake is useful for the prevention of dementia.

Lecithin/Choline and Other Potential Benefits

Despite very little scientific evidence, proponents of lecithin and choline have linked the supplements to weight loss. There's absolutely no substantiation for the use of lecithin as a weight loss treatment. One study, conducted with marathon runners, suggests that choline supplements may improve athletic performance. However, much more research needs to be done in this area.

Should You Supplement with Lecithin and Choline?

Since lecithin is not an essential nutrient, there's no deficiency associated with it. The only reason to take lecithin supplements is

Lecithin and Choline in Food

There are many food sources of natural lecithin, including cabbage, calf's liver, cauliflower, caviar, egg yolks, garbanzo beans (chick peas), lettuce, milk, peanuts, soy beans, split peas, rice, and lentils. It's also added to foods as an emulsifier to keep ingredients mixed together properly and to maintain a thick consistency. Mayonnaise and ice cream, for example, often contain added lecithin, and it's present in cooking sprays and many baked goods, too. It's possible to consume a diet that delivers 1 gram per day of choline. In addition, it's estimated that lecithin added during food processing increases the average daily consumption of choline by 1.5 milligrams per kilogram of body weight for adults.

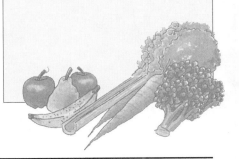

to get the choline that's its natural component. One can be deficient in choline, although there is only one published study examining the effects of inadequate choline intake in humans. That study reported decreased choline stores and liver damage when men consumed a choline-deficient diet for three weeks. Animal studies have shown that a choline-deficient diet results not only in liver dysfunction, but in growth retardation, kidney dysfunction, and bone abnormalities.

Infants need a dietary supply of choline, since there's a high need for choline-containing compounds during periods of rapid growth. In 1985, the American Academy of Pediatrics recommended that infant formula contain 7 milligrams of choline per 100 calories. This amount is based on the choline content of human milk. Children should not take the supplements unless under a doctor's supervision. Although there is no Recommended Dietary Allowance for either lecithin or choline, the National Academy of Sciences recently set the Adequate Intake level for choline at 550 milligrams per day for men and 425 milligrams for women. Most of us reach that level—the average daily intake of choline is about 400 to 900 milligrams, according to the NAS.

Since choline and folic acid (folate) are metabolically related, researchers investigated the impact of folate status on choline in the body. Folate deficiencies caused blood levels of choline to decrease, although no symptoms of choline deficiency were noticed among the study volunteers. Once body folate levels were increased via supplementation, choline rose to normal levels, or even higher. This suggests that the body cannot make enough choline when folate status is low. Therefore, people who consume a chronically low-folate diet may need additional choline—or should improve their folate intake. There are also some experts who believe that people who take niacin for the treatment of high cholesterol may need more lecithin and choline.

Research dosages of lecithin vary widely depending on the condition being studied. For neurological conditions, very high amounts—5 to 10 grams taken three times per day—have been used; for liver disease, a typical dose is 350 to 500 milligrams taken three times daily. Taking large amounts of lecithin or choline does produce side effects, including vomiting, gastro-intestinal upset, sweating, excessive salivation, and hypotension (low blood pressure). Long-term megadoses of lecithin or choline may cause more serious effects, including liver damage, mental depression, and nervous system disorders. One very obvious side effect of too much choline (10 grams per day or more) is a "fishy" body odor, which doesn't occur with lecithin.

What to Know about Taking Lecithin and Choline Supplements

- Lecithin is generally available in softgel or granular form. Softgels contain varying amounts of lecithin, usually around 1,200 milligrams. Lecithin supplements vary widely in their choline content, but are usually around 3 to 4 percent choline by weight. In most cases paying extra for a higher concentration of choline isn't worth it.

- Lecithin granules can be sprinkled over foods or mixed into drinks and allow you to use as much or as little as desired. One teaspoon of granules contains about 1,200 milligrams of lecithin. Store granules in the refrigerator, or they'll become rancid quickly.

- Choline supplements are available in softgel form as either choline chloride or choline bitartrate, and frequently contain approximately 60 milligrams of pure choline. Liver "complex" supplements contain varying amounts of choline.

- For better absorption, lecithin and choline should be taken with meals.

- Phosphatidylcholine supplements are much more costly than plain choline supplements and are not worth the money.

- Since dietary supplements (or claims for them) are not reviewed by the Food and Drug Administration, quality control and potency problems may exist with lecithin and choline supplements.

Caution!

- Lecithin and choline supplements are not necessary for healthy people. Those who want to try them for liver disorders should do so only under their doctor's supervision. All other uses are considered preliminary or experimental.

- Consult your doctor regarding the appropriateness of lecithin or choline supplements before you take them for neurological or liver conditions.

- If you have a medical condition or are pregnant or lactating, talk to your doctor before taking any supplement.

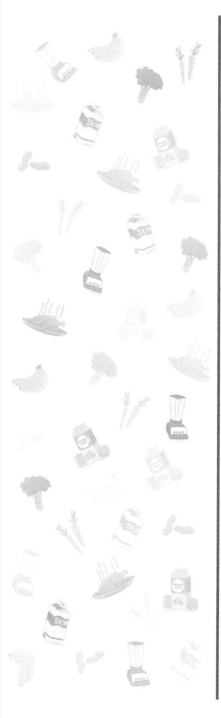

ADEQUATE INTAKES (AI)[a] FOR CHOLINE*

AGE/SEX	CHOLINE (MG)**
Males	
9–13 years	375
14+ years	550
Females	
9–13 years	375
14–18 years	400
19+ years	425
Pregnant women	450
Lactating women	550

Reprinted by permission of The National Academy of Sciences, 1998. Courtesy of the National Academy Press, Washington D.C.

*There are no RDAs for choline due to insufficient information.

**mg = milligrams.

[a] = Although AIs have been set for choline, there are few data to assess whether a dietary supply of choline is needed at all stages of the life cycle, and it may be that the choline requirement can be met by endogenous synthesis at some of these stages.

TOLERABLE UPPER INTAKE LEVEL (UL)[a] FOR CHOLINE

AGE	CHOLINE (G)*
0–½ year	ND[b]
½–1 year	ND
1–3 years	1.0
4–8 years	1.0
9–13 years	2.0
14–18 years	3.0
19+ years	3.5
Pregnancy	
≤18 years	3.0
19–50 years	3.5
Lactation	
≤18 years	3.0
19–50 years	3.5

Reprinted by permission of The National Academy of Sciences, 1998. Courtesy of the National Academy Press, Washington D.C.

*g = grams.

[a] = The maximum level of daily nutrient intake that is likely to pose no risk of adverse effects. Unless otherwise specified, the UL represents total intake from food, water, and supplements.

[b] = Not determinable due to lack of data or adverse effects in this age group and concern with regard to lack of ability to handle excess amounts. Source of intake should be from food only to prevent high levels of intake.

Chondroitin

Chondroitin (pronounced con-DROY-tin) is a natural bodily substance found in and around the cells of cartilage. It's basically a chain of glucosamine (another "building block" of cartilage also available in supplement form), with sugar molecules attached. Chondroitin sulfate, the form currently sold as a dietary supplement, is believed to provide strength and resilience to cartilage.

The Benefits of Chondroitin

Osteoarthritis

According to the Arthritis Foundation, osteoarthritis occurs when the cartilage that cushions the ends of bone joints breaks down, resulting in stiff joints, joint pain, and deformity. (Rheumatoid arthritis, on the other hand, is an autoimmune disease characterized by inflamed knuckles and joints and, often, misshapen hands. In addition, rheumatoid arthritis is a condition of the entire body that can cause fatigue, loss of appetite, and fever.)

There have been several human studies that suggest chondroitin is an effective treatment for osteoarthritis. In one study of 119 people, those who took 1,200 milligrams of chondroitin sulfate showed reduced rates of severe joint damage: only 8.8 percent of them developed severely damaged joints during the study, compared to 30 percent of those in the placebo group. And, in many of the studies, those subjects who received chondroitin rated their arthritis improvement and pain relief higher than those receiving either a prescription pain reliever or a placebo.

How does chondroitin work? It's unknown, but there are a few theories. Chondroitin is thought to give cartilage elasticity, which may improve joint function. It may also block enzymes that break down cartilage, thereby slowing the progression of osteoarthritis. Chondroitin may also increase the amount of lubricating fluid in the joints. Finally, chondroitin may have a mild anti-inflammatory effect. Some proponents of chondroitin (as well as marketers of the supplement) claim that it may even prevent joint damage and repair

Caution!

- The research on chondroitin is still preliminary. Given the questions surrounding chondroitin's abilities as an arthritis treatment, the best bet may be to take a combined glucosamine–chondroitin supplement. Not everyone who takes chondroitin will experience benefits.
- If you take blood-thinning medications, including aspirin, consult your doctor before taking chondroitin supplements.
- If you have osteoarthritis, do not stop or decrease current medication dosages without consulting your doctor.
- If you have a medical condition or are pregnant or lactating, talk to your doctor before taking any supplement.

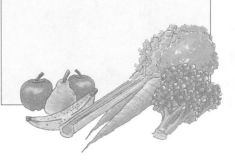

damaged cartilage, thereby reversing arthritis. However, there is no scientific evidence to support these claims.

Until recently, no long-term studies on chondroitin benefits and safety had been performed. Now, a detailed long-term study of chondroitin (and glucosamine) on osteoarthritis of the knee has been initiated by the National Institutes of Health.

Should You Supplement with Chondroitin?

Currently, it's unclear whether chondroitin is most effective when coupled with glucosamine or when taken alone. Some experts say that since much of the research on chondroitin used an injectable form and not a pill form, the usefulness of chondroitin supplements is questionable, and that the real benefits come from the glucosamine with which it's often combined. This remains to be seen. However, as more and more researchers begin using the oral form of chondroitin in their studies, additional information about chondroitin as a single supplement should be available in the next couple of years.

The usual dosage for osteoarthritis is 1,200 milligrams of chondroitin per day (400 milligrams taken three times daily). This dosage is considered safe and has only been associated with mild gastrointestinal side effects in some studies. Children should not take these supplements.

What to Know about Taking Chondroitin Supplements

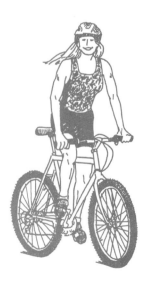

- Chondroitin sulfate is available as a single supplement in 250-milligram and 400-milligram capsules. It's also available combined with glucosamine and various other compounds in varying dosages.
- Chondroitin sulfate is extracted from animal tissue, most often from cattle tracheas, but sometimes from shark cartilage, too (the cheaper way to make it). Some experts recommend avoiding chondroitin supplements made from shark cartilage, citing inconsistent quality and amount of chondroitin in the supplement.

- Chondroitin has not been shown to provide relief for people with rheumatoid arthritis.
- Since dietary supplements (or claims for them) are not reviewed by the Food and Drug Administration, quality control and potency problems may exist with chondroitin supplements.

Glucosamine

Glucosamine (pronounced glue-KOSE-uh-mean) is made in the body from sugar and is a component of substances called proteoglycans and glycosaminoglycans. These substances are major components or "building blocks" of cartilage. As such, glucosamine is found naturally in the body's joints and connective tissues, where it's used for cartilage repair and maintenance. It's also believed that glucosamine stimulates cartilage cell growth.

The Benefits of Glucosamine

Glucosamine and Osteoarthritis

Initial research with animals suggested that glucosamine supplements might be useful for people with osteoarthritis, the most common form of arthritis, which results in stiff joints, joint pain, and deformity.

In the early 1980s a small number of studies conducted in Europe and Asia found that some osteoarthritis patients received short-term symptomatic pain relief from taking glucosamine supplements. More recently, a 1992 study of 252 people with osteoarthritis of the knee showed that taking 500 milligrams of glucosamine sulfate three times per day brought significant pain relief compared to a placebo.

Studies comparing the effectiveness of glucosamine to nonsteroidal anti-inflammatory drugs (NSAIDs) have also been performed. In a four-week study of 199 participants with osteoarthritis in at least one knee, improvements were noted in both those who took 400 milligrams of ibuprofen (an NSAID) three times per day and those who took 500 milligrams of glucosamine sulfate three

Buying Tip

In early 2000 ConsumerLab, Inc., conducted tests of glucosamine–chondroitin supplements, as well as glucosamine-only and chondroitin-only supplements. Almost half of the combination products, and both of the chondroitin-only products, failed quality tests because of low levels of chondroitin. Interestingly, according to ConsumerLab, chondroitin costs manufacturers about four times more than glucosamine, which may explain why it was lacking in so many products. Check the ConsumerLab Web site (*www.consumerlab.com*) to see how specific brands fared in the tests before purchasing a chondroitin supplement.

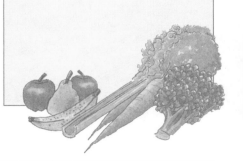

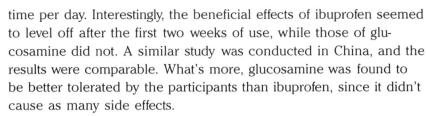

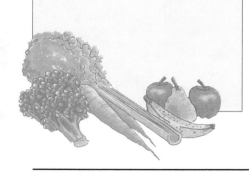

time per day. Interestingly, the beneficial effects of ibuprofen seemed to level off after the first two weeks of use, while those of glucosamine did not. A similar study was conducted in China, and the results were comparable. What's more, glucosamine was found to be better tolerated by the participants than ibuprofen, since it didn't cause as many side effects.

Recent preliminary research also suggests that the supplement might slow down cartilage loss, helping to keep arthritis from getting worse. How? Apparently glucosamine stimulates collagen production and reduces the breakdown of healthy tissue. Additional research is needed to determine if glucosamine supplements actually can reverse the degenerative processes associated with arthritis. However, taking the supplements will not increase the amount of glucosamine in the joints.

Until recently, no long-term studies on glucosamine safety or benefits had been performed. Now, a detailed long-term study of glucosamine (and osteoarthritis of the knee) has been initiated by the National Institutes of Health, but results won't be available for a couple of years.

Should You Supplement with Glucosamine?

Although glucosamine seems promising for osteoarthritis, not everyone who takes it will experience benefits, and any results at all take at least six to eight weeks to occur. The usual dosage for osteoarthritis is 1,500 milligrams glucosamine (500 milligrams taken three times a day). If this amount relieves symptoms, the dosage can be gradually decreased.

Glucosamine is available as a "hydrochloride" (HCl) and as a "sulfate." Both forms have performed equally well in studies. The glucosamine that's present in supplements is extracted from natural sources such as ground-up crab, lobster, or shrimp shells. Although glucosamine is frequently sold in combination with a substance called chondroitin, some researchers suggest it isn't necessary to take both, especially since much of the research on chondroitin used an injectable form and not pill form. In addition, no studies have shown that the efficacy of glucosamine is enhanced by taking it with SAMe supplements. (For more information on SAMe, see page 274.)

Side effects from glucosamine supplementation include headache, gastrointestinal upset, swelling, and itching, which are reversible when the dosage is decreased or supplements are discontinued. Recently, a preliminary animal study showed that taking glucosamine sulfate caused insulin resistance, or decreased insulin action. Further studies are necessary to determine if the effects also occur in humans. It is not recommended for children.

What to Know about Taking Glucosamine Supplements

- Glucosamine is available in tablet and capsule forms in widely varying dosages. A glucosamine-containing drink is also available.
- Glucosamine has not been shown to provide relief for people with rheumatoid arthritis.
- Glucosamine should be taken along with NSAIDs and prescribed osteoarthritis medications to get maximum pain relief. Talk to your doctor before taking glucosamine supplements.
- Many of the combined glucosamine/chondroitin products in a ConsumerLab test did not contain the amount of active ingredient stated on the product labels. Check *www.consumerlab.com* to see how specific brands fared before purchasing a supplement.
- Since dietary supplements (or claims for them) are not reviewed by the Food and Drug Administration, quality control and potency problems may exist with glucosamine supplements.

Kelp

Kelp refers to several flat, brown-colored seaweed species called *Laminaria* and *Macrocystis*, which grow on rocks in the cold ocean waters of the Northern Hemisphere. A sea vegetable, kelp is a con-

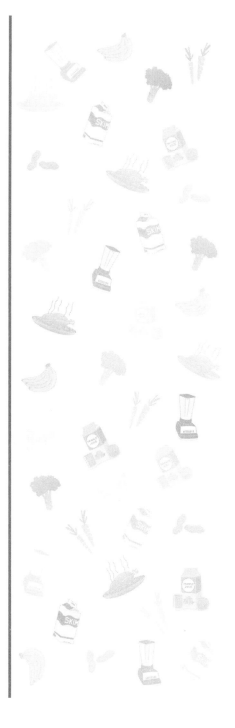

centrated source of numerous minerals, including iodine, potassium, magnesium, calcium, and iron.

The Benefits of Kelp

As a great source of iodine, kelp is useful in making thyroid hormones, which are essential for maintaining normal metabolism, and for normal growth and development of a healthy fetus and infant.

Where to Find Kelp

Kelp can be eaten fresh or dried. Some people use it as a side dish, while others use kelp to flavor soups, stews, and salads. Kelp can often be found in Asian markets, health food stores, via mail order, and on the Internet.

Should You Supplement with Kelp?

Goiter is the classic iodine deficiency disease. When the iodine level in the blood is low, the cells of the thyroid gland enlarge in an attempt to trap as many particles of iodine as possible. If the gland enlarges until it's visible at the neck, it is called a goiter.

Iodine deficiency can also impair growth and neurological development—which can lead to brain damage. Depending on its severity and the stage of development at which the deficiency occurs, a lack of iodine can lead to a number of health problems ranging from mild intellectual impairment to severe mental retardation (cretinism), growth stunting, apathy, and impaired speech, hearing, or movement. Although cretinism is rare, the more "mild" deficiency symptoms are all too common in undeveloped areas of the world.

However, since the iodization of salt in the United States, iodine deficiency is rare in this country and additional sources of iodine, such as kelp, are unnecessary. Kelp can still be taken as a source of other nutrients, although all of the nutrients it contains can be obtained from other foods as well.

It's important to note that extremely high intakes of kelp could provide toxic levels of iodine. Symptoms of mild iodine toxicity include mouth sores, a metallic taste, diarrhea, vomiting, a rash,

Caution!

- Supplementing with kelp is not necessary, since all of the minerals it contains can be consumed in a normal diet that includes iodized salt.
- If you have a medical condition or are pregnant or lactating, talk to your doctor before taking any supplement.

DAILY
Multivitamin
100 TABLETS

and difficulty breathing. Chronic, excessive iodine intakes (about 15 times the recommended levels of 150 to 200 micrograms per day), though, can actually cause goiter—the same problem caused by iodine deficiency. And, preliminary research suggests that high iodine intakes may be linked to thyroid cancer. In any case, children should not take kelp supplements.

What to Know about Taking Kelp Supplements

- Kelp supplements are available in tablet, capsule, and liquid forms, and typically provide 80 to 330 micrograms of iodine per serving.
- Since dietary supplements (or claims for them) are not reviewed by the Food and Drug Administration, quality control and potency problems may exist with kelp supplements.

MSM (Methylsulfonylmethane)

Methylsulfonylmethane (pronounced METH-el-SULF-el-methane), MSM for short, is a sulfur compound found in small amounts in the human body and in some foods. MSM is a product of the breakdown of dimethylsulfoxide, or DMSO, which comes from trees and has medicinal uses (such as the treatment of interstitial cystitis, a chronic bladder condition). MSM is sold as a dietary supplement primarily for the treatment of osteoarthritis pain. Although there are other benefits touted by MSM backers and the many MSM supplement marketers, MSM supplements are not recommended for anyone because of the lack of supporting research. With only two studies to suggest any effectiveness of MSM on arthritis, even this is not a confirmed benefit.

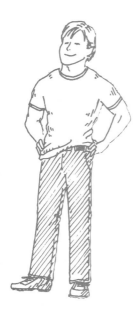

Pyruvate

Pyruvate (pronounced PIE-roo-vate) is produced in the body as a result of sugar metabolism. It supplies the body with pyruvic acid,

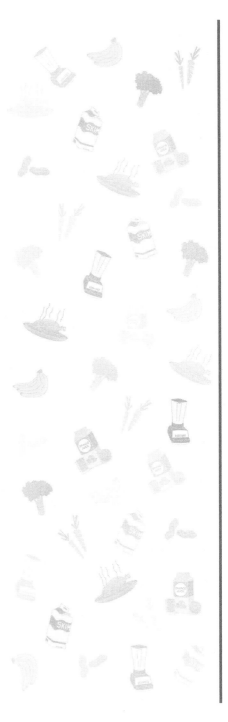

which has a number of important roles in producing and utilizing energy. Pyruvate supplements (some of which contain small amounts of dihydroxyacetone, which is converted to pyruvate in the body) have become increasingly popular because of the wide variety of claims associated with them. Promoters of pyruvate credit the supplements with everything from weight and fat loss to improved exercise endurance to cholesterol lowering, but the evidence supporting these claims is pretty thin.

Given that pyruvate is made in the body and therefore is not an essential nutrient, and that no deficiency condition exists, pyruvate supplements would only serve potentially therapeutic purposes. Weight loss seems to be the area of most promise for pyruvate supplementation, yet even those studies are considered preliminary. And, in all of the areas where pyruvate supplementation is claimed to be beneficial, there are problems with the research— in terms of both quality and quantity. What's more, much of the research on pyruvate supplements has been conducted by one researcher, involved small numbers of people, and hasn't been duplicated by other researchers or with larger groups. Finally, no studies have shown that the small amounts of pyruvate in commercially available supplements have any beneficial effects whatsoever.

The long-term safety of pyruvate supplements—especially the huge amounts used in the studies—has not been shown. And, should any contaminants be contained in the supplement, taking such large doses would increase the chance of harmful substances accumulating in the body. Because the body of research does not currently substantiate any of the claimed benefits of pyruvate supplements, they're not recommended for anyone.

Shark Cartilage

Shark cartilage is the connective tissue that serves as a shark's skeleton. It's made up of proteins (40 percent), calcium, sulfur, chondroitin sulfate, and collagen. Shark cartilage first made headlines in 1993 when CBS TV's *60 Minutes* aired a program highlighting the book *Sharks Don't Get Cancer*, by biochemist I.

William Lane, Ph.D. The program discussed a Cuban study that found many cancer patients "felt better" after taking shark cartilage, but the National Cancer Institute (NCI) called the study "incomplete and unimpressive." Even so, shark cartilage was soon touted as a powerful cancer fighter in humans. It has also been claimed to help relieve arthritis pain, inflammation, and psoriasis.

The Benefits of Shark Cartilage

Shark Cartilage and Cancer

Ironically, while manufacturers of shark cartilage supplements promote the myth that sharks don't get cancer, the fact of the matter is that sharks *do* get cancer, even in the very cartilage marketed as a cancer cure! However, shark cartilage may still have a role in fighting cancer in humans. Since the 1970s, many test-tube and animal studies have shown that shark cartilage can slow or stop the growth of blood vessels that feed tumors. Shark cartilage may also help protect against cancer by preventing damage to the genetic material in healthy cells.

To date, there has been very little conclusive research in humans. In a 1998 study in the *Journal of Clinical Oncology*, 47 men and women with advanced cancer took 1 gram of shark cartilage per kilogram of body weight every day for 12 weeks. After three months, there was no measurable change in tumor size, aggressiveness of the disease, or quality of life.

Experts haven't given up on the potential benefits of shark cartilage, however. In 1999 the NCI funded a multicenter study involving several hundred lung cancer patients. Researchers are testing a liquid shark cartilage extract in conjunction with chemotherapy and radiation therapy. The results won't be available for a few years.

Shark Cartilage and Arthritis

Several studies conducted in Europe with osteoarthritis patients have shown that chondroitin sulfate, an ingredient in shark cartilage, improves joint mobility and reduces pain (see "Chondroitin," page 265).

Caution!

- Most shark cartilage capsules do not contain enough active ingredients to have any effect. Don't use them until there is more data with humans.
- If you are considering taking shark cartilage, talk to your doctor first.
- Since shark cartilage contains calcium, intakes greater than 50 grams per day could lead to calcium toxicity.

Who Should NOT Take Shark Cartilage Supplements

- Individuals with cardiovascular disease
- Anyone having or having had surgery, since it can delay healing
- Athletes who are training intensely
- Children, because it can slow normal growth
- Women who are planning to be or are pregnant, because shark cartilage could slow fetus growth
- Women who are lactating

Should You Supplement with Shark Cartilage?

Shark cartilage is not an essential nutrient—you don't *need* it to survive. It is estimated that more than 50,000 Americans used shark cartilage in 1992, and in 1995 there were more than 40 brand names of shark cartilage products sold in the United States. However, the amount of shark cartilage that patients in studies took each day (numerous spoonfuls dissolved in juice or flavored water three times per day) would cost about $1,000 per month. To get the equivalent amount in capsule form, you would have to take 100 or more 500-milligram capsules a day.

Information on the side effects of shark cartilage supplementation is limited, but it appears to be relatively safe in small doses. Reported side effects include dysgeusia (a bad taste in the mouth), fatigue, diarrhea, nausea, dyspepsia (problems with digestion), fever, dizziness, hypercalcemia, discomfort at the injection site, and swelling of the scrotum.

What to Know about Taking Shark Cartilage Supplements

- Shark cartilage can be taken orally as a pill, powder, or liquid extract. It can also be given as a topical agent, enema, intravenous infusion, or an injection into the skin, abdomen, or muscle.
- Dose recommendations vary and supplements can be costly.
- Since dietary supplements are not reviewed by the FDA, quality control and potency problems may exist with shark cartilage supplements.

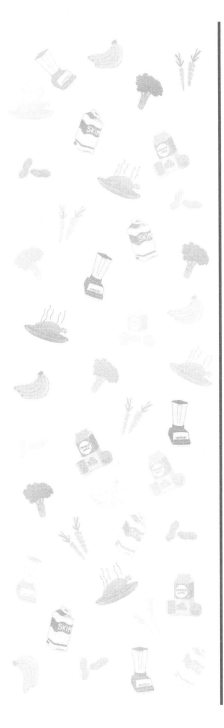

SAMe (S-Adenosylmethionine)

SAMe (pronounced "Sammy") is the "nickname" for S-adenosylmethionine—a form of the amino acid methionine. SAMe occurs naturally in the body and is used for many essential functions, including making cartilage, the tissue found in joints. Books about SAMe supplements tout it for treating everything from mood disorders such as depression, to osteoarthritis, to liver damage. The supplement has been available in the United States since March 1999 and has been a top seller, despite controversy over the quality and quantity of scientific research on the supplement's efficacy and safety.

The Benefits of SAMe

SAMe and Osteoarthritis

Although the mechanism by which SAMe works in the body is not fully understood, it's believed that SAMe rebuilds damaged cartilage lining the joints by stimulating the production of proteoglycans, a "building block" of cartilage. This, in turn, may cushion the joint and provide some pain relief, instead of just covering up the pain, as nonsteroidal anti-inflammatory drugs (NSAIDs) do. Also, unlike NSAIDs, SAMe does not cause gastric bleeding and ulcers. The Arthritis Foundation supports the use of SAMe, stating that "there is sufficient information to support the claim that SAMe provides pain relief" for osteoarthritis. However, the foundation says that claims that the supplement contributes to "joint health" are not scientifically supported thus far.

In other countries, SAMe has been prescribed for arthritis for many years. For osteoarthritis pain reduction, 400 milligrams to 1,200 milligrams of SAMe daily may be helpful.

SAMe and Depression

SAMe appears to increase the levels of certain neurotransmitters, the chemical "messengers" of the brain, and may thereby affect moods and emotions. A review of the various studies done using SAMe for depression revealed that in nine studies, SAMe compared favorably with antidepressant drugs, including imipramine, amitryptaline, and clomipramine. For mild to moderate depression, some clinical trials indicate that 400 milligrams of SAMe per day is sufficient, while others suggest that up to 1,600 milligrams might be necessary.

Low SAMe levels have been found in the cerebral spinal fluid of people with psychiatric and neurological disorders, and low blood levels of SAMe are associated with mood disorders. However,

Caution!

- SAMe is a treatment option for people suffering from osteoarthritis or depression, but for healthy people there don't appear to be benefits to taking SAMe. Its long-term safety and efficacy are unknown.
- Depression is a complicated condition, and self-diagnosis is dangerous. Before taking SAMe supplements, talk to your doctor.
- If you have a family history of heart disease, talk to your doctor before taking SAMe.
- If you have a medical condition or are pregnant or lactating, talk to your doctor before taking any supplement.
- People with bipolar depression, obsessive–compulsive disorder, or addictive tendencies should not take SAMe.

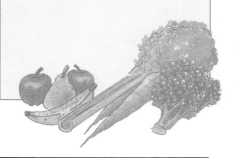

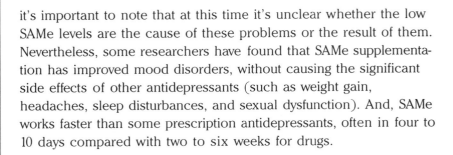

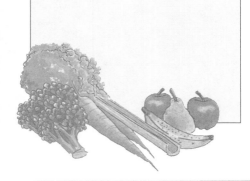

it's important to note that at this time it's unclear whether the low SAMe levels are the cause of these problems or the result of them. Nevertheless, some researchers have found that SAMe supplementation has improved mood disorders, without causing the significant side effects of other antidepressants (such as weight gain, headaches, sleep disturbances, and sexual dysfunction). And, SAMe works faster than some prescription antidepressants, often in four to 10 days compared with two to six weeks for drugs.

Should You Supplement with SAMe?

The initial research on SAMe as a treatment for osteoarthritis and depression appears encouraging. However, there are still plenty of unanswered questions about the supplement. First, since many of the research studies on SAMe were short (lasting only a few weeks in some cases), the long-term safety and efficacy of the supplement are unknown. Second, many of the SAMe studies involved few participants, while those for prescription antidepressants usually involve thousands of patients and last for months. Other research flaws found in early SAMe studies are serious enough to make the conclusions invalid in some cases.

There are risks associated with taking SAMe. For people with bipolar depression (sometimes called "manic depression"), obsessive–compulsive disorder, or addictive tendencies, SAMe can cause their conditions to worsen. Another major concern with SAMe is that it's converted to the amino acid homocysteine in the body. Recent studies have showed that the higher the levels of homocysteine, the greater the risk of cardiovascular disease. Homocysteine can be changed into methionine, the amino acid that is the precursor to SAMe, but in order for that to take place, both folate and vitamin D are needed. Therefore, people who take SAMe may want to consider taking a multivitamin supplement, too. It should not be given to children.

Appendices

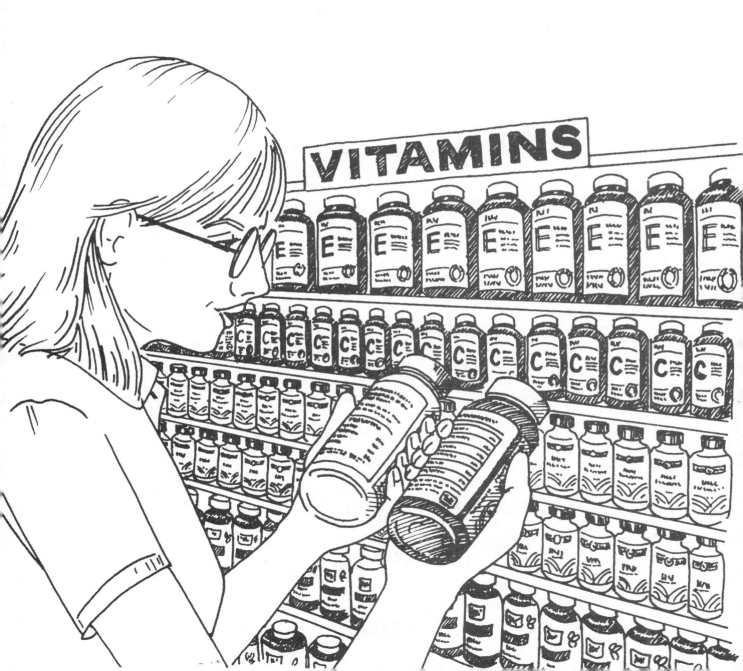

Dietary Reference Intakes (DRIs): Recommended Intakes for Individuals, Vitamins
Food and Nutrition Board, Institute of Medicine, National Academies

Life Stage Group	Vitamin A (µg/d)[a]	Vitamin C (mg/d)	Vitamin D (µg/d)[b,c]	Vitamin E (mg/d)[d]	Vitamin K (µg/d)	Thiamin (mg/d)	Riboflavin (mg/d)	Niacin (mg/d)[e]	Vitamin B6 (mg/d)	Folate (µg/d)[f]	Vitamin B12 (µg/d)	Pantothenic Acid (mg/d)	Biotin (µg/d)	Choline[g] (mg/d)
Infants														
0–6 mo	400*	40*	5*	4*	2.0*	0.2*	0.3*	2*	0.1*	65*	0.4*	1.7*	5*	125*
7–12 mo	500*	50*	5*	5*	2.5*	0.3*	0.4*	4*	0.3*	80*	0.5*	1.8*	6*	150*
Children														
1–3 y	300	15	5*	6	30*	0.5	0.5	6	0.5	150	0.9	2*	8*	200*
4–8 y	400	25	5*	7	55*	0.6	0.6	8	0.6	200	1.2	3*	12*	250*
Males														
9–13 y	600	45	5*	11	60*	0.9	0.9	12	1.0	300	1.8	4*	20*	375*
14–18 y	900	75	5*	15	75*	1.2	1.3	16	1.3	400	2.4	5*	25*	550*
19–30 y	900	90	5*	15	120*	1.2	1.3	16	1.3	400	2.4	5*	30*	550*
31–50 y	900	90	5*	15	120*	1.2	1.3	16	1.3	400	2.4	5*	30*	550*
51–70 y	900	90	10*	15	120*	1.2	1.3	16	1.7	400	2.4[h]	5*	30*	550*
>70 y	900	90	15*	15	120*	1.2	1.3	16	1.7	400	2.4[h]	5*	30*	550*
Females														
9–13 y	600	45	5*	11	60*	0.9	0.9	12	1.0	300	1.8	4*	20*	375*
14–18 y	700	65	5*	15	75*	1.0	1.0	14	1.2	400[i]	2.4	5*	25*	400*
19–30 y	700	75	5*	15	90*	1.1	1.1	14	1.3	400[i]	2.4	5*	30*	425*
31–50 y	700	75	5*	15	90*	1.1	1.1	14	1.3	400[i]	2.4	5*	30*	425*
51–70 y	700	75	10*	15	90*	1.1	1.1	14	1.5	400	2.4[h]	5*	30*	425*
>70 y	700	75	15*	15	90*	1.1	1.1	14	1.5	400	2.4[h]	5*	30*	425*
Pregnancy														
≤18 y	750	80	5*	15	75*	1.4	1.4	18	1.9	600[j]	2.6	6*	30*	450*
19–30 y	770	85	5*	15	90*	1.4	1.4	18	1.9	600[j]	2.6	6*	30*	450*
31–50 y	770	85	5*	15	90*	1.4	1.4	18	1.9	600[j]	2.6	6*	30*	450*
Lactation														
≤18 y	1,200	115	5*	19	75*	1.4	1.6	17	2.0	500	2.8	7*	35*	550*
19–30 y	1,300	120	5*	19	90*	1.4	1.6	17	2.0	500	2.8	7*	35*	550*
31–50 y	1,300	120	5*	19	90*	1.4	1.6	17	2.0	500	2.8	7*	35*	550*

NOTE: This table (taken from the DRI reports, see www.nap.edu) presents Recommended Dietary Allowances (RDAs) in **bold type** and Adequate Intakes (AIs) in ordinary type followed by an asterisk (*). RDAs and AIs may both be used as goals for individual intake. RDAs are set to meet the needs of almost all (97 to 98 percent) individuals in a group. For healthy breastfed infants, the AI is the mean intake. The AI for other life stage and gender groups is believed to cover needs of all individuals in the group, but lack of data or uncertainty in the data prevent being able to specify with confidence the percentage of individuals covered by this intake.

[a] As retinol activity equivalents (RAEs). 1 RAE = 1 µg retinol, 12 µg β-carotene, 24 µg α-carotene, or 24 µg β-cryptoxanthin. The RAE for dietary provitamin A carotenoids is two-fold greater than retinol equivalents (RE), whereas the RAE for preformed vitamin A is the same as RE.

[b] cholecalciferol. 1 µg cholecalciferol = 40 IU vitamin D.

[c] In the absence of adequate exposure to sunlight.

[d] As α-tocopherol. α-Tocopherol includes RRR-α-tocopherol, the only form of α-tocopherol that occurs naturally in foods, and the 2R-stereoisomeric forms of α-tocopherol (RRR-, RSR-, RRS-, and RSS-α-tocopherol) that occur in fortified foods and supplements. It does not include the 2S-stereoisomeric forms of α-tocopherol (SRR-, SSR-, SRS-, and SSS-α-tocopherol), also found in fortified foods and supplements.

[e] As niacin equivalents (NE). 1 mg of niacin = 60 mg of tryptophan; 0–6 months = preformed niacin (not NE).

[f] As dietary folate equivalents (DFE). 1 DFE = 1 µg food folate = 0.6 µg of folic acid from fortified food or as a supplement consumed with food = 0.5 µg of a supplement taken on an empty stomach.

[g] Although AIs have been set for choline, there are few data to assess whether a dietary supply of choline is needed at all stages of the life cycle, and it may be that the choline requirement can be met by endogenous synthesis at some of these stages.

[h] Because 10 to 30 percent of older people may malabsorb food-bound B12, it is advisable for those older than 50 years to meet their RDA mainly by consuming foods fortified with B12 or a supplement containing B12.

[i] In view of evidence linking folate intake with neural tube defects in the fetus, it is recommended that all women capable of becoming pregnant consume 400 µg from supplements or fortified foods in addition to intake of food folate from a varied diet.

[j] It is assumed that women will continue consuming 400 µg from supplements or fortified food until their pregnancy is confirmed and they enter prenatal care, which ordinarily occurs after the end of the periconceptional period—the critical time for formation of the neural tube.

Dietary Reference Intakes (DRIs): Tolerable Upper Intake Levels (UL[a]), Vitamins
Food and Nutrition Board, Institute of Medicine, National Academies

Life Stage Group	Vitamin A (μg/d)[b]	Vitamin C (mg/d)	Vitamin D (μg/d)	Vitamin E (mg/d)[c,d]	Vitamin K	Thiamin	Riboflavin	Niacin (mg/d)[d]	Vitamin B$_6$ (mg/d)	Folate (μg/d)[d]	Vitamin B$_{12}$	Pantothenic Acid	Biotin	Choline (g/d)	Carotenoids[e]
Infants															
0–6 mo	600	ND[f]	25	ND	ND	ND	ND	ND	ND	ND	ND	ND	ND	ND	ND
7–12 mo	600	ND	25	ND	ND	ND	ND	ND	ND	ND	ND	ND	ND	ND	ND
Children															
1–3 y	600	400	50	200	ND	ND	ND	10	30	300	ND	ND	ND	1.0	ND
4–8 y	900	650	50	300	ND	ND	ND	15	40	400	ND	ND	ND	1.0	ND
Males, Females															
9–13 y	1,700	1,200	50	600	ND	ND	ND	20	60	600	ND	ND	ND	2.0	ND
14–18 y	2,800	1,800	50	800	ND	ND	ND	30	80	800	ND	ND	ND	3.0	ND
19–70 y	3,000	2,000	50	1,000	ND	ND	ND	35	100	1,000	ND	ND	ND	3.5	ND
>70 y	3,000	2,000	50	1,000	ND	ND	ND	35	100	1,000	ND	ND	ND	3.5	ND
Pregnancy															
≤18 y	2,800	1,800	50	800	ND	ND	ND	30	80	800	ND	ND	ND	3.0	ND
19–50 y	3,000	2,000	50	1,000	ND	ND	ND	35	100	1,000	ND	ND	ND	3.5	ND
Lactation															
≤18 y	2,800	1,800	50	800	ND	ND	ND	30	80	800	ND	ND	ND	3.0	ND
19–50 y	3,000	2,000	50	1,000	ND	ND	ND	35	100	1,000	ND	ND	ND	3.5	ND

[a] UL = The maximum level of daily nutrient intake that is likely to pose no risk of adverse effects. Unless otherwise specified, the UL represents total intake from food, water, and supplements. Due to lack of suitable data, ULs could not be established for vitamin K, thiamin, riboflavin, vitamin B$_{12}$, pantothenic acid, biotin, or carotenoids. In the absence of ULs, extra caution may be warranted in consuming levels above recommended intakes.

[b] As preformed vitamin A only.

[c] As α-tocopherol; applies to any form of supplemental α-tocopherol.

[d] The ULs for vitamin E, niacin, and folate apply to synthetic forms obtained from supplements, fortified foods, or a combination of the two.

[e] β-Carotene supplements are advised only to serve as a provitamin A source for individuals at risk of vitamin A deficiency.

[f] ND = Not determinable due to lack of data of adverse effects in this age group and concern with regard to lack of ability to handle excess amounts. Source of intake should be from food only to prevent high levels of intake.

Dietary Reference Intakes (DRIs): Recommended Intakes for Individuals, Elements
Food and Nutrition Board, Institute of Medicine, National Academies

Life Stage Group	Calcium (mg/d)	Chromium (µg/d)	Copper (µg/d)	Fluoride (mg/d)	Iodine (µg/d)	Iron (mg/d)	Magnesium (mg/d)	Manganese (mg/d)	Molybdenum (µg/d)	Phosphorus (mg/d)	Selenium (µg/d)	Zinc (mg/d)
Infants												
0–6 mo	210*	0.2*	200*	0.01*	110*	0.27*	30*	0.003*	2*	100*	15*	2*
7–12 mo	270*	5.5*	220*	0.5*	130*	11*	75*	0.6*	3*	275*	20*	3
Children												
1–3 y	500*	11*	340	0.7*	90	7	80	1.2*	17	460	20	3
4–8 y	800*	15*	440	1*	90	10	130	1.5*	22	500	30	5
Males												
9–13 y	1,300*	25*	700	2*	120	8	240	1.9*	34	1,250	40	8
14–18 y	1,300*	35*	890	3*	150	11	410	2.2*	43	1,250	55	11
19–30 y	1,000*	35*	900	4*	150	8	400	2.3*	45	700	55	11
31–50 y	1,000*	35*	900	4*	150	8	420	2.3*	45	700	55	11
51–70 y	1,200*	30*	900	4*	150	8	420	2.3*	45	700	55	11
>70 y	1,200*	30*	900	4*	150	8	420	2.3*	45	700	55	11
Females												
9–13 y	1,300*	21*	700	2*	120	8	240	1.6*	34	1,250	40	8
14–18 y	1,300*	24*	890	3*	150	15	360	1.6*	43	1,250	55	9
19–30 y	1,000*	25*	900	3*	150	18	310	1.8*	45	700	55	8
31–50 y	1,000*	25*	900	3*	150	18	320	1.8*	45	700	55	8
51–70 y	1,200*	20*	900	3*	150	8	320	1.8*	45	700	55	8
>70 y	1,200*	20*	900	3*	150	8	320	1.8*	45	700	55	8
Pregnancy												
≤18 y	1,300*	29*	1,000	3*	220	27	400	2.0*	50	1,250	60	13
19–30 y	1,000*	30*	1,000	3*	220	27	350	2.0*	50	700	60	11
31–50 y	1,000*	30*	1,000	3*	220	27	360	2.0*	50	700	60	11
Lactation												
≤18 y	1,300*	44*	1,300	3*	290	10	360	2.6*	50	1,250	70	14
19–30 y	1,000*	45*	1,300	3*	290	9	310	2.6*	50	700	70	12
31–50 y	1,000*	45*	1,300	3*	290	9	320	2.6*	50	700	70	12

NOTE: This table presents Recommended Dietary Allowances (RDAs) in **bold type** and Adequate Intakes (AIs) in ordinary type followed by an asterisk (*). RDAs and AIs may both be used as goals for individual intake. RDAs are set to meet the needs of almost all (97 to 98 percent) individuals in a group. For healthy breastfed infants, the AI is the mean intake. The AI for other life stage and gender groups is believed to cover needs of all individuals in the group, but lack of data or uncertainty in the data prevent being able to specify with confidence the percentage of individuals covered by this intake.

SOURCES: *Dietary Reference Intakes for Calcium, Phosphorous, Magnesium, Vitamin D, and Fluoride* (1997); *Dietary Reference Intakes for Thiamin, Riboflavin, Niacin, Vitamin B6, Folate, Vitamin B12, Pantothenic Acid, Biotin, and Choline* (1998); *Dietary Reference Intakes for Vitamin C, Vitamin E, Selenium, and Carotenoids* (2000); and *Dietary Reference Intakes for Vitamin A, Vitamin K, Arsenic, Boron, Chromium, Copper, Iodine, Iron, Manganese, Molybdenum, Nickel, Silicon, Vanadium, and Zinc* (2001). These reports may be accessed via www.nap.edu.

Dietary Reference Intakes (DRIs): Tolerable Upper Intake Levels (UL[a]), Elements
Food and Nutrition Board, Institute of Medicine, National Academies

Life Stage Group	Arsenic[b]	Boron (mg/d)	Calcium (g/d)	Chromium	Copper (µg/d)	Fluoride (mg/d)	Iodine (µg/d)	Iron (mg/d)	Magnesium (mg/d)[c]	Manganese (mg/d)	Molybdenum (µg/d)	Nickel (mg/d)	Phosphorus (g/d)	Selenium (µg/d)	Silicon[d]	Vanadium (mg/d)[e]	Zinc (mg/d)
Infants																	
0–6 mo	ND[f]	ND	ND	ND	ND	0.7	ND	40	ND	ND	ND	ND	ND	45	ND	ND	4
7–12 mo	ND	ND	ND	ND	ND	0.9	ND	40	ND	ND	ND	ND	ND	60	ND	ND	5
Children																	
1–3 y	ND	3	2.5	ND	1,000	1.3	200	40	65	2	300	0.2	3	90	ND	ND	7
4–8 y	ND	6	2.5	ND	3,000	2.2	300	40	110	3	600	0.3	3	150	ND	ND	12
Males, Females																	
9–13 y	ND	11	2.5	ND	5,000	10	600	40	350	6	1,100	0.6	4	280	ND	ND	23
14–18 y	ND	17	2.5	ND	8,000	10	900	45	350	9	1,700	1.0	4	400	ND	ND	34
19–70 y	ND	20	2.5	ND	10,000	10	1,100	45	350	11	2,000	1.0	4	400	ND	1.8	40
>70 y	ND	20	2.5	ND	10,000	10	1,100	45	350	11	2,000	1.0	3	400	ND	1.8	40
Pregnancy																	
≤18 y	ND	17	2.5	ND	8,000	10	900	45	350	9	1,700	1.0	3.5	400	ND	ND	34
19–50 y	ND	20	2.5	ND	10,000	10	1,100	45	350	11	2,000	1.0	3.5	400	ND	ND	40
Lactation																	
≤18 y	ND	17	2.5	ND	8,000	10	900	45	350	9	1,700	1.0	4	400	ND	ND	34
19–50 y	ND	20	2.5	ND	10,000	10	1,100	45	350	11	2,000	1.0	4	400	ND	ND	40

[a] UL = The maximum level of daily nutrient intake that is likely to pose no risk of adverse effects. Unless otherwise specified, the UL represents total intake from food, water, and supplements. Due to lack of suitable data, ULs could not be established for arsenic, chromium, and silicon. In the absence of ULs, extra caution may be warranted in consuming levels above recommended intakes.

[b] Although the UL was not determined for arsenic, there is no justification for adding arsenic to food or supplements.

[c] The ULs for magnesium represent intake from a pharmacological agent only and do not include intake from food and water.

[d] Although silicon has not been shown to cause adverse effects in humans, there is no justification for adding silicon to supplements.

[e] Although vanadium in food has not been shown to cause adverse effects in humans, there is no justification for adding vanadium to food and vanadium supplements should be used with caution. The UL is based on adverse effects in laboratory animals and this data could be used to set a UL for adults but not children and adolescents.

[f] ND = Not determinable due to lack of data of adverse effects in this age group and concern with regard to lack of ability to handle excess amounts. Source of intake should be from food only to prevent high levels of intake.

SOURCES: *Dietary Reference Intakes for Calcium, Phosphorous, Magnesium, Vitamin D, and Fluoride (1997); Dietary Reference Intakes for Thiamin, Riboflavin, Niacin, Vitamin B6, Folate, Vitamin B12, Pantothenic Acid, Biotin, and Choline (1998); Dietary Reference Intakes for Vitamin C, Vitamine E, Selenium, and Carotenoids (2000); and Dietary Reference Intakes for Vitamin A, Vitamin K, Arsenic, Boron, Chromium, Copper, Iodine, Iron, Manganese, Molybdenum, Nickel, Silicon, Vanadium, and Zinc (2001).* These reports may be accessed via www.nap.edu.

Additional Resources

American Association of Naturopathic Physicians
8201 Greensboro Drive, Suite 300
McLean, Virginia 22102
703/610-9037
www.naturopathic.org

American College for Advancement in Medicine
23121 Verdugo, Suite 204
Laguna Hills, CA 92653
949/583-7666
www.acam.org

American Council on Science and Health
www.acsh.org

American Diabetes Association
www.diabetes.org

American Dietetic Association
216 West Jackson Boulevard
Chicago, IL 60606-6995
800/877-1600
www.eatright.org

Cancer Information Service
Office of Cancer Communications
National Cancer Institute
Building 31, Room 10A16
9000 Rockville Pike
Bethesda, MD 20892
http://cis.nci.nih.gov

Center for Nutrition Policy and Promotion, USDA
1120 20th Street, NW, Suite 200, North Lobby
Washington, DC 20036
www.usda.gov.cnpp

ConsumerLab, Inc.
www.consumerlab.com

Food and Drug Administration
200 C Street, SW
Washington, DC 20204
www.fda.gov

Food and Nutrition Information Center
National Agricultural Library, USDA
10301 Baltimore Boulevard, Room 304
Beltsville, MD 20705-2351
www.fns.usda.gov.fns

National Health Information Center
U.S. Department of Health and Human Services
P.O. Box 1133
Washington, DC 20013-1133
www.healthfinder.gov

National Council Against Health Fraud
www.ncahf.org

National Heart, Lung, and Blood Institute
P.O. Box 30105
Bethesda, MD 20824-0105
www.nhlbi.nih.gov

National Institutes of Health
www.nih.gov

QuackWatch/Stephen Barrett, M.D.
www.quackwatch.com

Tufts University Guide to Nutrition Web Sites
www.navigator.tufts.edu
This site may be a good place to start, since it evaluates the accuracy of a variety of nutrition-related sites on the Web.

University of Pennsylvania Cancer Center
www.oncolink.upenn.edu

Glossary

Acetylcholine: A neurotransmitter made from choline.

Age-related macular degeneration (ARMD): The leading cause of blindness in the United States.

Aggregate: Used in relation to blood cells, it refers to the clustering or clumping together of blood cells, especially platelets or red blood cells. For example, platelets that tend to aggregate stick together in clumps.

Amino acid: Often called the "building blocks of protein," the 20 amino acids are classified as "essential" or "nonessential." Amino acids are necessary for a wide variety of functions, including building and maintaining muscles, tendons, skin, ligaments, organs, blood, glands, nails, and hair. They also aid in the production of hormones, neurotransmitters, antibodies that fight disease, and enzymes that trigger bodily functions.

Anemia: A deficiency either in the number of red blood cells or in the amount of hemoglobin that the cells contain.

Angina: An episode of chest pain often caused by a temporary restriction of oxygenated blood to the heart muscle.

Anthocyanin: Pigment found in red, blue, and purple foods such as blueberries and grapes.

Antioxidant: These special compounds protect against oxidation, or cellular damage caused by free radicals (see "free radical"). Examples of antioxidants include vitamins C and E, selenium, and many phytochemicals. Antioxidants in foods may help reduce the risk of a number of chronic diseases, such as cancer, stroke, diabetes, heart and lung disease, and cataracts.

Arteriosclerosis: Commonly known as "hardening of the arteries," this condition causes artery walls to thicken and lose elasticity. Often, fibrous tissue, fatty substances, and/or minerals build up along the artery walls. Blocked arteries can lead to heart attack, stroke, or poor circulation in the legs.

Artery: A blood vessel that carries blood away from the heart to the body.

Atherosclerosis: A form of arteriosclerosis in which fatty deposits build up on the inner arterial walls, hindering blood flow and leading to heart disease, angina, heart attack, stroke, and other health problems.

Beriberi: A disease caused by thiamin deficiency.

Bile: A fat-digesting substance produced in the liver and stored in the gallbladder.

Bran: The thin inner husk of grains such as wheat, rice, and oats. Bran is a good source of fiber, vitamins, and minerals.

Carcinogen: A cancer-causing substance.

Caries: Decay of the teeth.

Carotenoid: More than 600 different natural pigments in the diet. These pigments give fruits and vegetables their yellow, orange, and red colors (in green leafy vegetables such as spinach, the carotenoid pigments are masked by green chlorophyll).

Cartilage: The flexible, yet protective tissue found in the joints, spine, throat, ears, nose, and other areas.

Cataract: Cloudy spots on the lens of the eye that can interfere with vision. Cataracts are commonly seen in older adults as a result of the aging process.

Celiac sprue: A malabsorption disorder caused by intolerance to a protein found in certain grains (especially wheat).

Chelation: The process of treating minerals to change their electrical charge, usually by binding them to an amino acid. Chelation supposedly helps the body absorb minerals better, but this hasn't been proven.

Cholesterol: A fatty substance that is necessary for life, but only in moderate amounts. Cholesterol is a major component of all cell membranes, and our bodies use it to make hormones, bile acids, and vitamin D in the skin. Dietary cholesterol is found only in animal products.

Cirrhosis: A disease of the liver characterized by scarring and inflammation. Although it's frequently associated with alcohol abuse, this is not the only cause of the condition.

Coenzyme: A substance (usually a vitamin or mineral) that acts with an enzyme.

Cofactor: A substance (usually a vitamin or mineral) that is an essential component of an enzyme.

Colitis: Inflammation of the colon; characterized by abdominal pain, tenderness, fever, and sometimes bleeding.

Collagen: A fibrous protein that holds cells together and also helps form bones, cartilage, joints, and other tissues.

Complementary protein: Two protein-containing plant foods that alone are deficient in at least one essential amino acid, but together make up for what the other is lacking, making up a complete protein.

Complete protein: A protein that contains all the essential amino acids in the proper proportions for humans. Animal foods are complete proteins, but two complementary proteins can also make up a complete protein.

Constipation: Also called "irregularity," it's having fewer bowel movements than normal, or having stools that are difficult to eliminate.

Coronary heart disease: Condition in which the main arteries of the heart (the coronary arteries) are blocked by fatty deposits, and blood flow to the heart is decreased.

Cretinism: A severe type of mental retardation caused by a deficiency in thyroid hormone, usually resulting from a lack of iodine.

Crohn's disease: A serious inflammatory disease of the large and/or small intestine.

Cystic fibrosis: A genetic disorder of the mucus-producing glands in the pancreas, lungs, intestines, and liver.

Deficiency: A significant shortage of a nutrient in the body.

Diabetes: A condition in which insufficient amounts of the hormone insulin or a resistance to insulin causes decreased utilization of sugar by the cells. This leads to an excess of sugar in the blood and the resulting presence of sugar in the urine. Type 1 diabetes occurs from birth; Type 2 occurs later in life and is therefore often called "adult-onset" diabetes.

Diabetic neuropathy: A condition that sometimes occurs in people with diabetes, characterized by numbness, tingling, and pain in the nerves of the feet and legs, which sometimes spreads to the arms.

Diarrhea: Frequent and abundant loose, watery stools.

Diastolic blood pressure: The lower number in a blood pressure reading, it is the measurement of pressure between heartbeats.

Dietary fiber: The indigestible parts of plant foods.

Diuretic: A drug that stimulates increased fluid excretion from the kidneys.

Diverticulosis: A condition in which bulges, or sacs, form on the walls of the intestines. When food particles become trapped in the sacs and cause inflammation, pain, and bleeding, the condition is called diverticul*itis*.

Down's syndrome: One of the most common developmental disorders in the United States, this genetic disorder affects nearly 1 in 150 conceptions every year.

Edema: Fluid retention that causes swelling. The arms, hands, legs, feet, and ankles are typical sites for edema, but it can occur anywhere in the body.

Electrolyte: An electrically charged mineral that dissolves in water. Positive or negative charges allow electrolytes to easily move back and forth across the body's cell membranes. This is essential because as they move in and out of cells, they carry things with them, such as nutrients, water, and waste products. The functions of electrolytes in the body include maintaining the body's water balance, carrying nerve impulses, and helping muscles contract and relax. Electrolytes also keep the body from becoming too acidic or alkaline.

Enrich: To restore nutrients that were lost during food processing. In most cases, this refers to grains and grain products.

Enzyme: Protein molecules that cause or speed up many of the chemical reactions that take place in the body. Some of these reactions include breaking down proteins, releasing energy, and disarming dangerous substances in the body.

Essential amino acid: An amino acid you must get from food.

Essential fatty acid: The polyunsaturated fatty acids that cannot be produced by the human body and must be obtained from food. These include alpha-linolenic acid (ALA), in the family of omega-3 fatty acids, and linoleic acid (LA), in the family of omega-6 fatty acids. ALA is found in foods such as cold-water fatty fish, walnuts, flaxseed, and leafy green vegetables. LA is found in vegetable oils such as safflower and corn oils.

Essential nutrient: A nutrient that is necessary for life and that must be obtained from food because the body either does not produce it or doesn't produce it in large enough quantities.

Estrogen: A female sex hormone that's produced mainly in the ovaries. Estrogen helps regulate reproduction and other processes.

Fat-soluble vitamin: Fat-soluble vitamins, including vitamins A, D, E, and K, are water-avoiding and therefore must travel through the body attached to protein carriers. They are accumulated in the body.

Fluorosis: Characterized by mottled tooth enamel (white horizontal lines on the teeth), fluorosis develops on permanent teeth while they're still forming. Although fluorosis may be aesthetically objectionable, it has no effect on tooth function.

Fortify: To add nutrients that are not normally present, or in amounts not normally present, in the food.

Free radical: A highly unstable and reactive oxygen molecule that is generated by the body's immune system through the use of oxygen, or in reaction to environmental pollutants including air pollutants, radiation, cigarette smoke, pesticides, herbicides, some food additives, and a wide variety of drugs. Free radicals attack cells, causing both structural and functional damage. Free radicals have been implicated in the development of a number of diseases and conditions, including cancer, cardiovascular disease, cataracts, Alzheimer's disease, and other ailments.

Gallstone: "Stone" in the gallbladder or biliary passages that is composed of cholesterol and calcium.

Gelatin Digesting Unit (GDU): A measure of the pain-reducing and inflammation-reducing power of the pineapple-derived enzyme bromelain. 1 GDU equals 1.5 milk clotting unit (MCU), another measure for bromelain.

Goiter: A swollen thyroid gland, usually caused by a lack of iodine.

Gram (g): A metric measure of weight. One gram equals 1,000 milligrams; 1 ounce equals 28.35 grams.

Heme iron: The iron-containing part of hemoglobin that's found in all animal products, especially red meat, liver, and organ meats.

Hemochromatosis: A genetic disease of iron metabolism in which iron accumulates in body tissues.

Hemoglobin: The oxygen-carrying component of red blood cells. It moves oxygen from the lungs to the body's cells and carries carbon dioxide (a waste product) from the cells back to the lungs to be exhaled.

Hepatitis: Inflammation of the liver due to a viral or bacterial infection, or alcohol or drug abuse.

High-density lipoprotein (HDL): A lipoprotein that carries cholesterol away from all parts of the body to the liver to be excreted from the body. Also called the "good" cholesterol. High HDL levels are protective against heart disease.

Homocysteine: An amino acid–like substance. High levels of homocysteine are linked to heart disease.

Hormone: A chemical messenger. Hormones, such as insulin, are secreted by a variety of glands in the body. Each affects a specific target tissue or organ, resulting in a specific response.

Hormone replacement therapy (HRT): The use of supplemental estrogen and progesterone hormones to relieve the symptoms of menopause.

Hypercholesterolemia: A disorder characterized by excessive amounts of cholesterol in the blood.

Hypertension: High blood pressure, typically greater than 140 mm/90 mm.

Hypoglycemia: Low blood sugar.

Hypokalemia: A deficiency of potassium.

Insoluble fiber: The form of fiber that does not dissolve in water and aids in the prevention of constipation, diverticulosis, hemorrhoids, and some forms of cancer, such as colon and rectal. Examples of insoluble fiber include cellulose, hemicellulose, and lignin. Whole grains and cereals (especially wheat bran), the skins of fruits, and many vegetables (cauliflower, green beans, and potatoes) are good sources of insoluble fiber.

Insulin: A hormone that transfers blood sugar to the body's cells.

Insulin resistance: A condition in which the body's cells don't respond adequately to insulin, and higher blood sugar levels, increased insulin production, and even diabetes can result.

Intermittent claudication: A condition characterized by painful cramps in the calf that make walking difficult. Caused by poor circulation, intermittent claudication usually occurs after walking or other exercise.

International Unit (IU): A unit of measurement for vitamin potency.

Intravenous: Within or into a vein.

Iron deficiency anemia: Anemia caused by a deficiency of iron, usually due to blood loss, increased iron needs during pregnancy or infancy, or low iron intake.

Irritable bowel syndrome (IBS): A common disorder of the intestines that leads to crampy pain, gassiness, bloating, and changes in bowel habits, such as diarrhea and constipation.

Isoflavone: Phytoestrogens that are found primarily in soy products.

Lactose: The naturally occurring sugar found in milk and other dairy products.

Lactose intolerance: A condition that occurs when the milk sugar, lactose, is not digested and reaches the large intestine, where naturally present bacteria ferment it, leading to a variety of symptoms. These symptoms (cramps, gas, bloating, diarrhea, and abdominal pain) usually appear within 30 minutes to two hours after eating or drinking lactose-containing foods. Symptoms vary from person to person and depend on the type and amount of food eaten.

Lipid: A fatty substance. Cholesterol and triglycerides are blood lipids.

Lipoprotein: Molecules that carry fats through the blood.

Low-density lipoprotein (LDL): A lipoprotein that carries harmful cholesterol in the body, that is also known as the "bad" cholesterol. LDL cholesterol tends to accumulate on artery walls. A high LDL level is a major risk factor for heart disease.

Menkes disease: A hereditary disorder affecting copper absorption, which leads to brain damage, growth retardation, and death in infants.

Metabolism: The many chemical reactions involved in breaking down food and converting it to energy.

Microgram (mcg): A metric measure of weight; 1,000 micrograms equals 1 milligram.

Migraine headache: A severe headache that results from the abnormal dilation of the blood vessel on the scalp, neck, or around the eye. Nausea, vomiting, visual problems, and sensitivity to light can accompany the pain.

Milk clotting unit (MCU): A measure for the pain-reducing and inflammation-reducing power of the pineapple-derived enzyme bromelain. 1.5 MCU equals 1 GDU.

Milligram (mg): A metric measure of weight; 1,000 milligrams equals 1 gram.

Mineral: Substances found in the earth's crust that have many important functions in the human body. Minerals are essential for nearly every bodily process, including enzyme creation, regulation of the heart, bone formation, digestion, and oxygen transport.

Mitochondria: Structures found in every cell that convert glucose (blood sugar) into energy.

Natural vitamins: Sometimes called "natural-source" vitamins, these contain extracts from foods or plants instead of synthetic sources. There are no completely natural vitamins; many labeled as "natural" contain a large percentage of synthetic vitamin or are processed in a laboratory.

Neural tube defect (NTD): One of the most serious and common birth defects in the United States. Neural tube defects occur in the neural tube, which develops into the spinal cord. If the defect occurs at the top of the tube, the result is fatal because the baby is born with anencephaly (no brain). If the defect occurs farther down on the tube, the baby is born with spina bifida (an open spine). Damage to the exposed spinal cord usually results in a child who is either wheelchair-bound or on crutches.

Neuron: Nerve cell.

Neurotransmitter: Chemical that helps the brain, body, and nervous system function by carrying messages to and from the brain.

Nonessential amino acid: An amino acid that the body can make, so it isn't necessary to get it from food.

Nonheme iron: Dietary iron from plant sources; it's not as well absorbed as iron from animal sources.

Nonsteroidal anti-inflammatory drug (NSAID): A drug that reduces pain and inflammation. Aspirin and ibuprofen are common NSAIDs.

Nutrient: Any of the many food substances that nourish the body.

Obesity: An excess of body fat, which can strain the heart and increase risk of high blood pressure and diabetes.

Osteoarthritis: A disease characterized by the breakdown of cartilage, which cushions the ends of bone joints, resulting in stiff joints, joint pain, and deformity.

Osteomalacia: A vitamin D deficiency, often referred to as "adult rickets," characterized by a decreased mineral content of the bones, leaving them more prone to fractures. Some people with this disease complain of deep bone pain.

Osteoporosis: A debilitating disease caused by low bone mass and the structural deterioration of bone tissue, leading to porous, fragile bones and an increased susceptibility to fractures of the hip, spine, and wrist.

Oxalic acid: A compound that combines with certain nutrients, such as iron and calcium, so that the nutrients cannot be absorbed. Oxalic acid is found in peanuts, rhubarb, spinach, and cranberries.

Oxidation: A chemical reaction that provides energy for cell processes and activities. Free radicals are produced during the oxidation process.

Parkinson's disease: A nervous system disorder that causes tremors, slowed movement, and other symptoms.

Pellagra: A niacin deficiency disease.

Peptide: A small protein made from just a few amino acids.

Phenylketonuria: A rare genetic defect in which the amino acid phenylalanine cannot be broken down in the body. The accumulation of phenylalanine can cause mental retardation, seizures, and hyperactivity.

Phospholipid: A fatty-like substance containing phosphoric acid; a component of cell membranes.

Phytic acid: Also called "phytate," this natural component in foods binds, or blocks, some nutrients (usually minerals), thereby diminishing the nutrient's absorption.

Phytochemical: Chemical compound found in plants that is not a vitamin or mineral and therefore is not considered essential for life.

Phytoestrogen: A phytochemical that is the plant version of the female hormone estrogen. Researchers are looking at a potential role of phytoestrogens in the fight against cancer, heart disease, and osteoporosis. They're also investigating the use of phytoestrogens in the treatment of menopausal symptoms such as hot flashes and night sweats.

Placebo: Sometimes called a "sugar pill" or "dummy pill," a placebo is an ineffective substance used in scientific testing as a control measure, to allow comparisons with the effects of the ingredient being tested.

Polyunsaturated fatty acid: These fats are often liquid at room temperature and come mostly from plant foods. Examples of foods rich in polyunsaturated fats include walnuts and safflower, corn, and sunflower oils. Polyunsaturated fats can help lower LDL, or the "bad" cholesterol.

Prebiotic: Nondigestible food substance that acts as food for "friendly" or beneficial bacteria present in the gut.

Preformed: A vitamin already in its active form.

Premenstrual syndrome (PMS): A group of physical and emotional symptoms that occur before each menstrual period in some women. Symptoms may include irritability, water retention, headache, and cramping.

Probiotic: Meaning "pro-life." This is a food that introduces "friendly" or beneficial bacteria into the gut in order to favorably alter the balance of bacteria there.

Provitamin: The precursor to a vitamin. The body changes it into an active form through normal metabolic activity.

Psoriasis: A common, chronic skin condition characterized by thickened, red, scaly patches.

Retinol Equivalent (RE): A unit of measurement for vitamin A potency.

Rheumatoid arthritis: An autoimmune disease characterized by inflamed knuckles and joints and, often, misshapen hands. Rheumatoid arthritis affects the entire body and can therefore cause fatigue, loss of appetite, and fever.

Rickets: A bone disease caused by vitamin D deficiency, in which the bone doesn't harden properly, causing pain, bowed legs, or spinal misalignment.

Rotavirus: The virus responsible for the majority of diarrhea cases in infants and young children.

Scurvy: Vitamin C deficiency characterized by swollen, bleeding gums; loosening of the teeth; hemorrhaging, including bleeding into the joints; tender and painful extremities; poor wound healing; weakness and fatigue; and psychological disturbances.

Serotonin: A neurotransmitter that promotes sleep and regulates pain perception, among other functions.

Soluble fiber: The "sticky" form of fiber that thickens the contents of the intestines, thereby slowing the digestion/absorption process and making you feel full for a longer period of time. Soluble fiber also appears to play a protective role against diabetes and heart disease. Examples of soluble fiber include pectin, gums, and mucilages. It's also found in peas, dried beans, some fruits and vegetables (oranges, apples, and carrots), oats and oat bran, psyllium, and barley.

Sublingual: Underneath the tongue. Some supplements, such as zinc and vitamin B_{12}, are meant to be held under the tongue until they're dissolved.

Systolic blood pressure: The top number in a blood pressure reading; it is the pressure when your heart is contracting.

Tannin: A component of tea that can decrease iron absorption.

Therapeutic dose: The amount of a substance needed to produce a desired health effect, beyond the amount needed to prevent deficiency.

Thioctic acid: Another name for lipoic acid.

Thrombosis: The formation of a blood clot; a common cause of heart attacks.

Thyroid gland: A small, butterfly-shaped gland found in your neck that produces hormones that regulate metabolism.

Trace mineral: Mineral needed by the body in very small amounts.

Transferrin: A protein in blood that carries the mineral iron.

Triglyceride: A type of fat that comes from food or is made in the body from carbohydrates. Calories from food that are not immediately used are converted to triglycerides and stored in fat cells.

Vegan: Strict vegetarians who eat no animal products at all.

Vitamins: Compounds that are generally much smaller in size than carbohydrates, proteins, or fats. They do not provide any energy, but are necessary for a number of bodily processes.

Water-soluble vitamin: Water-soluble vitamins, such as C and the B vitamins, are water-loving and travel freely throughout the bloodstream. When not in use, they circulate among all the organs in the body, including the kidneys.

Wernicke–Korsakoff syndrome: A disorder of the nervous system caused by excessive alcohol intake or a severe vitamin B deficiency (particularly thiamin). Symptoms include weakness, inability to walk without help, and confusion.

Wilson's disease: A hereditary condition that results in the toxic accumulation of copper, leading to liver and brain damage.

Index

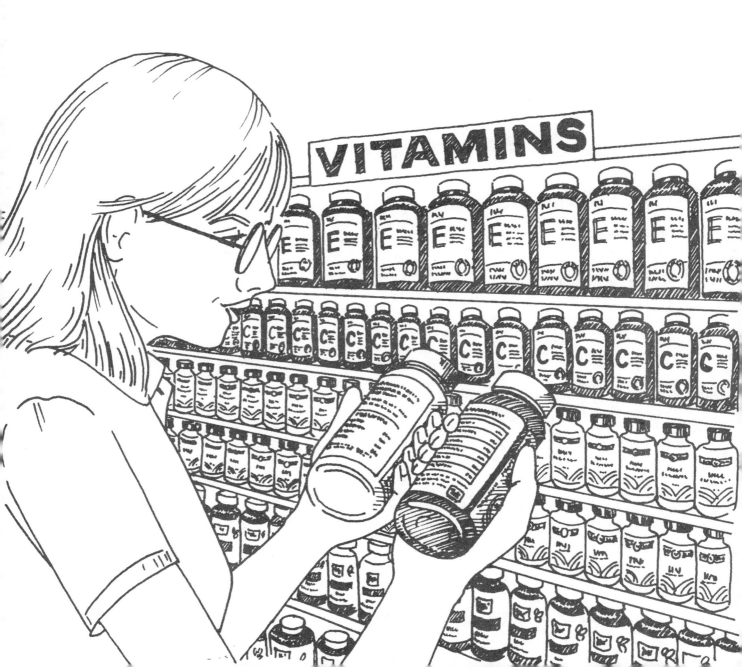

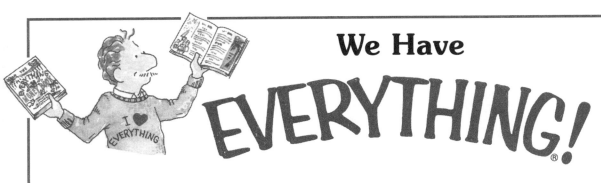

We Have EVERYTHING!

Everything® **After College Book**
$12.95, 1-55850-847-3

Everything® **Angels Book**
$12.95, 1-58062-398-0

Everything® **Astrology Book**
$12.95, 1-58062-062-0

Everything® **Baby Names Book**
$12.95, 1-55850-655-1

Everything® **Baby Shower Book**
$12.95, 1-58062-305-0

Everything® **Baby's First Food Book**
$12.95, 1-58062-512-6

Everything® **Barbeque Cookbook**
$12.95, 1-58062-316-6

Everything® **Bartender's Book**
$9.95, 1-55850-536-9

Everything® **Bedtime Story Book**
$12.95, 1-58062-147-3

Everything® **Bicycle Book**
$12.00, 1-55850-706-X

Everything® **Build Your Own Home Page**
$12.95, 1-58062-339-5

Everything® **Business Planning Book**
$12.95, 1-58062-491-X

Everything® **Casino Gambling Book**
$12.95, 1-55850-762-0

Everything® **Cat Book**
$12.95, 1-55850-710-8

Everything® **Chocolate Cookbook**
$12.95, 1-58062-405-7

Everything® **Christmas Book**
$15.00, 1-55850-697-7

Everything® **Civil War Book**
$12.95, 1-58062-366-2

Everything® **College Survival Book**
$12.95, 1-55850-720-5

Everything® **Computer Book**
$12.95, 1-58062-401-4

Everything® **Cookbook**
$14.95, 1-58062-400-6

Everything® **Cover Letter Book**
$12.95, 1-58062-312-3

Everything® **Crossword and Puzzle Book**
$12.95, 1-55850-764-7

Everything® **Dating Book**
$12.95, 1-58062-185-6

Everything® **Dessert Book**
$12.95, 1-55850-717-5

Everything® **Dog Book**
$12.95, 1-58062-144-9

Everything® **Dreams Book**
$12.95, 1-55850-806-6

Everything® **Etiquette Book**
$12.95, 1-55850-807-4

Everything® **Family Tree Book**
$12.95, 1-55850-763-9

Everything® **Fly-Fishing Book**
$12.95, 1-58062-148-1

Everything® **Games Book**
$12.95, 1-55850-643-8

Everything® **Get-A-Job Book**
$12.95, 1-58062-223-2

Everything® **Get Published Book**
$12.95, 1-58062-315-8

Everything® **Get Ready for Baby Book**
$12.95, 1-55850-844-9

Everything® **Golf Book**
$12.95, 1-55850-814-7

Everything® **Guide to Las Vegas**
$12.95, 1-58062-438-3

Everything® **Guide to New York City**
$12.95, 1-58062-314-X

Everything® **Guide to Walt Disney World®, Universal Studios®, and Greater Orlando, 2nd Edition**
$12.95, 1-58062-404-9

Everything® **Guide to Washington D.C.**
$12.95, 1-58062-313-1

Everything® **Herbal Remedies Book**
$12.95, 1-58062-331-X

Everything® **Home-Based Business Book**
$12.95, 1-58062-364-6

Everything® **Homebuying Book**
$12.95, 1-58062-074-4

Everything® **Homeselling Book**
$12.95, 1-58062-304-2

Everything® **Home Improvement Book**
$12.95, 1-55850-718-3

Everything® **Hot Careers Book**
$12.95, 1-58062-486-3

Everything® **Internet Book**
$12.95, 1-58062-073-6

Everything® **Investing Book**
$12.95, 1-58062-149-X

Everything® **Jewish Wedding Book**
$12.95, 1-55850-801-5

Everything® **Job Interviews Book**
$12.95, 1-58062-493-6

Everything® **Lawn Care Book**
$12.95, 1-58062-487-1

Everything® **Leadership Book**
$12.95, 1-58062-513-4

Everything® **Low-Fat High-Flavor Cookbook**
$12.95, 1-55850-802-3

Everything® **Magic Book**
$12.95, 1-58062-418-9

Everything® **Microsoft® Word 2000 Book**
$12.95, 1-58062-306-9

**For more information, or to order, call 800-872-5627
or visit everything.com**

Adams Media Corporation, 260 Center Street, Holbrook, MA 02343

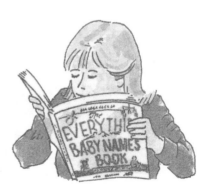

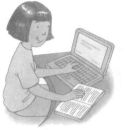
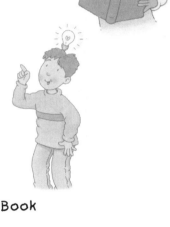
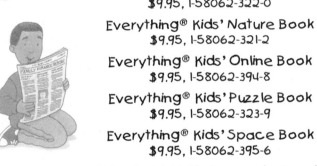
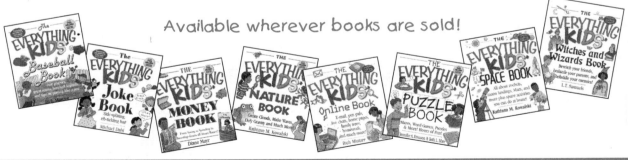